Vascular Anesthesia

Editors

HEATHER K. HAYANGA
MEGAN P. KOSTIBAS

ANESTHESIOLOGY CLINICS

www.anesthesiology.theclinics.com

Consulting Editor
LEE A. FLEISHER

December 2022 • Volume 40 • Number 4

ELSEVIER

1600 John F. Kennedy Boulevard • Suite 1800 • Philadelphia, Pennsylvania, 19103-2899

http://www.theclinics.com

ANESTHESIOLOGY CLINICS Volume 40, Number 4
December 2022 ISSN 1932-2275, ISBN-13: 978-0-323-93945-4

Editor: Joanna Collett
Developmental Editor: Arlene Campos

Anesthesiology Clinics (ISSN 1932-2275) is published quarterly by Elsevier Inc., 360 Park Avenue South, New York, NY 10010-1710. Months of issue are March, June, September, and December. Periodicals postage paid at New York, NY and at additional mailing offices. Subscription prices are $100.00 per year (US student/resident), $375.00 per year (US individuals), $464.00 per year (Canadian individuals), $986.00 per year (US institutions), $1016.00 per year (Canadian institutions), $100.00 per year (Canadian student/resident), $225.00 per year (foreign student/resident), $498.00 per year (foreign individuals), and $1016.00 per year (foreign institutions). To receive student and resident rate, orders must be accompanied by name of affiliated institution, date of term, and the *signature* of program/residency coordinator on institutions letterhead. Orders will be billed at individual rate until proof of status is received. Foreign air speed delivery is included in all *Clinics'* subscription prices. All prices are subject to change without notice. POSTMASTER: Send address changes to *Anesthesiology Clinics,* Elsevier Health Sciences Division, Subscription Customer Service, 3251 Riverport Lane, Maryland Heights, MO 63043. Customer Service (orders, claims, online, change of address): Elsevier Health Sciences Division, Subscription Customer Service, 3251 Riverport Lane, Maryland Heights, MO 63043. **Tel:1-800-654-2452 (U.S. and Canada); 314-447-8871 (outside U.S. and Canada). Fax: 314-447-8029. E-mail: journalscustomerservice-usa@elsevier.com (for print support); journalsonlinesupport-usa@elsevier.com (for online support).**

Reprints. For copies of 100 or more of articles in this publication, please contact the Commercial Reprints Department, Elsevier Inc., 360 Park Avenue South, New York, NY 10010-1710. Tel.: 212-633-3874; Fax: 212-633-3820; E-mail: reprints@elsevier.com.

Anesthesiology Clinics, is also published in Spanish by McGraw-Hill Inter-americana Editores S. A., P.O. Box 5-237, 06500 Mexico D. F., Mexico.

Anesthesiology Clinics, is covered in *MEDLINE/PubMed (Index Medicus), Current Contents/Clinical Medicine, Excerpta Medica, ISI/BIOMED,* and *Chemical Abstracts.*

Contributors

CONSULTING EDITOR

LEE A. FLEISHER, MD, FACC, FAHA
Robert D. Dripps Professor and Chair of Anesthesiology and Critical Care, Professor of Medicine, Perelman School of Medicine, University of Pennsylvania, Philadelphia, Pennsylvania

EDITORS

HEATHER K. HAYANGA, MD, MPH
Associate Professor, Division of Cardiovascular and Thoracic Anesthesiology, Department of Anesthesiology, West Virginia University, Morgantown, West Virginia

MEGAN P. KOSTIBAS, MD
Assistant Professor, Department of Anesthesiology and Critical Care Medicine, Johns Hopkins School of Medicine, Baltimore, Maryland

AUTHORS

REBECCA A. ARON, MD
Associate Professor, Department of Anesthesiology, The University of Nebraska Medical Center, Omaha, Nebraska

EDWARD A. BITTNER, MD, PHD, MSEd, FCCM
Program Director, Critical Care-Anesthesiology Fellowship, Department of Anesthesia, Critical Care and Pain Medicine, Associate Professor of Anaesthesia, Harvard Medical School, Massachusetts General Hospital, Boston, Massachusetts

MICHAEL P. CALGI, BS
University of Virginia School of Medicine, Charlottesville, Virginia

ANNA L. CARPENTER, MD
Assistant Professor, Department of Anesthesiology, Division of Chronic Pain Medicine, Center for Integrative Pain Management, West Virginia University, Morgantown, West Virginia

STEPHANIE CHA, MD
Department of Anesthesiology and Critical Care Medicine, Assistant Professor, Johns Hopkins School of Medicine, Baltimore, Maryland

SREEKANTH CHERUKU, MD, MPH
Associate Professor, Department of Anesthesiology and Pain Management, UT Southwestern Medical Center, Dallas, Texas

BRIAN C. CHO, MD
Assistant Professor, Division of Cardiothoracic Anesthesiology, Johns Hopkins School of Medicine, Baltimore, Maryland

RYAN T. DOWNEY, MD
Assistant Professor, Department of Radiology, The University of Nebraska Medical Center, Omaha, Nebraska

CALLIE EBELING, MD
Assistant Professor, Department of Anesthesiology and Pain Management, UT Southwestern Medical Center, Dallas, Texas

LEE A. GOEDDEL, MD, MPH
Department of Anesthesiology and Critical Care Medicine, Assistant Professor, Johns Hopkins School of Medicine, Baltimore, Maryland

MICHAEL C. GRANT, MD, MSE
Department of Anesthesiology and Critical Care Medicine, Associate Professor, Johns Hopkins School of Medicine, Baltimore, Maryland

RICHARD GYI, DO
Fellow, Anesthesiology, Johns Hopkins Hospital, Baltimore

SALIM HABIB, MD
Visiting Scholar, Department of Vascular Surgery, University of Pittsburgh Medical Center, Pittsburgh, Pennsylvania

MUHAMMAD SAAD HAFEEZ, MBBS
Visiting Scholar, Department of Vascular Surgery, University of Pittsburgh Medical Center, Pittsburgh, Pennsylvania

NADIA B. HENSLEY, MD
Assistant Professor, Division of Cardiothoracic Anesthesiology, Johns Hopkins School of Medicine, Baltimore, Maryland

CAITLIN W. HICKS, MD, MS
Division of Vascular Surgery and Endovascular Therapy, Johns Hopkins School of Medicine, Baltimore, Maryland

NICOLE HOLLIS, MD
Assistant Professor, Department of Anesthesiology, West Virginia University, Morgantown, West Virginia

ALANA KEEGAN, MD
General Surgery, Sinai Hospital of Baltimore, Baltimore, Maryland

JESSE KIEFER, MD, MSEd
Department of Anesthesiology and Critical Care Medicine, University of Pennsylvania, Perelman School of Medicine, Philadelphia, Pennsylvania

MEGAN P. KOSTIBAS, MD
Assistant Professor, Department of Anesthesiology and Critical Care Medicine, Johns Hopkins School of Medicine, Baltimore, Maryland

CORINNE M. LAYNE-STUART, DO
Assistant Professor, Department of Anesthesiology, Division of Chronic Pain Medicine, Center for Integrative Pain Management, West Virginia University, Morgantown, West Virginia

LAEBEN CHOLA LESTER, MD
Assistant Professor, Department of Anesthesiology and Critical Care Medicine, Johns Hopkins School of Medicine, Baltimore, Maryland

MICHAEL MAZZEFFI, MD, MPH, MSC, FASA
Department of Anesthesiology, University of Virginia Health, Charlottesville, Virginia

VENKAT REDDY MANGUNTA, MD
Assistant Professor, Department of Anesthesiology, Division of Cardiovascular Anesthesia, Division of Critical Care Medicine, University of Virginia, School of Medicine, University of Virginia Health System,Charlottesville, Virginia, USA

JOHN S. MCNEIL, MD
Assistant Professor, Department of Anesthesiology, University of Virginia School of Medicine, Charlottesville, Virginia

DANIEL NYHAN, MD
Johns Hopkins Department of Anesthesiology and Critical Care Medicine, Baltimore, Maryland

JEAN-PIERRE P. OUANES, DO
Assistant Clinical Professor, Cornell Medicine, Anesthesiology Site Director, Hospital for Special Surgery, West Palm Beach, Florida

JOSHUA ROACH, MD
Department of Anesthesiology and Critical Care Medicine, Johns Hopkins School of Medicine, Baltimore, Maryland

MILAD SHARIFPOUR, MD, MS
Medical Director, Division of Vascular Anesthesia, Department of Anesthesiology, Staff Anesthesiologist, Intensivist, Cedars Sinai Medical Center, Los Angeles, California

CHARLIE SLOWEY, MB, BCh, BAO
Johns Hopkins Department of Anesthesiology and Critical Care Medicine, Baltimore, Maryland

D. KEEGAN STOMBAUGH, MD
Assistant Professor, Department of Anesthesiology, Division of Cardiovascular Anesthesia, Division of Critical Care Medicine, University of Virginia, School of Medicine, University of Virginia Health System, Charlottesville, Virginia, USA

KATHIRVEL SUBRAMANIAM, MD, MPH, FASE
Department of Anesthesiology and Perioperative Medicine, University of Pittsburgh Medical Center, Pittsburgh, Pennsylvania

VICENTE GARCIA TOMAS, MD
Assistant Professor, Chief, Division of Regional Anesthesiology and Acute Pain Medicine, Northwestern University Feinberg School of Medicine, Chicago, Illinois

THEODORE H. YUO, MD, MSC
Assistant Professor of Surgery, Division of Vascular Surgery, Department of Surgery, University of Pittsburgh School of Medicine, UPMC Presbyterian Hospital, Pittsburgh, Pennsylvania

Contents

The vascular system is one of the earliest recognized anatomical systems. It is composed of 3 parts; arterial, capillary, and venous, each with their own unique anatomy and physiology. Blood flow through this system is compromised in aging, atherosclerosis and peripheral vascular disease, and the practicing anesthesiologist must understand both the physiology and pathophysiology of the vascular tree.

We summarize epidemiologic trends, outcomes, and preoperative guidelines for vascular surgery patients from 2010 to 2022. Vascular surgery continues to evolve in technology and engineering to treat a surgical population that suffers from a high prevalence of comorbidities. Preoperative optimization seeks to characterize the burden of disease and to achieve medical control in the timeline available before surgery. Risk assessment, evaluation, optimization, and prediction of major adverse cardiac events is an evolving science where the Vascular Surgery Quality Initiative has made an impact. Ongoing investigation may demonstrate value for preoperative echocardiography, functional capacity, frailty, and mobility assessments.

Vascular diseases and their sequelae increase perioperative risk for noncardiac surgical patients. In this review, the authors discuss vascular diseases, their epidemiology and pathophysiology, risk stratification, and management strategies to reduce adverse perioperative outcomes.

Patient blood management (PBM) is an evidence-based, multidisciplinary approach aimed at appropriately allocating blood products to patients requiring transfusion while simultaneously minimizing inappropriate transfusions. The 3 pillars of patient blood management are optimizing erythropoiesis, minimizing blood loss, and optimizing physiological reserve of anemia. Benefits seen from PBM include limiting hospital costs and mitigating harm from numerous risks of transfusion.

Today's vascular surgeon must navigate their practice through a field of ever-advancing technology while maintaining knowledge of open techniques that remain equally important in the care of their patients. In this article, the authors provide insight into the perioperative decision-making that goes into choosing a surgical plan for each patient based on their disease process, anatomy, nonmodifiable risk factors, and other comorbidities.

Vascular surgical patients present unique challenges for anesthesiologists, because of their medical vulnerabilities as well as their tendency for rapid intraoperative hemodynamic changes. Intraoperative monitors have been used for decades to reduce adverse outcomes, improve mortality, and create optimal surgical conditions. Understanding the indications and appropriate management of monitoring modalities is essential for optimizing patient care, and preventing harm associated with misinterpretation. We aim to review monitoring technologies used in complex vascular procedures, as well as the current guidelines, clinical trial outcomes, and basic mechanisms of each monitoring modality.

Abdominal aortic aneurysm is a potentially lethal condition that is decreasing in frequency as tobacco use declines. The exact etiology remains unknown, but smoking and other perturbations seem to trigger an inflammatory state in the tunica media. Male sex and advanced age are clear demographic risk factors for the development of abdominal aortic aneurysms. The natural history of this disease varies, but screening remains vital as it is rarely diagnosed on physical examination, and elective repair (most commonly done endovascularly) offers significant morbidity and mortality advantages over emergent intervention for aortic rupture.

Thoracic aortic aneurysms and thoracoabdominal aneurysms are often found incidentally. Complications include dissection or rupture. Most of the thoracic aortic aneurysms and thoracoabdominal aneurysms develop in patients with risk factors for atherosclerosis. Younger patients without significant cardiovascular risk factors may have a genetic basis and include syndromes such as Marfan, Ehlers–Danlos, and Loeys–Dietz and bicuspid aortic valve. Most thoracic aneurysms grow slowly over time and factors that accelerate growth rate include dissection, aneurysm size, bicuspid valve disease, and Marfan syndrome. Size cutoffs where complications occur determine when surgery or intervention should be considered.

Acute aortic dissection is a highly morbid condition with high mortality that requires emergent surgical evaluation and repair. The intraoperative management of acute aortic dissection requires the anesthesiologist to do far more than administer anesthesia and begins before the patient arrives at the operative theater. High-fidelity communication with the surgeon, knowledge of the surgical plan, knowledge of the anatomy of the dissection, and a nuanced understanding of aortic dissection pathophysiology are all critical aspects of anesthetic management.

Open thoracoabdominal and abdominal aortic aneurysm repairs are some of the most challenging cases for anesthesiologists because of the potential for rapid blood loss combined with clamping and reperfusion, potential use of left heart bypass, the potential need for lung isolation, and potential placement and management of a spinal drain. In addition, patients often present with other significant comorbidities and a detailed understanding of the disease process, the complex physiology throughout the case, and the intricacies of organ protection are critical.

Aortic aneurysms—both abdominal and thoracic—are a significant cause of death and disability in the United States. Endovascular aneurysm repair has since become the preferred operative treatment of most thoracic and abdominal aneurysms because of a lower rate of complications and better outcomes compared with the open approach. Patients who present for endovascular aneurysm repair often have comorbid conditions related to their aortic pathology. These conditions should be evaluated and optimized before the procedure.

Carotid revascularization is performed to prevent cerebrovascular events in patients with symptomatic (>50%) and asymptomatic high degree (>70%) carotid stenosis. As this operation carries significant risks for perioperative stroke, careful selection of patients who will benefit from the procedure is essential. Certain plaque characteristics, including texture, are associated with increased tendency for rupture and can be used to identify high-risk patients. Medical therapy, carotid endarterectomy, and carotid stenting are the mainstays for patient management. With careful selection of patients, all anesthesia techniques (general anesthesia, monitored anesthesia care, and regional anesthesia) can be used safely for these revascularization procedures.

Patients undergoing vascular surgery tend to have significant systemic co-morbidities. Vascular surgery itself is also associated with greater cardiac morbidity and overall mortality than other types of noncardiac surgery. Regional anesthesia is amenable as the primary anesthetic technique for vascular surgery or as an adjunct to general anesthesia. When used as the primary anesthetic, regional anesthesia techniques avoid complications associated with general anesthesia in this challenging patient population. In this article, the authors describe regional anesthetic techniques for carotid endarterectomy, arteriovenous fistula creation, lower extremity bypass surgery, and amputation.

Patients that require major vascular surgery suffer from widespread atherosclerosis and have multiple comorbidities that place them at increased risk for postoperative complications and require admission to the intensive care unit (ICU). Postoperative critical care of these patients is focused on hemodynamic optimization, and early identification and management of complications to improve outcomes.

Cardiovascular disease affects close to half of the United States population and many of these patients will develop chronic pain syndromes as a result of their disease process. This article provides an overview of several pain syndromes that result, directly or indirectly, from cardiovascular disease including peripheral arterial disease, angina, thoracic outlet syndrome, postamputation pain, complex regional pain syndrome, and poststroke pain. Psychological and medical comorbidities that affect the medical decision-making process in the treatment of chronic pain associated with cardiovascular disease are also discussed.

ANESTHESIOLOGY CLINICS

SERIES OF RELATED INTEREST

Critical Care Clinics

THE CLINICS ARE AVAILABLE ONLINE!
Access your subscription at:
www.theclinics.com

FORTHCOMING ISSUES

March 2023
Current Topics in Critical Care for the
Anesthesiologist
Athanasios Chalkias, Mary Jarzebowski
and Kathryn Rosenblatt, Editors

September 2023
Geriatric Anesthesia
Shamsuddin Akhtar, Editor

December 2023
Endoscopic Sedation
Matthew D. McEvoy and Basem
Abdelmalak, Editors

RECENT ISSUES

September 2022
Orthopedic Anesthesiology
Patton Lisk and Karen Vlaskov, Editors

June 2022
Total Well-being
Alison J. Brainard and Lyndsay M. Hoy,
Editors

March 2022
Enhanced Recovery After Surgery and
Perioperative Medicine
Michael J. Scott, Anton Krige, and
Michael P.W. Grocott, Editors

Foreword

Vascular Anesthesiology: Managing the High-Risk Patient

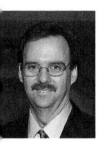

Lee A. Fleisher, MD
Consulting Editor

Patients undergoing vascular surgery have atherosclerotic disease that affects most of the body's organs, including their heart. Over the past several decades, surgical interventions for peripheral vascular disease have become less invasive while the medical management of these patients has improved. When I completed my vascular anesthesia fellowship, the care for these patients was among the most complex, and extensive preoperative evaluation was common. In this issue of *Anesthesiology Clinics*, the editors have provided some basic epidemiology and physiology of vascular disease and discuss the entire perioperative care from preoperative evaluation, intraoperative management and monitoring, and postoperative critical care.

In order to commission an issue on vascular anesthesia care, I invited two cardiovascular anesthesiologists. Dr Megan Kostibas is an Assistant Professof of Anesthesiology and Critical Care Medicine at the Johns Hopkins University School of Medicine. She earned her MD from the University of Texas Health Science Center at San Antonio. She completed her anesthesiology residency and cardiothoracic anesthesiology and critical care medicine fellowships at Johns Hopkins. Dr Kostibas serves as the program director of the Adult Cardiothoracic and Intervention Echocardiography Fellowship. Dr Heather K. Hayanga is an Associate Professor in the Division of Cardiovascular and Thoracic Anesthesiology at the West Virginia University. She earned her MD at the University of Cincinnati College of Medicine, and a Master of Public Health in healthy policy and comparative health systems from the Johns Hopkins Bloomberg School of Public Health. She completed her Anesthesiology

Anesthesiology Clin 40 (2022) xiii–xiv
https://doi.org/10.1016/j.anclin.2022.09.001
1932-2275/22/© 2022 Published by Elsevier Inc.

Residency and Fellowship in Adult Cardiothoracic Anesthesiology at Johns Hopkins Hospital. Together, they have edited an important issue.

Lee A. Fleisher, MD, FACC
3400 Spruce Street, Dulles 680
Philadelphia, PA 19104, USA

E-mail address:
Lee.Fleisher@pennmedicine.upenn.edu

Preface

The Changing Face of Anesthesiology Practice for Vascular Surgery Patients

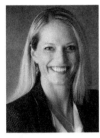   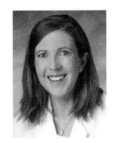

Heather K. Hayanga, MD, MPH   Megan P. Kostibas, MD
Editors

In a long and storied history, vascular surgery dates back to the second century AD. During this time, it is reported that the Greek surgeon, Antyllus, performed surgeries on aortic aneurysms. In more modern times, the legendary surgeons, Drs Michael Debakey and Denton Cooley, performed the first replacement of a thoracic aneurysm with a homograft in the 1950s. Contributions by Drs Nikolai Korotkov, Charles Theodore Dotter, Edward Dietrich, and many others have continued to advance the field and make up the foundations of this surgical specialty. There have been refinements in surgical technique, imaging, endovascular approaches and targeted drug therapies.

Alongside those surgical advances, anesthetic management and training have continued to evolve. Cardiovascular disease claims more than 17.9 million lives each year, constitute the leading cause of death globally.[1] As the 65 and older population continues to grow, those with vascular disease will increasingly continue to require vascular interventions and treatment.

The last issue of *Anesthesiology Clinics* dedicated to the care of vascular surgery patients was in 2014. In the following articles of this special issue of *Anesthesiology Clinics*, expert anesthesiologists and surgeons have included the latest understanding of pathophysiology, preoperative optimization, surgical technique, intraoperative anesthetic management, potential complications, postoperative management, and outcomes. Planning starts in the preoperative period with a focus on perioperative optimization, such as prehabilitation and optimization of preoperative anemia. Using risk calculators, we can predict morbidity and mortality and limit complications and it is hoped, limit perioperative complications. Intraoperative management has shown improvement with technology, such as the use of transesophageal echocardiography, numerous neuromonitoring options, and advanced perfusion techniques. Other

Anesthesiology Clin 40 (2022) xv–xvi
https://doi.org/10.1016/j.anclin.2022.08.003
1932-2275/22/© 2022 Published by Elsevier Inc.

advancements in anesthetic management, such as enhanced recovery pathways, intraoperative blood salvage, and spinal cord perfusion pressure monitoring, have shown promise in improved patient safety and care. The routine use of intensive postoperative monitoring permits early recognition of potential complications.

We wish to express our utmost appreciation to our anesthesiology and surgical colleagues, who have dedicated their time and dedicated knowledge toward the articles in this unique collection. Also, a special thank you to Dr Lee Fleisher, who has entrusted us with the honor of editing this issue. Last but not least, we are very grateful to Arlene Campos and Joanna Collett, who have given continued guidance and patience.

Heather K. Hayanga, MD, MPH
Division of Cardiovascular and
Thoracic Anesthesiology
Department of Anesthesiology
West Virginia University
1 Medical Center Drive
Morgantown, WV 26506-9134, USA

Megan P. Kostibas, MD
Department of Anesthesiology and Critical Care Medicine
Johns Hopkins School of Medicine
1800 Orleans Street
Baltimore, MD 21287, USA

E-mail addresses:
heather.hayanga@wvumedicine.org (H.K. Hayanga)
mkostib1@jhmi.edu (M.P. Kostibas)

REFERENCE

1. World Health Organization. Cardiovascular diseases fact sheet. Available at: https://www.who.int/en/news-room/fact-sheets/detail/cardiovascular-diseases-(cvds). Accessed July 10, 2022.

The Vascular System
Anatomical, Physiological, Pathological, and Aging Considerations

Charlie Slowey, MB, BCh, BAO*, Daniel Nyhan, MD

KEYWORDS

- Vessel biology • Vessel histology • Atherosclerosis • Peripheral vascular disease
- Arterial system • Capillary system • Venous system

KEY POINTS

- The vascular system is one of the earliest systems documented in human history.
- All components of the vascular system contain intrinsic methods to regulate tone and thus flow.
- The splanchnic venous blood reservoir is the compensatory mechanism by which intra-vascular hypovolemia is initially corrected.
- The clinical landscape of atherosclerosis is currently changing with the use of plaque stabilizing drugs leading paradoxically to more complications from plaque erosion and the recognition of new emerging risk factors.
- Peripheral vascular disease has 2 clinical causes: primary atherosclerosis in large vessels and chronic thrombi in smaller vessels. Medial wall calcification contributes to thrombus formation in smaller vessels.

INTRODUCTION

Since the earliest forms of medicine, blood vessels have been recognized to carry substances from one site of the body to another. Egyptian physicians describing the pulse[1] in 1500 BCE continually misidentified blood vessels as 2 different systems; the arterial system believed to carry mostly gaseous material and little liquid, and the venous system carrying mostly liquid and which originated from the liver.[1] It wasn't until William Harvey's *An Anatomical Exercise on the Motion of the Heart and Blood in Living Beings* publication in 1628 that the circulation was understood to be a closed loop system originating and terminating in the heart.[2] Here we will describe the anatomy and physiology of the vascular tree, and discuss very briefly common pathologies.

Author Statement: All authors have no conflicts of interest and no funding sources to identify. Johns Hopkins Department of Anesthesiology and Critical Care Medicine, 600 North Wolf Street, Baltimore, MD 21287, USA
* Corresponding author.
E-mail address: cslowey1@jh.edu

Anesthesiology Clin 40 (2022) 557–574
https://doi.org/10.1016/j.anclin.2022.08.004   anesthesiology.theclinics.com

Abbreviations	
VSMC	Vascular Smooth Muscle Cells
NO	Nitric Oxide
NADPH	Nicotinamide Adenine Dinucleotide Phosphate
PWV	Pulse Wave Velocity
PP	Pulse Pressure
MACE	Major Adverse Cardiac Event
ECM	Extracellular Matrix
VSM	Vascular Smooth Muscle
VVC	Vascular Ventricular Coupling
VAC	Ventricular Arterial Coupling
FHS	Framingham Heart Study
LDL	Low Density Lipoprotein
MRI	Magnetic Resonance Imaging
NETs	Neutrophil Extracellular Traps
STEMI	ST-Elevation Myocardial Infarction
NSTEMI	Non ST-Elevation Myocardial Infarction
PVD	Peripheral Vascular Disease

Anatomy of Blood Vessels

Arterial system

The arterial system consists of 8 branching segments proximal to the capillary system.[3] However, functionally there are only 3 relevant categories of vessels in the arterial system; large conduit arteries (diameter>300 μm), resistance arteries (diameter 50–300 μm), and arterioles (diameter 10–50 μm). All vessels consist of 3 layers; the interna (or intima), the media, and the adventitia[4](**Fig. 1**). The interna consists of the endothelium, which is semipermeable and whose endothelial cells [EC] synthesizes various "paracrine" vasoactive agents,[5–7] and the internal elastic lamina which separates the endothelium from the media. The latter functions as a fenestrated barrier allowing various cells and substances passage between layers.[8] The media contains transversely arranged vascular smooth muscle cells (VSMC) that mediate vascular tone and a matrix of collagen and elastic lamellae.[9] Tone and caliber are modulated by the neurotransmitter activation of subunit receptors.[10] The media changes in size and content with the branching of the arterial system, in proximal branches elastin predominates and in the terminal conduit arteries VSMC predominates.[11] In resistance arteries and arterioles the media has progressively less VSMC before transitioning to the capillary system.[12] The external elastic lamina resides between media and adventitia. The adventitia is the outermost layer and is comprised of collagen, elastin, and fibroblasts. This outer layer protects the artery from damage.[4] The vasa vasorum (blood vessels that supply blood vessels) and nerves that innervate the media reside within the adventitia.[13,14]

Capillary system

Capillaries are the smallest vessel in the human body (diameter 4–10 μm).[9] Comprising of an endothelial layer surrounded by connective tissue, they allow nutrient and metabolite exchange by diffusion.[14] There are 3 functional categories of capillaries: continuous (skin, lungs, blood brain barrier), fenestrated (intestinal villi), and discontinuous/sinusoid (liver, bone marrow) with progressively increasing diffusion capacity allowing larger substances across its membrane.[15]

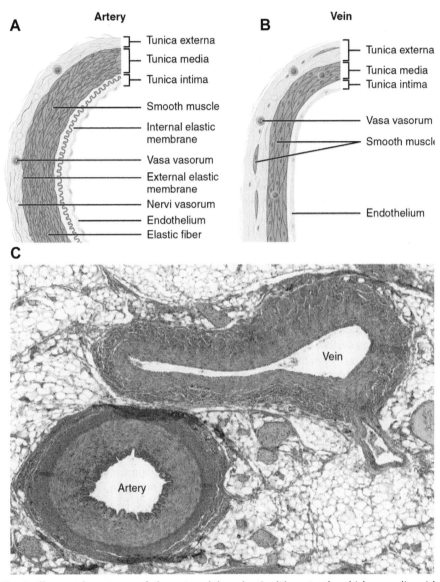

Fig. 1. Illustrated anatomy of the artery (*A*) and vein (*B*), note the thicker media with increased elastic laminae. (*C*) shows a side-by-side histological view of an artery and vein. (Comparison of Artery and Vein, by OpenStax College. Licensed under the Creative Commons Attribution 3.0 Unported license.)

Venous system

The venous system has 5 distinct morphologies; venules, muscular venules, small veins, medium veins, and large veins[9] although the delineation is not as clear as in the arterial system and is highly variable. The venous system branches in "reverse" to that of the arterial system, that is, the venules consist of little more than an endothelial layer with a basement membrane consisting of pericytes.[9] As the venous system converges a

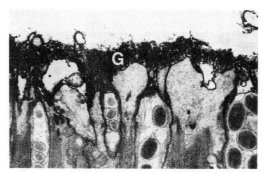

Fig. 2. Histological appearance of the capillary glycocalyx under electron microscopy with tendril like proteoglycans. Glycocalyx layer labeled 'G'. (The Biological bulletin, by Marine Biological Laboratory (Woods Hole, Mass.), August 1985. University of Chicago Press - Journals.)

tunica media appears (muscular venules), then 3 distinct tunics (small veins), valves (medium veins), and finally large named veins[13](see **Fig. 1**). One significant difference between venous and arterial systems is the vasa vasorum capacitance being larger in the venous system. This is due to deoxygenated venous blood with obligatory increased compensatory blood flow and increased vasa vasorum size.[16] The venous system is a high capacitance system with relatively smaller amounts of muscular intima and elastic lamina.[13] It contains 70% of all blood volume[17,18] with the splanchnic venous system used as the "blood reservoir" of the body.[19]

The glycocalyx

The glycocalyx is a negatively charged sugar–protein barrier that coats all healthy vessel endothelium[20] (**Fig. 2**). It has a net negative charge and repels negatively charged molecules including red and white blood cells, and platelets.[21] The discovery of the glycocalyx has caused the revision of the classic Sterling law of fluid dynamics to include the glycocalyx capacity to provide additional intraluminal "oncotic" pressure that limits the movement of fluid to the interstitial space.[22] The glycocalyx protects the endothelium from mechanical shear stress of blood flow[23] and from oxidative stress by scavenging free radicals.[21] It can be damaged by ischemia,[24] hyperglycemia,[25] hypervolemia through release of atrial natriuretic peptide,[26] and systemic inflammation.[27] Damage to the glycocalyx leads to capillary leak, platelet aggregation, edema, increased inflammation, hypercoagulability and loss of vascular responsiveness.[27] Some evidence indicates that certain therapies help maintain the glycocalyx; antioxidants including nitric oxide,[28] glucocorticoids,[29] albumin,[30] and sevoflurane.[31] The emerging literature suggests that protecting the glycocalyx layer may become a consideration in anesthesiology.

Physiology of Blood Vessels

Arterial system

Blood flow. Blood flow characteristics differ in conduit and resistance arteries, and in arterioles. The conduit arteries are elastic in nature and blood flows in a pulsatile manner based on the oscillatory ejections of the left ventricle (the ejected stroke volume is accommodated by the elastic characteristics of the central great arteries [Windkessel effect]). In conduit arteries blood flows in a "distending wave" or pressure pulsation[32] and it is this pulsation that is felt when a pulse is palpated. Two factors

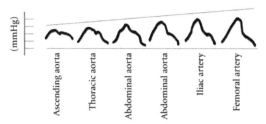

Fig. 3. Illustration showing widened pulse pressure as the flow wave progresses through the arterial tree. (Cohen DL, Townsend RR. Central Blood Pressure and Chronic Kidney Disease Progression.; 2011. Volume 2011, Article ID 407801, https://doi.org/10.4061/2011/407801.)

affect pulse pressure; stroke volume and vascular compliance.[33] In physiological conditions, the central arterial circulation has relatively high elastin content and is compliant/nonstiff. Elastin content and compliance decrease in progressively more distal arterial vessels. The net result is that one observes higher pulse pressures in more distal arteries (radial vs dorsalis pedis) (**Fig. 3**).[34] This pulse pressure lessens to almost no pressure variation after flowing through the resistance arteries due to their numerous branches and by extrinsically and intrinsically regulating their tone.[35] By the time flow of a theoretical "wave" reaches the arterioles, the flow has become continuous.[36]

Tone. Arterial tone is modulated by the autonomic innervation and contraction of VSMC. Although there are numerous receptors that can modulate VSMC tone including purinergic receptors,[37] calcitonin receptor-like receptors,[38] and neuropeptide Y receptors,[39] we will focus on the adrenergic receptor family and the muscarinic acetylcholine receptor. Adrenoreceptors include α1, α2, β1, and β2 subtypes. The alpha 1 receptor mediates increased tone by increasing calcium release from the sarcoplasmic reticulum[40] and this receptor is stimulated by the autonomic release of norepinephrine or direct acting alpha agonists such as phenylephrine.[41] Alpha 2 receptors have a similar function; however, these are located in resistance arteries and arterioles, and not in larger arteries.[42] Both beta 1 and beta 2 adrenergic receptors are present on vessel walls; however, beta 2 predominates in vascular smooth muscle[43] and both cause vasodilation.[44] Muscarinic acetylcholine receptor agonists cause both vasoconstriction and vasodilation by activating different muscarinic subtypes. Activation of muscarinic M2 and M3 receptors on vascular smooth muscle cause vasoconstriction by the inhibition of nitric oxide production.[45]

Capillary system
Flow. The capillary system contains no muscular media nor does it contain sensory innervation.[15] As such it must auto-regulate its flow on a local level by dilating or constricting upstream arterioles.[36] Historically the metabolic theory of autoregulation prevailed, that is, local tissue produces metabolites that cause vasodilation of arterioles resulting in increased oxygen and nutrient delivery to capillaries.[46] It is now believed that extracellular nitric oxide [NO] and its inhibition by the free radical superoxide (O_2^-) control local blood flow. They act as counter mechanisms. NO-induced relaxation increases blood flow and thus the availability of the metabolic substrates; oxygen and glucose. In turn, cellular metabolism involving the cytosolic NAD(P)H oxidase[47] generates superoxide radical neutralizing nitric oxide with resultant local vasoconstriction.[48] This local agonism–antagonism leads to cyclical opening/closing of

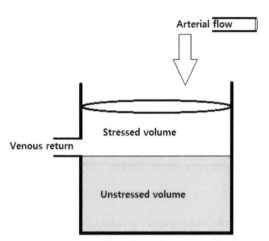

Fig. 4. Tub analogy of venous return. With a fluid bolus, the stressed volume would increase leading to greater venous return. With vasopressor administration, the venous return spout is effectively "lowered"; meaning that unstressed volume is returned to the central circulation.

capillaries termed vasomotion, and although a single capillary is either open or closed, a group of capillaries has an average constant blood flow.[36]

Venous system

A 2-compartment model has been proposed to describe the physiology of the venous system. The first compartment or *"stressed volume"* resides within skeletal muscle and large conduit veins emptying directly into the vena cava. The second or *"unstressed volume"* refers to the splanchnic venous reservoir and is not part of the central circulation.[49] These 2 compartments act differently when subjected to volume load. With arteriole dilation, flow in the stressed venous system increases, presuming arterial pressure has not decreased.[50] In contrast, on arteriole dilation blood flow *and volume* of the unstressed splanchnic reservoir increases. The opposite also holds true. Indeed, it is the decrease in blood flow to the unstressed venous system and resulting the mobilization of blood from the splanchnic reservoir into the central circulation through the hepatic veins[51] that compensates for early hypovolemia during times of stress and exercise[52] (**Fig. 4**). This phenomenon has been well documented both in a clinical setting (the increase of cardiac output after high aortic cross-clamping[53]) and directly (using whole body technetium-99 scans indicate that thoracic blood volume increases after diaphragmatic aortic cross clamping[54]). The venous system contains adrenoreceptors primarily on splanchnic and cutaneous veins, and alpha agonist induced venoconstriction can unload the unstressed volume in the splanchnic reservoir into the central circulation.[55] However in severe hypovolemic states, vasopressor-induced hepatic vasoconstriction can create a "barrier" effect to unloading this unstressed volume.[56]

Aging and Central Vascular Stiffness

The physiology of pulse wave transmission in the vessel wall has been described above. Antegrade pulse waves are reflected back toward the central circulation at points of what has been described as "physiological discontinuity," that is, branch points and abrupt changes in vessel diameter, resulting in a retrograde pulse wave. In healthy vessels, the velocity of both the antegrade and retrograde waves is low

[Pulse Wave Velocity [PWV] <3 m/s] and the retrograde pulse wave reaches the central circulation during diastole. The result is that pulse pressures [PP] increase progressively from the central to the peripheral circulation (see **Fig. 3**). Arterial disease and aging per se result in increased stiffening of vessels and increased PWV. This results in an attenuation and eventual reversal of the central to peripheral PP gradient.

Techniques to measure PWV and other indices of vascular stiffness [e.g., Augmentation Index, AI] are now well established and these have been used extensively in epidemiological studies to demonstrate that increased central vascular stiffness is an independent risk factor for predicting major adverse cardiac events (MACE) (a composite of total death, myocardial infarction, stroke, hospitalization because of heart failure, and any revascularization event). Indeed, data also exist suggesting that this notion may also apply perioperatively.[57]

The mechanisms underlying changes in vascular stiffness are important because an understanding of these mechanisms is fundamental to developing targeted therapies that interrogate these pathways. They include changes in the extracellular matrix

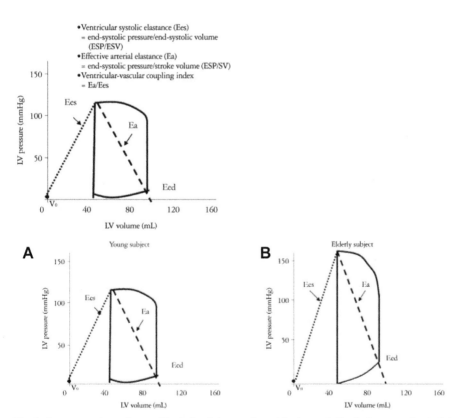

Fig. 5. Pressure volume loop with derived slopes of ventricular systolic elastance and arterial elastance. The ratio of these remains constant over a wide range of hemodynamic perturbations and this is termed ventricular vascular coupling. Compare A (a young patient) with B (an elderly patient) and note that the slope of ventricular and arterial elastance changes however the ratio remains the same. Adapted with permission from[59] (Shim CY. Arterial-Cardiac Interaction: The Concept and Implications. J Cardiovasc Ultrasound. 2011 Jun;19(2):62-66. https://doi.org/10.4250/jcu.2011.19.2.62.)

[ECM], in vascular smooth muscle [VSM], and the interactions between both. ECM changes include changes in elastin/collagen ratio, type of collagen [cross-linking], and the oxidative-reductive milieu. VSM changes include increases in stiffness of the VSM itself. This area is discussed in detail elsewhere.[58]

Under physiological conditions, the performances of the vasculature and the left ventricle are coupled with optimize overall cardiovascular function [vascular-ventricular or vascular-arterial coupling, VVC or VAC]. This coupling demonstrates remarkable parallel compensatory ability in that VVC remains intact over a large range of perturbations, a critical feature in maintaining cardiovascular homeostasis **(Fig. 5)**.[59]

Atherosclerosis

Atherosclerosis refers to the fibrous/fatty material that accumulates in the intima of arteries. Derived from the Greek work for "gruel"—it is the appearance of lipid material in the core of an atheromatous plaque that gives this entity its name. We will briefly discuss risk factors and the salient mechanisms underlying atheroma initiation, progression, and ensuing complications.

Atherosclerosis risk factors
Long established atherosclerosis risk factors (hypertension, male gender, smoking, diabetes, hypercholesterolemia, and age[60]), and their prediction of MACE have been elucidated from innumerable long-running studies including the Framingham Heart Study (FHS), now in its 74th year and its offshoot cohort studies in the US.[60] With the accumulation of longitudinal data by the FHS, risk factor identification has expanded beyond "traditional factors" to include left ventricular hypertrophy on electrocardiogram,[61] low exercise level,[62] obesity,[63] and finally the delineation of risk for high levels of LDL cholesterol.[64] As the FHS continues and more advanced investigative techniques become available including echocardiography,[65] exercise testing,[66] biomarker sampling,[67,68] arterial tonometry,[69] coronary artery calcium level measurement,[70] cardiac MRI,[71] and genetic[72,73] and epigenetic[74] sequencing which all contribute to the understanding of atherosclerosis initiation and progression but are beyond the scope of this review. A key concept here is whether the identification of additional/new risk factors adds predictive value over and above already established risk factors and are thus independent predictors. For a comprehensive review of the investigations of the FHS see review[60] by Andersson and colleagues The landscape of atherosclerosis risk is changing in the United States due to the early initiation of primary preventive measures. Paradoxically, these interventions are helping unmask additional potential underlying mechanisms and risk factors (inflammation,[75] genetic factors,[76] and air pollution[77]).

Atheroma initiation
Translocation of Apo-lipoprotein B [Apo-B] containing lipoproteins through the glycocalyx and into the intima layer causes a low-grade chronic inflammatory response and initiates atheroma formation.[78] Translocation occurs through the binding of lipid molecules to adhesion molecules and chemo-attractants that are produced when a high saturated fat/cholesterol-containing diet is consumed.[79] Once these molecules enter the intima they bind to negatively charged proteoglycans promoting the retention of lipoprotein molecules in the intima.[80] Inflammatory modification of plasma-derived lipoproteins and their uptake by macrophages results in foam cell formation. For example, free radical oxygen species oxidize LDL-c, a species that acts as a ligand for scavenger receptors that facilitate foam cell formation by overloading macrophages with cholesterol ester[81] **(Fig. 6)**[82]. Inflammatory mediators are commonly

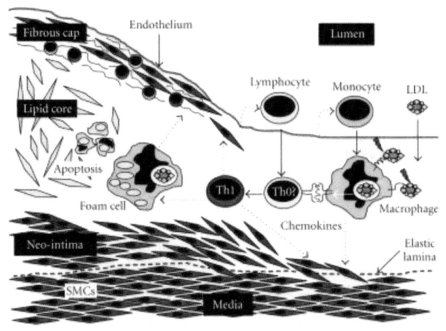

Fig. 6. Atheroma initiation and progression. Note vascular smooth muscle cell (SMC) translocation from media to intima. LDL: low-density lipoprotein, Th0: T-helper cell 0, Th1: T-helper cell 1. Open access use using creative commons license 3.0 from.83

found in atherosclerotic lesions; however, whether this is an initiating factor or a product of ongoing plaque formation is unclear.[83] It is also now increasingly recognized that plague progression while initiated and driven by proinflammatory mediators, is also profoundly influenced by the efficacy/lack of efficacy of proresolving mechanisms in these lesions.[84] Although discussed briefly later in discussion, a detailed discussion of the relative contributions of these counter mechanisms to plaque stability/instability, plague erosion and the morphological features that may predict plague behavior are beyond the scope of this review.

Atheroma progression
Once formed in the intima foam cells continue to accumulate over years. Formerly believed to originate only from macrophages, foam cells have been shown experimentally to also originate from vascular smooth muscle cells that themselves originate in the intima or are translocated from the media.[85] Along with foam cells, inflammatory leukocytes[86] and T lymphocytes localize within these lesions contributing to lesion progression.[83] Macrophages and vascular smooth muscle cells undergo programmed cell death and contribute to the lipid-rich nidus of an atheroma[87] which in turn promotes instability and plaque rupture[88] (see **Fig. 6**). Atheroma calcification is due to dysregulated calcium deposition and impaired clearance.[58] However, it is the *micro-calcifications* in the fibrous luminal cap that increase stress on the atheroma and promote rupture.[89] As calcifications enlarge, whether through natural deposition or through medical intervention, the fibrous cap of the atheroma stabilizes and stresses are decreased leading to plaque stability.[90] This is one of the mechanisms underlying the benefits of statin therapy.[91]

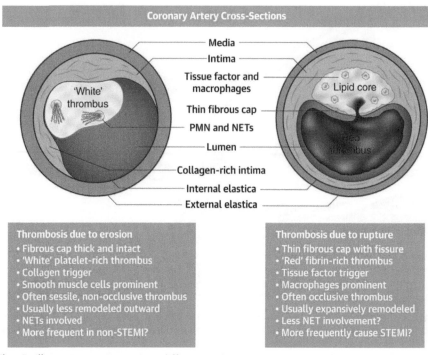

Coronary Artery Cross-Sections

Media
Intima
Tissue factor and macrophages
Thin fibrous cap
PMN and NETs
Lumen
Collagen-rich intima
Internal elastica
External elastica

'White' thrombus

Lipid core

'Red' thrombus

Thrombosis due to erosion
- Fibrous cap thick and intact
- 'White' platelet-rich thrombus
- Collagen trigger
- Smooth muscle cells prominent
- Often sessile, non-occlusive thrombus
- Usually less remodeled outward
- NETs involved
- More frequent in non-STEMI?

Thrombosis due to rupture
- Thin fibrous cap with fissure
- 'Red' fibrin-rich thrombus
- Tissue factor trigger
- Macrophages prominent
- Often occlusive thrombus
- Usually expansively remodeled
- Less NET involvement?
- More frequently cause STEMI?

Fig. 7. Illustration representing differences between rupture and erosion of arterial atheroma. NET, neutrophil extracellular trap; STEMI, ST elevation myocardial infarction. (Reused with permission from.[97])

Atheroma complications

Atheroma complications can be divided into 2: thrombosis and plaque erosion. Thrombosis occurs following rupture of so-called "vulnerable plaques"[92]—plaques with lipid-rich cores, thin fibrous caps(<60 μm), and microcalcifications as discussed above. Plaque rupture and exposure of thrombogenic material (namely tissue factor) in the core to the arterial lumen promotes thrombogenesis through thrombin-mediated generation of fibrin from fibrinogen and platelet aggregation.[93] Recent work has implicated neutrophil extracellular traps(NETs)[94] (strands of DNA that attract tissue factor and leukocyte granular enzymes) that also contribute to thrombus formation and exacerbate intimal injury.[95] Plaque erosion is increasingly recognized as an important mechanism underlying the evolving clinical manifestations of coronary artery disease, specifically the apparent decrease in STEMI and increase in NSTEMI prevalence.[96] This may be, in part, a function of the increased use of atheroma stabilizing drugs.[91] The lesions that undergo erosion are structurally different from those that undergo rupture; lesions that erode tend to have thick caps, a rich extracellular matrix and little lipid[97] (**Fig. 7**)[98]. There is a 2-hit hypothesis describing the mechanism underlying plaque erosion; first endothelial cell desquamation in areas of turbulent flow (for example, distal to arterial stenosis). Second, exposure and activation of toll-like receptor 2,[99] resultant attraction of NETs,[100] and impairment of neighboring endothelial cell repair.[101] This pathologic state produces the same clinical picture of decreased distal flow in an artery; however, the onset is much less rapid compared to plaque thrombosis.

Peripheral Arterial Disease

Peripheral arterial disease (PVD) is a global health issue affecting >200 million people worldwide and is increasing in both low, middle, and high income countries.[102] The American College of Cardiology/American Heart Association divides the presentation of peripheral arterial disease into 4 categories: asymptomatic, claudication, critical limb ischemia, and acute limb ischemia.[103]

PVD presentation

The presentation of peripheral vascular disease can be subdivided into the above-mentioned categories. Asymptomatic PVD is the presence of stenotic flow-limiting lesions despite no symptoms. Claudication is reported as fatigue, discomfort, or pain that occurs in specific muscle groups during an effort that is due to ischemia. Critical limb ischemia describes limb pain at rest which is often worse in the supine position and improves with dependent positioning of the affected limb. Acute limb ischemia presents classically with the 5 "P's": pain, paralysis, paresthesia, pulselessness, and pallor although many would include a sixth 'P" – polar denoting "cold limb."[103]

PVD causes primary atherosclerosis

In a recent investigation, Narula and colleagues[104] conducted histopathological studies of 299 arteries in patients with critical limb ischemia. They found that primary atherosclerosis causing luminal narrowing was present more often (67.6% vs 38.5%) in proximal arteries compared to peripheral arteries of the lower limbs (femoral and popliteal arteries). This luminal narrowing along with acute thrombosis leading to ischemia has been mechanistically discussed in the section "Atherosclerosis."

PVD causes chronic thrombi

Narula and colleagues[104] also showed that chronic thrombi are common in infrapopliteal arteries causing luminal narrowing and there was less significant primary atherosclerosis. This suggests that chronic thromboembolism from proximal arteries is a cause of infrapopliteal critical limb ischemia. One additional mechanism may contribute to thrombus formation and ischemia: medial wall calcification. Medial calcification occurs independently from atherosclerosis and its resultant intimal calcification. It is present in the human aorta at 20 years of age and progresses as the human body ages.[105] Medial calcification is thought to occur from the transition of vascular smooth muscle cells to an osteogenic phenotype propagating deposition of calcium on an elastic lamellae nidus.[106] Patients with diabetes mellitus[107] and chronic renal injury[108] are particularly susceptible. This induces arterial stiffness, stasis of blood and ultimately thrombus formation.[109] Narula and colleagues found that these medial calcifications were present in 71.1% of arteries contributing to critical limb ischemia with infrapopliteal arteries 3.4 times more likely to have medial calcification.

PVD treatment

Treatment is determined by PVD type and presentation. For all prevention is key to limiting complications being most beneficial for the asymptomatic; statins, antihypertensives, glucose reduction, and foot care if diabetic, antiplatelet agents, and smoking cessation are all class 1 recommendations from the American Heart Association guidelines on the prevention of PVD-related complications for patients with asymptomatic PVD. Supervised exercise programs along with cilostazol for symptom management are recommended for claudication patients, surgery is only recommended for this group if their symptoms are vocationally or lifestyle limiting.[103] The scope of discussion of surgical treatment (endovascular vs open and timing) is beyond the scope of this review.

Critical and acute limb ischemia are treated with either thrombolysis (mainly catheter directed) or surgical revascularization and is usually surgically driven.

SUMMARY

The vascular system is one of the oldest recognized biological systems, its importance to human health was first described by Egyptian physicians. Its sole purpose is to transport substances, both advantageous and deleterious, to various tissues and organs of the body. There are both intrinsic mechanisms and extrinsic factors that govern blood flow and thus oxygen delivery and metabolite clearance. Contemporary lifestyles especially in Western cultures have resulted in an epidemic of vascular disease (coronary artery disease, peripheral vascular disease, and so forth). These are increasing despite the best preventive and pharmacologic measures.

CLINICS CARE POINTS

- Arterial pulse pressure increases from the central to the peripheral arterial tree. Aging results in the eventual reversal gradient and thus overall increased work of the heart in the elderly patient.
- The capillary system autoregulates are mediated predominantly by the oxidation of nitric oxide.
- The venous system acts as both a conduit and reservoir of deoxygenated blood and can increase circulating blood volume in times of stress, hypovolemia, and exercise.
- Atherosclerosis is initiated by apolipoprotein-B, progresses over time, and eventually leads to a local decrease in the caliber of the blood vessel and thus blood flow.
- Both the risk factors and the pathologic mechanism of decreased blood flow caused by atherosclerosis are changing due to earlier medical interventions.
- Peripheral vascular disease is caused by atherosclerosis in proximal large caliber vessels and a combination of primary atherosclerosis and embolic showering in distal vessels.
- Peripheral vascular disease treatment is primarily through prevention and surgical intervention in its later stages.

REFERENCES

1. Aird WC. Discovery of the cardiovascular system: from Galen to William Harvey: Discovery of the cardiovascular system. J Thromb Haemost 2011;9:118–29.
2. Bolli R. William harvey and the discovery of the circulation of the blood. Circ Res 2019;124(8):1169–71.
3. Iberall AS. Anatomy and steady flow characteristics of the arterial system with an introduction to its pulsatile characteristics. Math Biosci 1967;1(3):375–95.
4. Tennant M, McGeachie JK. Blood vessel structure and function: a brief update on recent advances. ANZ J Surg 1990;60(10):747–53.
5. Edgell CJ, McDonald CC, Graham JB. Permanent cell line expressing human factor VIII-related antigen established by hybridization. Proc Natl Acad Sci U S A 1983;80(12):3734–7.
6. McIntyre TM, Zimmerman GA, Satoh K, et al. Cultured endothelial cells synthesize both platelet-activating factor and prostacyclin in response to histamine, bradykinin, and adenosine triphosphate. J Clin Invest 1985;76(1):271–80.

7. Wilcox JN, Smith KM, Williams LT, et al. Platelet-derived growth factor mRNA detection in human atherosclerotic plaques by in situ hybridization. J Clin Invest 1988;82(3):1134–43.
8. Sandow SL, Gzik DJ, Lee RMKW. Arterial internal elastic lamina holes: relationship to function? J Anat 2009;214(2):258–66.
9. Taylor AM, Bordoni B. Histology, blood vascular system. In: StatPearls. StatPearls Publishing; 2022. Available at: http://www.ncbi.nlm.nih.gov/books/NBK553217/. Accessed March 23, 2022.
10. Sheng Y, Zhu L. The crosstalk between autonomic nervous system and blood vessels. Int J Physiol Pathophysiol Pharmacol 2018;10(1):17–28.
11. Laurent S, Boutouyrie P. The structural factor of hypertension: large and small artery alterations. Circ Res 2015;116(6):1007–21.
12. Korsgaard N, Aalkjaer C, Heagerty AM, et al. Histology of subcutaneous small arteries from patients with essential hypertension. Hypertension 1993;22(4):523–6.
13. Junqueira LCU, Carneiro J, Junqueira LCU. Basic histology: text & atlas. 10. Lange; 2003.
14. Tucker WD, Arora Y, Mahajan K. Anatomy, Blood Vessels. In: StatPearls. StatPearls Publishing; 2022. http://www.ncbi.nlm.nih.gov/books/NBK470401/. [Accessed 22 March 2022]. Accessed.
15. Godwin L, Tariq MA, Crane JS. Histology, Capillary. In: StatPearls. StatPearls Publishing; 2022. Available at: http://www.ncbi.nlm.nih.gov/books/NBK546578/. Accessed March 23, 2022.
16. Brook WH. Vasa vasorum of veins in dog and man. Angiology 1977;28(5):351–60.
17. Hainsworth R. Vascular capacitance: its control and importance. Rev Physiol Biochem Pharmacol 1986;105:101–73.
18. Rothe CF. Reflex control of veins and vascular capacitance. Physiol Rev 1983;63(4):1281–342.
19. Gelman S. Venous function and central venous pressure: a physiologic story. Anesthesiology 2008;108(4):735–48.
20. Rehm M, Zahler S, Lötsch M, et al. Endothelial glycocalyx as an additional barrier determining extravasation of 6% hydroxyethyl starch or 5% albumin solutions in the coronary vascular bed. Anesthesiology 2004;100(5):1211–23.
21. Reitsma S, Slaaf DW, Vink H, et al. The endothelial glycocalyx: composition, functions, and visualization. Pflugers Arch 2007;454(3):345–59.
22. Adamson RH, Lenz JF, Zhang X, et al. Oncotic pressures opposing filtration across non-fenestrated rat microvessels. J Physiol 2004;557(Pt 3):889–907.
23. Pries AR, Secomb TW, Gaehtgens P. The endothelial surface layer. Pflugers Arch 2000;440(5):653–66.
24. Chappell D, Jacob M, Hofmann-Kiefer K, et al. Antithrombin reduces shedding of the endothelial glycocalyx following ischaemia/reperfusion. Cardiovasc Res 2009;83(2):388–96.
25. Nieuwdorp M, Mooij HL, Kroon J, et al. Endothelial glycocalyx damage coincides with microalbuminuria in type 1 diabetes. Diabetes 2006;55(4):1127–32.
26. Bruegger D, Jacob M, Rehm M, et al. Atrial natriuretic peptide induces shedding of endothelial glycocalyx in coronary vascular bed of guinea pig hearts. Am J Physiol Heart Circ Physiol 2005;289(5):H1993–9.
27. Becker BF, Chappell D, Bruegger D, et al. Therapeutic strategies targeting the endothelial glycocalyx: acute deficits, but great potential. Cardiovasc Res 2010;87(2):300–10.

28. Bruegger D, Rehm M, Jacob M, et al. Exogenous nitric oxide requires an endothelial glycocalyx to prevent postischemic coronary vascular leak in guinea pig hearts. Crit Care Lond Engl 2008;12(3):R73.

29. Chappell D, Jacob M, Hofmann-Kiefer K, et al. Hydrocortisone preserves the vascular barrier by protecting the endothelial glycocalyx. Anesthesiology 2007;107(5):776–84.

30. Jacob M, Bruegger D, Rehm M, et al. Contrasting effects of colloid and crystalloid resuscitation fluids on cardiac vascular permeability. Anesthesiology 2006; 104(6):1223–31.

31. Annecke T, Rehm M, Bruegger D, et al. Ischemia-reperfusion-induced unmeasured anion generation and glycocalyx shedding: sevoflurane versus propofol anesthesia. J Invest Surg 2012;25(3):162–8.

32. Dart AM, Kingwell BA. Pulse pressure–a review of mechanisms and clinical relevance. J Am Coll Cardiol 2001;37(4):975–84.

33. Magder S. The meaning of blood pressure. Crit Care Lond Engl 2018;22(1):257.

34. Cohen DL, Townsend RR. Central Blood Pressure and Chronic Kidney Disease Progression 2011. Available at: https://www.ncbi.nlm.nih.gov/pmc/articles/PMC3056344/.

35. Tykocki NR, Boerman EM, Jackson WF. Smooth Muscle Ion Channels and Regulation of Vascular Tone in Resistance Arteries and Arterioles. Compr Physiol 2017;7(2):485–581.

36. Hall JE. Guyton and Hall textbook of medical physiology. 13th edition. Elsevier; 2016.

37. Ralevic V, Burnstock G. Receptors for purines and pyrimidines. Pharmacol Rev 1998;50(3):413–92.

38. McLatchie LM, Fraser NJ, Main MJ, et al. RAMPs regulate the transport and ligand specificity of the calcitonin-receptor-like receptor. Nature 1998; 393(6683):333–9.

39. Håkanson R, Wahlestedt C, Ekblad E, et al. Neuropeptide Y: coexistence with noradrenaline. Functional implications. Prog Brain Res 1986;68:279–87.

40. Vanhoutte PM, Rimele TJ. Calcium and alpha-adrenoceptors in activation of vascular smooth muscle. J Cardiovasc Pharmacol 1982;4(Suppl 3):S280–6.

41. Guyenet PG. The sympathetic control of blood pressure. Nat Rev Neurosci 2006;7(5):335–46.

42. Daniel EE, Brown RD, Wang YF, et al. α-Adrenoceptors in canine mesenteric artery are predominantly 1A subtype: pharmacological and immunochemical evidence. J Pharmacol Exp Ther 1999;291(2):671.

43. Osswald W, Guimarães S. Adrenergic mechanisms in blood vessels: Morphological and pharmacological aspects. In: Reviews of physiology, biochemistry and pharmacology96. Springer Berlin Heidelberg; 1983. p. 53–122. https://doi.org/10.1007/BFb0031007.

44. Begonha R, Moura D, Guimarães S. Vascular β-adrenoceptor-mediated relaxation and the tone of the tissue in canine arteries. J Pharm Pharmacol 2011;47(6): 510–3.

45. Bolton TB, Lim SP. Action of acetylcholine on smooth muscle. Z Kardiol 1991; 80(Suppl 7):73–7.

46. Rowell LB. Ideas about control of skeletal and cardiac muscle blood flow (1876-2003): cycles of revision and new vision. J Appl Physiol Bethesda Md 1985 2004;97(1):384–92.

47. Cosentino F, Sill JC, Katusić ZS. Role of superoxide anions in the mediation of endothelium-dependent contractions. Hypertens Dallas Tex 1979 1994;23(2): 229–35.
48. Gryglewski RJ, Palmer RM, Moncada S. Superoxide anion is involved in the breakdown of endothelium-derived vascular relaxing factor. Nature 1986; 320(6061):454–6.
49. Mason DT, Bartter FC. Autonomic regulation of blood volume. Anesthesiology 1968;29(4):681–92.
50. Emerson TE. Changes of venous return and other hemodynamic parameters during bradykinin infusion. Am J Physiol 1967;212(6):1455–60.
51. Rothe CF, Gaddis ML. Autoregulation of cardiac output by passive elastic characteristics of the vascular capacitance system. Circulation 1990;81(1):360–8.
52. Rowell LB. Human cardiovascular control. Oxford University Press; 1993.
53. Gregoretti S, Henderson T, Parks DA, et al. Haemodynamic changes and oxygen uptake during crossclamping of the thoracic aorta in dexmedetomidine pretreated dogs. Can J Anaesth J Can Anesth 1992;39(7):731–41.
54. Gelman S, Khazaeli MB, Orr R, et al. Blood volume redistribution during crossclamping of the descending aorta. Anesth Analg 1994;78(2):219–24.
55. Karim F, Hainsworth R. Responses of abdominal vascular capacitance to stimulation of splanchic nerves. Am J Physiol 1976;231(2):434–40.
56. Gelman S, Mushlin PS. Catecholamine-induced changes in the splanchnic circulation affecting systemic hemodynamics. Anesthesiology 2004;100(2):434–9.
57. Nyhan D, Berkowitz DE. Perioperative Blood Pressure Management: Does Central Vascular Stiffness Matter? Anesth Analg 2008;107(4):1103–6.
58. Ruiz JL, Hutcheson JD, Aikawa E. Cardiovascular calcification: current controversies and novel concepts. Cardiovasc Pathol Off J Soc Cardiovasc Pathol 2015;24(4):207–12.
59.. Shim CY. Arterial-cardiac interaction: the concept and implications. 2011. https://www.ncbi.nlm.nih.gov/pmc/articles/PMC3150697/. [Accessed 27 April 2022].
60. Andersson C, Johnson AD, Benjamin EJ, et al. 70-year legacy of the framingham heart study. Nat Rev Cardiol 2019;16(11):687–98.
61. Kannel WB, Dawber TR, Kagan A, et al. Factors of risk in the development of coronary heart disease–six year follow-up experience. The Framingham Study. Ann Intern Med 1961;55:33–50.
62. Kannel WB. Habitual level of physical activity and risk of coronary heart disease: the Framingham study. Can Med Assoc J 1967;96(12):811–2.
63. Hubert HB, Feinleib M, McNamara PM, et al. Obesity as an independent risk factor for cardiovascular disease: a 26-year follow-up of participants in the Framingham Heart Study. Circulation 1983;67(5):968–77.
64. Castelli WP, Abbott RD, McNamara PM. Summary estimates of cholesterol used to predict coronary heart disease. Circulation 1983;67(4):730–4.
65. Levy D, Garrison RJ, Savage DD, et al. Prognostic implications of echocardiographically determined left ventricular mass in the Framingham Heart Study. N Engl J Med 1990;322(22):1561–6.
66. Lauer MS, Okin PM, Larson MG, et al. Impaired heart rate response to graded exercise. Prognostic implications of chronotropic incompetence in the Framingham Heart Study. Circulation 1996;93(8):1520–6.
67. Shoamanesh A, Preis SR, Beiser AS, et al. Circulating biomarkers and incident ischemic stroke in the Framingham Offspring Study. Neurology 2016;87(12): 1206–11.

68. Wang TJ, Gona P, Larson MG, et al. Multiple biomarkers and the risk of incident hypertension. Hypertens Dallas Tex 1979 2007;49(3):432–8.
69. Mitchell GF, Hwang SJ, Vasan RS, et al. Arterial stiffness and cardiovascular events: the Framingham Heart Study. Circulation 2010;121(4):505–11.
70. Tsao CW, Preis SR, Peloso GM, et al. Relations of long-term and contemporary lipid levels and lipid genetic risk scores with coronary artery calcium in the framingham heart study. J Am Coll Cardiol 2012;60(23):2364–71.
71. Tsao CW, Gona PN, Salton CJ, et al. Left Ventricular Structure and Risk of Cardiovascular Events: A Framingham Heart Study Cardiac Magnetic Resonance Study. J Am Heart Assoc 2015;4(9):e002188.
72. Dehghan A, Bis JC, White CC, et al. Genome-wide association study for incident myocardial infarction and coronary heart disease in prospective cohort studies: the CHARGE consortium. PLoS One 2016;11(3):e0144997.
73. Natarajan P, Bis JC, Bielak LF, et al. Multiethnic exome-wide association study of subclinical atherosclerosis. Circ Cardiovasc Genet 2016;9(6):511–20.
74. Ligthart S, Marzi C, Aslibekyan S, et al. DNA methylation signatures of chronic low-grade inflammation are associated with complex diseases. Genome Biol 2016;17(1):255.
75. Xiao L, Harrison DG. Inflammation in Hypertension. Can J Cardiol 2020;36(5): 635–47.
76. Aragam KG, Natarajan P. Polygenic Scores to Assess Atherosclerotic Cardiovascular Disease Risk: Clinical Perspectives and Basic Implications. Circ Res 2020;126(9):1159–77.
77. Münzel T. Up in the air: links between the environment and cardiovascular disease. Cardiovasc Res 2019;115(13):e144–6.
78. Ference BA, Ginsberg HN, Graham I, et al. Low-density lipoproteins cause atherosclerotic cardiovascular disease. 1. Evidence from genetic, epidemiologic, and clinical studies. A consensus statement from the European Atherosclerosis Society Consensus Panel. Eur Heart J 2017;38(32):2459–72.
79. Cybulsky MI, Gimbrone MA. Endothelial expression of a mononuclear leukocyte adhesion molecule during atherogenesis. Science 1991;251(4995):788–91.
80. Skålén K, Gustafsson M, Rydberg EK, et al. Subendothelial retention of atherogenic lipoproteins in early atherosclerosis. Nature 2002;417(6890):750–4.
81. Navab M, Ananthramaiah GM, Reddy ST, et al. The oxidation hypothesis of atherogenesis: the role of oxidized phospholipids and HDL. J Lipid Res 2004; 45(6):993–1007.
82. Milioti N, Bermudez-Fajardo A, Penichet ML, et al. Antigen-Induced Immunomodulation in the Pathogenesis of Atherosclerosis. 2008. Available at: https://www.ncbi.nlm.nih.gov/pmc/articles/PMC2423423/.
83. Nus M, Mallat Z. Immune-mediated mechanisms of atherosclerosis and implications for the clinic. Expert Rev Clin Immunol 2016;12(11):1217–37.
84. Bäck M, Yurdagul A, Tabas I, et al. Inflammation and its resolution in atherosclerosis: mediators and therapeutic opportunities. Nat Rev Cardiol 2019;16(7): 389–406.
85. Bennett MR, Sinha S, Owens GK. Vascular smooth muscle cells in atherosclerosis. Circ Res 2016;118(4):692–702.
86. Robbins CS, Hilgendorf I, Weber GF, et al. Local proliferation dominates lesional macrophage accumulation in atherosclerosis. Nat Med 2013;19(9):1166–72.
87. Geng YJ, Libby P. Evidence for apoptosis in advanced human atheroma. Colocalization with interleukin-1 beta-converting enzyme. Am J Pathol 1995;147(2): 251–66.

88. Huang H, Virmani R, Younis H, et al. The Impact of Calcification on the Biomechanical Stability of Atherosclerotic Plaques. Circulation 2001;103(8):1051–6.
89. Kelly-Arnold A, Maldonado N, Laudier D, et al. Revised microcalcification hypothesis for fibrous cap rupture in human coronary arteries. Proc Natl Acad Sci 2013;110(26):10741–6.
90. Imoto K, Hiro T, Fujii T, et al. Longitudinal structural determinants of atherosclerotic plaque vulnerability. J Am Coll Cardiol 2005;46(8):1507–15.
91. Ludman A, Venugopal V, Yellon DM, et al. Statins and cardioprotection — More than just lipid lowering? Pharmacol Ther 2009;122(1):30–43.
92. Bentzon JF, Otsuka F, Virmani R, et al. Mechanisms of plaque formation and rupture. Circ Res 2014;114(12):1852–66.
93. Libby P, Buring JE, Badimon L, et al. Atherosclerosis. *Nat Rev Dis Primer.* 2019; 5(1):56.
94. Martinod K, Wagner DD. Thrombosis: tangled up in NETs. Blood 2014;123(18): 2768–76.
95. Folco EJ, Mawson TL, Vromman A, et al. Neutrophil extracellular traps induce endothelial cell activation and tissue factor production through interleukin-1α and cathepsin G. Arterioscler Thromb Vasc Biol 2018;38(8):1901–12.
96. Fahed AC, Jang IK. Plaque erosion and acute coronary syndromes: phenotype, molecular characteristics and future directions. Nat Rev Cardiol 2021;18(10): 724–34.
97. Quillard T, Franck G, Mawson T, et al. Mechanisms of erosion of atherosclerotic plaques. Curr Opin Lipidol 2017;28(5):434–41.
98.. Sarnak Mark J, Amann K, Bangalore Sripal, et al. Chronic kidney disease and coronary artery disease. Am Coll Cardiol Found 2019. https://doi.org/10.1016/j. jacc.2019.08.1017. Accessed May 13, 2022. https://www.researchgate.net/ publication/336196155_Chronic_Kidney_Disease_and_Coronary_Artery_ Disease_JACC_State-of-the-Art_Review.
99. Franck G, Mawson T, Sausen G, et al. Flow perturbation mediates neutrophil recruitment and potentiates endothelial injury via TLR2 in mice: implications for superficial erosion. Circ Res 2017;121(1):31–42.
100. Megens RTA, Vijayan S, Lievens D, et al. Presence of luminal neutrophil extracellular traps in atherosclerosis. Thromb Haemost 2012;107(3):597–8.
101. Quillard T, Araújo HA, Franck G, et al. TLR2 and neutrophils potentiate endothelial stress, apoptosis and detachment: implications for superficial erosion. Eur Heart J 2015;36(22):1394–404.
102. Sampson UK, Fowkes FGR, McDermott MM, et al. Global and regional burden of death and disability from peripheral artery disease: 21 world regions, 1990 to 2010. Glob Heart 2014;9(1):145–58.
103. Hirsch AT, Haskal ZJ, Hertzer NR, et al. ACC/AHA guidelines for the management of patients with peripheral arterial disease (lower extremity, renal, mesenteric, and abdominal aortic): a collaborative report from the american associations for vascular surgery/society for vascular surgery, society for cardiovascular angiography and interventions, society for vascular medicine and biology, society of interventional radiology, and the ACC/AHA task force on practice guidelines (writing committee to develop guidelines for the management of patients with peripheral arterial disease)–summary of recommendations. J Vasc Interv Radiol JVIR 2006;17(9):1383–97 [quiz: 1398].

104. Narula N, Dannenberg AJ, Olin JW, et al. Pathology of peripheral artery disease in patients with critical limb ischemia. J Am Coll Cardiol 2018;72(18):2152–63.
105. Elliott RJ, McGrath LT. Calcification of the human thoracic aorta during aging. Calcif Tissue Int 1994;54(4):268–73.
106. Proudfoot D, Shanahan CM. Biology of calcification in vascular cells: intima versus media. Herz 2001;26(4):245–51.
107. Lehto S, Niskanen L, Suhonen M, et al. Medial artery calcification. A neglected harbinger of cardiovascular complications in non-insulin-dependent diabetes mellitus. Arterioscler Thromb Vasc Biol 1996;16(8):978–83.
108. Moe SM, Chen NX. Mechanisms of vascular calcification in chronic kidney disease: figure 1. J Am Soc Nephrol 2008;19(2):213–6.
109. Lanzer P, Boehm M, Sorribas V, et al. Medial vascular calcification revisited: review and perspectives. Eur Heart J 2014;35(23):1515–25.

Preoperative Evaluation and Cardiac Risk Assessment in Vascular Surgery

Lee A. Goeddel, MD, MPH*, Michael C. Grant, MD, MSE

KEYWORDS

- Vascular surgery • Preoperative assessment • Perioperative medicine
- Risk prediction • Echocardiography • Frailty assessment
- Preoperative optimization

KEY POINTS

- The rate of perioperative myocardial infarction in major vascular surgery remains high and estimated to be between 1% and 3% with increased risk of mortality.
- The Vascular Surgery Quality Initiative (VQI) has coordinated data gathering across the United States to improve postoperative outcomes.
- Epidemiologically, the prevalence of comorbidities such as hypertension, diabetes mellitus, and coronary artery disease continue to rise in the United States with evidence suggesting inadequate medical control of these comorbidities.
- The 2014 American Heart Association/American College of Cardiology (AHA/ACC) guidelines for cardiac evaluation before noncardiac surgery remain the primary guidance for preoperative evaluation, but new evidence suggests a needed update in risk prediction.
- Prediction of cardiac events after vascular surgery is inaccurate with the Revised Cardiac Risk Index and National Surgery Quality Improvement Program. The VQI shows utility and functional capacity assessment, echocardiography, mobility, and frailty will likely be increasingly incorporated.

INTRODUCTION

Vascular surgery continues to evolve at a rapid pace pushing the frontiers of technology and technique to treat life-limiting and life-threatening conditions of the human vasculature. With the aging population and concomitant increased prevalence of hypertension, diabetes, and atherosclerosis in the United States the prevalence of cardiovascular conditions also continues to grow. Patients who present for open or endovascular vascular therapies often have multiple medical comorbidities that present a challenge to safely undergo and recover from surgery. Preoperative

Department of Anesthesiology & Critical Care Medicine, Johns Hopkins School of Medicine, Zayed 6208J, 1800 Orleans, Baltimore, MD 21287, USA
* Corresponding author.
E-mail address: lgoedde1@jh.edu

Anesthesiology Clin 40 (2022) 575–585
https://doi.org/10.1016/j.anclin.2022.08.005
1932-2275/22/© 2022 Elsevier Inc. All rights reserved.
anesthesiology.theclinics.com

assessment is key to identify conditions that can be optimized before surgery. As vascular surgery has evolved so has the data collection on this patient population, mainly led by the Vascular Surgery Quality Initiative (VQI), a multicenter patient data registry. As the vascular processes underlying the need for vascular surgery also affect both the coronary and cerebral arteries, the risk of cardiac and cerebral injury is a consistent concern in this population. In open abdominal aortic aneurysm repair, mortality remains around 3%, for carotid endarterectomy, a myocardial infarction occurs at approximately 2.5%, and stroke 1%.[1] Despite improvements in perioperative care, the incidence of perioperative myocardial infarction remains significant and unchanged over the last decades with an average rate of 3% in open procedures with an associated Increased risk of cardiac arrest and death.[2]

Thorough preoperative evaluation identifies problems that will affect vascular surgery intervention and recovery. Preoperative optimization seeks to modify these problems when possible before surgery and account for them with sufficient resources throughout the perioperative phases of care. This review summarizes key guidelines and evidence to consider during the preoperative phase of care for vascular patients while also highlighting areas of active investigation.

TRENDS IN PREOPERATIVE EVALUATION

Diabetes, hyperlipidemia, hypertension, smoking, and chronic lung disease are associated with the development of the arterial vascular disease that ultimately becomes symptomatic and requires intervention. Given the typically short window of time between the presentation of illness and vascular surgery, there is rarely sufficient time to adequately optimize these comorbidities, which have been shown to significantly impact perioperative care and recovery. However, there are often opportunities to intervene and develop a comprehensive perioperative management plan.

Despite increasing prevalence of certain comorbidities, including diabetes, hypertension and hyperlipidemia in the population as well as improved control of those comorbidities through medical management alone at the turn of the century, data from the National Health and Nutrition Examination Survey (NHANES) cohort show declining glycemic and blood pressure control with a leveling off of lipid control in the 2010s.[3] Patients presenting for vascular surgery, in particular, tend to have a higher prevalence of comorbidities than the national average. Across the population, it is reasonable to assume that a large selection of patients presenting for vascular surgery will have suboptimal blood sugar, blood pressure, or lipid control. **Table 1** organizes the prevalence of comorbidities for open carotid endarterectomy and open abdominal aortic aneurysm repair as reported in the VQI and compared with other reported cohorts.[1,4]

In the limited time available before surgery, optimization of these chronic conditions is important but may be challenging - if not impossible. Perioperative blood glucose levels have been associated with postoperative wound infections that alone cause significant morbidity and even mortality. Based on the evidence of harm associated with hyperglycemia versus harm from overcorrection causing hypoglycemia, multiple professional societies have issued guidelines for blood glucose targets. With the different clinical scenarios present in the perioperative period, multiple guideline statements are necessary. **Table 2** summarizes the glucose management guidelines from societies involved in perioperative care.

Similarly, blood pressure management before and during surgery is challenging in vascular surgery. Perioperative blood pressure targets do not clearly exist in this population but guidelines have been proposed.[5] Multiple factors need to be individualized per patient and differ by surgery and clinical situation. A patient with uncontrolled

Table 1
Prevalence of comorbidities reported in patients presenting for open carotid endarterectomy and open abdominal aortic aneurysm repair

	Carotid Endarterectomy		Open AAA	
Registry	VQI	NSQUIP	NIS	VQI
No. of patients	89,079	1667	3196	3912
Prevalence of Comorbidities				
Current smoker	26%	45%	33%	91%
Hypertension	89%	79%	64%	85%
CAD	28%	–	7%	26%
CHF	11%	2%	9%	8%
COPD	23%	20%	35%	33%
CABG/PCI	35%	–	–	–
Diabetes	36%	12%	16%	17%
Renal insufficiency	9%	–	–	–
	Outcomes			
Mortality	5.5		5.2	3.3
Stroke				
Myocardial Infection				

Data from Arinze et al and Scully et al.

Table 2
Society guidelines for treating perioperative hyperglycemia

Society	Recommendation
Society of Ambulatory Anesthesia	Treatment goal: Intraoperative blood glucose <180 mg/dL
American Diabetes Association	Initiate insulin therapy if blood glucose> 180 mg/dL Treatment goal: Blood glucose between 140 and 180 mg/dL Goal of 110–140 mg/dL may be appropriate for some patients
American College of Physicians	Treatment goal: Blood glucose between 140 and 200 mg/dL Recommends against intensive insulin therapy in surgical/medical ICU
Society of Critical Care Medicine	Treatment goal: Maintain glucose <150 mg/dL for most ICU patients
Endocrine Society	Treatment goal: Premeal Blood glucose between <140 and random <180 mg/dL Higher target glucose <200 mg/dL is acceptable in patients with terminal illness and/or limited life expectancy or at high risk of hypoglycemia
Society of Thoracic Surgeons	Continuous infusion preferred over SC or intermittent bolus Treatment goal: <180 mg/dL during surgery ≦110 in fasting and premeal states

hypertension who manifests with symptoms consistent with hypertensive urgency or emergency should be addressed and treated before surgery. Otherwise, for patients with high blood pressure before surgery the "10% and 20%" rule is currently suggested for perioperative management stating that the blood pressure nadir should not go below 20% of baseline and max not above 10%.[5] This rule is based primarily on multiple retrospective observational studies that include vascular surgery patients. No prospective randomized trials to best inform blood pressure management have been performed.

CARDIAC EVALUATION AND ASSESSMENT OF RISK OF A MAJOR ADVERSE CARDIAC EVENT BEFORE VASCULAR SURGERY

Major adverse cardiac events (MACE) is a critical outcome of interest and has a higher rate of incidence than myocardial infarction. Of the 200 million yearly noncardiac surgeries, the 30-day cardiac complication rate is estimated at 5% to 8% within 30 days of surgery.[6] MACE can be rather confusing because it is defined differently across clinical studies. Typically, MACE includes postoperative myocardial infarction, but studies vary in the use and clinical definition of myocardial infarction. These definitions of myocardial infarction do not always follow the third of fourth universal definition of myocardial infarction but usually include elements of those definitions such as elevated troponin levels, electrocardiogram changes, and clinical symptomatology. MACE may also include other important clinical outcomes such as arrhythmia, and death. Within this body of literature, therefore, it is important to observe exactly how MACE is defined in each individual study.

As of 2022, the 2014 American Heart Association/American College of Cardiology (AHA/ACC) guideline on perioperative cardiovascular evaluation and management of patients undergoing noncardiac surgery remains the guiding document for the evaluation and assessment of patients before noncardiac surgery.[7] Although this resource is rich with multiple guidelines to direct care, the algorithm for assessment and management of the risk of MACE provides a clear step-by-step guide (**Fig. 1**). *Step 1* assesses the nature of the planned surgical procedure and the immediacy of it based on the clinical situation. If emergent, this guideline states to provide best management of blood pressure and perfusion to mitigate the risk of MACE. Should the procedure not require emergent care, *step 2* evaluates for the presence of a new or chronic condition that would qualify as an active cardiac condition requiring intervention or optimization before noncardiac surgery. The guidelines consider **Table 3** a list of active cardiac conditions. Should any of these conditions be present additional consultation with other specialists for optimization before surgery is likely warranted?

Should no active condition appear to be present the guidelines proceed to *step 3* and promote the use of a prediction calculator to assess the risk of perioperative MACE. The guidelines highlight the Revised Cardiac Risk Index Calculator[8] (RCRI) and the American College of Surgeons National Surgical Quality Improvement Program (NSQUIP) outcome calculator. Should the risk of MACE be less than 1% then no further evaluation before surgery is recommended? However, if the risk is calculated to be greater than 1%, *step 4* recommends that functional capacity be assessed. Based on previous research that showed sufficient functional capacity is associated with a lower rate of cardiac complications,[9] the guidelines suggest to proceed with surgery for self-reported functional capacity greater than 4 metabolic equivalents. Should functional capacity be less or unknown, additional testing including stress testing may be considered in *step 5:* "Will further testing impact decision making OR perioperative care?"

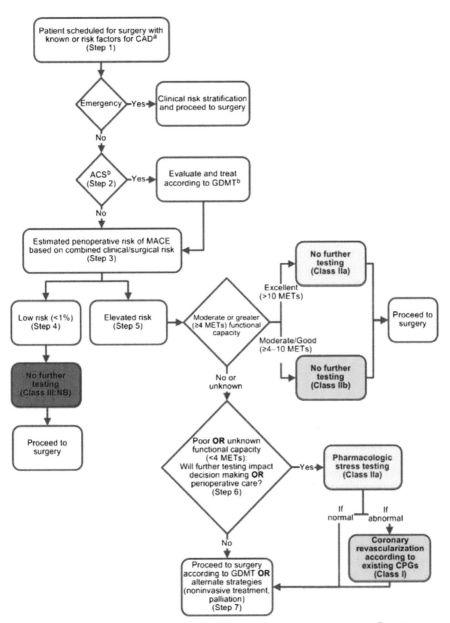

Fig. 1. From Previously published materials unchanged from the source: "From[7] with permission". Step-by-step algorithm for the cardiac evaluation of patients before noncardiac surgery. [a]See sections 2.2, 2.4, and 2.5 in the full-text CPG for recommendations for patients with symptomatic HF, VHD, or arrhythmias. [b]See UA/NSTEMI and STEMI CPGs (see **Table 2**).

IMPORTANT EVIDENCE SINCE THE 2014 GUIDELINES

Since the publication of the 2014 guidelines, there is additional evidence that brings aspects of the above steps into more clarity. In Step 3, the prediction step, the original guidelines specify that this area of research will evolve over time from the publication

Table 3
List of active cardiac conditions defined in the (ACC/AHA) guidelines for preoperative cardiac evaluation in noncardiac surgery

Active Cardiac Condition	Additional Information
Unstable coronary artery disease	
Symptomatic heart failure	
Unstable valvular heart disease	Progressive and symptomatic
Unstable arrhythmia	Unstable, acute, symptomatic, or malignant
Unstable pulmonary vascular disease	Symptomatic
Unstable adult congenital heart disease	Symptomatic

of the guidelines with additional investigation that should be incorporated into the algorithm. Three particular publications are of interest to highlight in this review. The first two demonstrate concern with the RCRI and NSQUIP. Glance and colleagues analyzed the data from 10,000 patients in the NSQUIP patient database and assessed the percent agreement of low versus high risk by the NSQUIP and RCRI, and found that these predictive approaches disagree regularly (29% of the time) on the classification of low versus high patients.[10] This level of disagreement highlights a major concern for potential inaccuracy inherent in one or both predictive mechanisms and introduces confusion to the evidence-based preoperative evaluation of patients. From an epidemiologic perspective, step 3 of the algorithm should have a high sensitivity to best identify patients at high risk to then undergo additional evaluation. If 30% of patients are misclassified as low risk, one or both of these predictive strategies may miss patients that should receive additional evaluation.

To further clarify these potential inaccuracies within the RCRI and NSQUIP as well as assess their predictive utility, Fronczek and colleagues[11] sought to externally validate the RCRI and the NSQUIP within a nested portion of the Vascular Events in Noncardiac Surgery (VISION) cohort. The VISION cohort was a multinational group of patients presenting for noncardiac surgery by age and history considered to be at elevated risk of postoperative cardiac complications. Importantly, this cohort had very detailed surveillance of complications in the days following surgery including daily troponin, electrocardigram, and clinical monitoring. This enabled the investigators to apply the third universal definition of myocardial infarction[12] along with death as the primary composite outcome measure in the population. Using a nested cohort of 1000 patients within the 20,000 total patients, the investigators assessed the accuracy of the RCRI and the NSQUIP to predict MACE. They found the predictive accuracy of both to be poor and ultimately no net benefit in either predictor. The c-statistic for the prediction of these models was RCRI was 0.6 for the RCRI compared with 0.64 for the NSQUIP. In this study, accuracy of RCRI prediction was improved by using the Canadian Cardiovascular Society adjustment to RCRI risk prediction, but these results are consistent with other previously reported concerns of poor external validation and underestimation of cardiac events attributed to the RCRI. Vascular surgery populations in particular have suffered these trends of inaccurate prediction.[11,13]

Given the inaccuracies in prediction seen with the RCRI and NSQUIP that particularly affect the vascular surgery population, the VQI developed its own predictive algorithm for myocardial infarction based on troponin elevation, clinical, or echocardiographic criteria.[14] This analysis built two separate prediction model strategies. One to apply to all surgeries and multiple others to address prediction within individual surgeries. The all-procedure model yielded a different level of accuracy by surgery with AUC ranging from 0.68 for open abdominal aortic aneurysm repair to 0.72 for endovascular aneurysm repair. Procedure-specific prediction models performed better. This risk calculator is available for online use through the VQI website; however, it is important to note that it is unclear how to incorporate the VQI risk prediction into the 2014 guidelines, and this prediction tool has not undergone rigorous external validation.

Overall, it is clear that preoperative risk prediction remains in the developmental phase. With the addition of more data through efforts like the VQI, risk prediction should become more accurate. Future directions may consider incorporating other data in prediction modeling strategies which may include measurements of preoperative frailty, mobility, functional capacity assessment, or echocardiography. Also, other patient-centered outcomes, like loss of independence and kidney injury[15] will also be considered in risk modeling.

TRANSTHORACIC ECHOCARDIOGRAPHY BEFORE VASCULAR SURGERY

Current appropriate use guidelines for transthoracic echocardiography (TTE) recommend against the routine use of the imaging modality before noncardiac surgery.[7,16] In the absence of symptoms or previously diagnoses a disease that would qualify, TTE is broadly considered an expensive and unnecessary ad hoc screening tool before surgery. Halm and colleagues studied 500 consecutive vascular surgery patients and found TTE to be associated with cardiovascular complications if the left ventricular ejection fraction (LVEF) was less than 40%, but as with other general populations, most of the patients presented with preserved LVEF.[17] Overall in both noncardiac and cardiac surgeries, over 80% of patients present to surgery with preserved LVEF.[18] LVEF then is not a useful population-based screening data point to guide perioperative care.

TTE provides other measurements of cardiac structure and function that may be of interest in preoperative evaluation but are currently under further investigation. The ideal echocardiographic measurement would be consistently measured, reproducible, easy to interpret, and provide insight to the mechanism of cardiovascular risk. Beyond LVEF, diastolic dysfunction has been shown to be associated with complications after vascular surgery,[19,20] but it is inconsistently measured and flow dependent. Measurements of LV geometry, and in particular left ventricular relative wall thickness, show significant promise. In the setting of preserved LVEF, left ventricular relative wall thickness was associated with decreased systolic performance under resting and exercising conditions,[21,22] and has been independently associated with important clinical outcomes after surgery including acute kidney injury,[23] length of stay,[23] and mortality.[24] RWT is also consistently measured on routine TTE. Other measurements of interest that may be of utility from preoperative TTE and warrant additional investigation are the myocardial performance index, or a simplified component of it that assesses systolic performance only, left ventricular systolic ejection time. Both of these measurements have been shown to quantify ventricular performance in a more granular fashion than LVEF and are particularly useful to understand ventricular performance in patients with preserved LVEF.[25–27] More investigation is warranted into their utility in the perioperative care of vascular surgery patients.

Best estimates suggest that TTE is performed or available in approximately 8% to 15% of patients before noncardiac surgery with approximately 80% of patients meeting appropriate use criteria for TTE.[28] As mentioned above, guidelines state that routine TTE before noncardiac surgery is not indicated and in the future will require documentation of an approved indication for reimbursement. As the 2014 guidelines serve as a useful guide for preoperative evaluation, and TTE is often available before surgery, we find it useful to consider the following 3-part framework to describe how TTE may fit into the preoperative evaluation algorithm: (1) TTE may newly identify or clarify whether a patient has an active cardiac condition that requires further optimization before surgery. (2) Pursuant to step 5 of the assessment algorithm mentioned above, TTE may impact decision-making or perioperative care. Beyond just the clarification of an active cardiac condition, a TTE may guide the allocation of additional resources in the care of complex patients. (3). Lastly, purely in the investigative phase now, echocardiography may in the future clarify risk assessment or actively guide perioperative management strategies.

TRENDS IN FUNCTIONAL CAPACITY, FRAILTY, MOBILITY, AND IN PREOPERATIVE ASSESSMENT

For the patients assessed to have an MACE risk of greater than 1%, Step 4 in the guidelines states to assess functional capacity to further clarify the risk of cardiac complication. This step is originally based on retrospective data that found an association between the functional capacity of less than four metabolic equivalents of oxygen aerobic capacity and an increase in cardiac complications.[9] Data from cardiopulmonary exercise stress testing have further quantified functional capacity via oxygen consumption and anerobic thresholds during exercise evaluation before surgery and has been used in risk assessment. Data relating these measures to postoperative complications seem to support the previously identified association between functional capacity and outcomes after surgery.[29] The Duke activity status index,[30] a self-reported survey of functional capacity was shown to outperform these physical quantitative measures in a large international prospective trial.[31] It is a series of yes or no questions of activity that are scored and weighted to physiologic calorimetry assessment. As a result, the Duke activity status index or another method to standardize the assessment of functional capacity may in the future be included into step 4 of the guidelines.

Frailty, commonly defined as lacking the physiologic resilience to undergo and recover from surgery, and mobility, clinically defined as the ability to freely move have not yet been formally included in preoperative assessment. Although they are not the same entities, much is shared between functional capacity, frailty, and mobility. Frailty assessment has been shown to similarly predict bad outcomes, particularly in low-risk surgery.[32–34] It may offer additional utility, however, translating preoperative frailty assessment to perioperative intervention is currently challenged by the heterogeneity of over 20 different frailty assessments. Ongoing research is currently assessing individual components of frailty, certain perioperative intervention, and associated outcome. Although it includes similar domains of information, mobility is commonly assessed by the Activity Measure for Post-Acute Care (AM-PAC) scale which is used to guide physical therapy and discharge to rehababilitation.[35] These widely available measurements may provide important information to improve the precision of prediction. In the future, both frailty and mobility assessments may add value to preoperative assessment and optimization.

SUMMARY

This review summarizes key guidelines and evidence within the preoperative phase of care for vascular surgery patients from 2010 to the present day. With a clear grasp of the epidemiologic trends, evidence, and most recent guidelines, anesthesiologists will continue to lead in the evidenced-based care of medically complex patients and drive innovation to improve outcomes. Vascular surgery continues to evolve along the cutting edge of technology and engineering to treat a surgical population that suffers from a high prevalence of comorbidities. Preoperative optimization seeks to characterize the extent of these abnormalities and to achieve medical control, when possible, in the time available before surgery. Risk assessment, evaluation, and optimization of MACE continue to be an evolving science in vascular surgery that appears to be moving beyond the RCRI and NSQUIP. The VQI risk calculator may offer a more accurate prediction. Ongoing investigation into preoperative echocardiography, functional capacity assessment, frailty assessment, and mobility assessment may show that these entities add clinical value to preoperative assessment and perioperative management.

CLINICS CARE POINTS

- Despite innovations in surgery and perioperative care the risk of complications remains high in vascular surgery. Knowledge of the most recent cohort data is important to clinical care.

- The National Health and Nutrition Examination Survey (NHANES) data show that the general US population has worse control of hypertension, hyperlipemia, and diabetes, a challenge for preoperative optimization in vascular surgery.

- It is critical to understand the clinical evidence and definition of outcomes in the prediction of major adverse cardiac events as one applies the most recent guidelines to clinical care.

DISCLOSURE

The authors have nothing to disclose.

REFERENCES

1. Arinze N, Farber A, Levin SR, et al. The Association of Body Mass Index with Outcomes after Carotid Endarterectomy. Ann Vasc Surg 2021;77:7–15.
2. Juo YY, Mantha A, Ebrahimi R, et al. Incidence of Myocardial Infarction After High-Risk Vascular Operations in Adults. JAMA Surg 2017;152(11):e173360.
3. Fang M, Wang D, Coresh J, et al. Trends in Diabetes Treatment and Control in U.S. Adults, 1999-2018. N Engl J Med 2021;384(23):2219–28.
4. Scully RE, Sharma G, Soo Hoo AJ, et al. Comparative analysis of open abdominal aortic aneurysm repair outcomes across national registries. J Vasc Surg 2022; 75(1):162–7.e1.
5. Meng L, Yu W, Wang T, et al. Blood Pressure Targets in Perioperative Care. Hypertension 2018;72(4):806–17.
6. Devereaux PJ, Sessler DI. Cardiac Complications in Patients Undergoing Major Noncardiac Surgery. N Engl J Med 2015;373(23):2258–69.
7. Fleisher LA, Fleischmann KE, Auerbach AD, et al. 2014 ACC/AHA guideline on perioperative cardiovascular evaluation and management of patients undergoing noncardiac surgery: executive summary: a report of the American College of Cardiology/American Heart Association Task Force on Practice Guidelines. Circulation 2014;130(24):2215–45.
8. Lee TH, Marcantonio ER, Mangione CM, et al. Derivation and prospective validation of a simple index for prediction of cardiac risk of major noncardiac surgery. Circulation 1999;100(10):1043–9.

9. Reilly DF, McNeely MJ, Doerner D, et al. Self-reported exercise tolerance and the risk of serious perioperative complications. Arch Intern Med 1999;159(18):2185–92.

10. Glance LG, Faden E, Dutton RP, et al. Impact of the Choice of Risk Model for Identifying Low-risk Patients Using the 2014 American College of Cardiology/American Heart Association Perioperative Guidelines. Anesthesiology 2018;129(5):889–900.

11. Fronczek J, Polok K, Devereaux PJ, et al. External validation of the Revised Cardiac Risk Index and National Surgical Quality Improvement Program Myocardial Infarction and Cardiac Arrest calculator in noncardiac vascular surgery. Br J Anaesth 2019.

12. Thygesen K, Alpert JS, Jaffe AS, et al. Third universal definition of myocardial infarction. J Am Coll Cardiol 2012;60(16):1581–98.

13. Polok K, Fronczek J, Szczeklik W. Myocardial Infarction After Vascular Surgery: A Systematic Troponin Surveillance and a Uniform Definition Is Needed. JAMA Surg 2018;153(5):496.

14. Bertges DJ, Neal D, Schanzer A, et al. The Vascular Quality Initiative Cardiac Risk Index for prediction of myocardial infarction after vascular surgery. J Vasc Surg 2016;64(5):1411–21.e1.

15. Donald GW, Ghaffarian AA, Isaac F, et al. Preoperative frailty assessment predicts loss of independence after vascular surgery. J Vasc Surg 2018;68(5):1382–9.

16. Fernando RJ, Goeddel LA, Shah R, et al. Analysis of the 2019 ACC/AATS/AHA/ASE/ASNC/HRS/SCAI/SCCT/SCMR/STS Appropriate Use Criteria for Multimodal Imaging in the Assessment of Structural Heart Disease. J Cardiothorac Vasc Anesth 2020;34(3):805–18.

17. Halm EA, Browner WS, Tubau JF, et al. Echocardiography for assessing cardiac risk in patients having noncardiac surgery. Study of Perioperative Ischemia Research Group. Ann Intern Med 1996;125(6):433–41.

18. Lerman BJ, Popat RA, Assimes TL, et al. Association of Left Ventricular Ejection Fraction and Symptoms With Mortality After Elective Noncardiac Surgery Among Patients With Heart Failure. JAMA 2019;321(6):572–9.

19. Matyal R, Hess PE, Subramaniam B, et al. Perioperative diastolic dysfunction during vascular surgery and its association with postoperative outcome. J Vasc Surg 2009;50(1):70–6.

20. Matyal R, Skubas NJ, Shernan SK, et al. Perioperative assessment of diastolic dysfunction. Anesth Analg 2011;113(3):449–72.

21. Aurigemma GP, Gaasch WH, McLaughlin M, et al. Reduced left ventricular systolic pump performance and depressed myocardial contractile function in patients > 65 years of age with normal ejection fraction and a high relative wall thickness. Am J Cardiol 1995;76(10):702–5.

22. Lam CS, Grewal J, Borlaug BA, et al. Size, shape, and stamina: the impact of left ventricular geometry on exercise capacity. Hypertension 2010;55(5):1143–9.

23. Goeddel LA, Erlinger S, Murphy Z, et al. Association Between Left Ventricular Relative Wall Thickness and Acute Kidney Injury After Noncardiac Surgery. Anesth analgesia 2022;135(3):605–16.

24. Zhu P, Dai Y, Qiu J, et al. Prognostic implications of left ventricular geometry in coronary artery bypass grafting patients. Quant Imaging Med Surg 2020;10(12):2274–84.

25. Alhakak AS, Teerlink JR, Lindenfeld J, et al. The significance of left ventricular ejection time in heart failure with reduced ejection fraction. Eur J Heart Fail 2021;23(4):541–51.
26. Biering-Sorensen T, Querejeta Roca G, Hegde SM, et al. Left ventricular ejection time is an independent predictor of incident heart failure in a community-based cohort. Eur J Heart Fail 2018;20(7):1106–14.
27. Carluccio E, Biagioli P, Alunni G, et al. Improvement of myocardial performance (Tei) index closely reflects intrinsic improvement of cardiac function: assessment in revascularized hibernating myocardium. Echocardiography 2012;29(3): 298–306.
28. Tank A, Hughey R, Ward RP, et al. Evaluation of Appropriate Use of Preoperative Echocardiography before Major Abdominal Surgery: A Retrospective Cohort Study. Anesthesiology 2021;135(5):854–63.
29. Moran J, Wilson F, Guinan E, et al. Role of cardiopulmonary exercise testing as a risk-assessment method in patients undergoing intra-abdominal surgery: a systematic review. Br J Anaesth 2016;116(2):177–91.
30. Hlatky MA, Boineau RE, Higginbotham MB, et al. A brief self-administered questionnaire to determine functional capacity (the Duke Activity Status Index). Am J Cardiol 1989;64(10):651–4.
31. Wijeysundera DN, Pearse RM, Shulman MA, et al. Assessment of functional capacity before major noncardiac surgery: an international, prospective cohort study. Lancet 2018;391(10140):2631–40.
32. He Y, Li LW, Hao Y, et al. Assessment of predictive validity and feasibility of Edmonton Frail Scale in identifying postoperative complications among elderly patients: a prospective observational study. Sci Rep 2020;10(1):14682.
33. McIsaac DI, MacDonald DB, Aucoin SD. Frailty for Perioperative Clinicians: A Narrative Review. Anesth Analg 2020;130(6):1450–60.
34. McIsaac DI, Taljaard M, Bryson GL, et al. Frailty as a Predictor of Death or New Disability After Surgery: A Prospective Cohort Study. Ann Surg 2020;271(2): 283–9.
35. Jette DU, Stilphen M, Ranganathan VK, et al. AM-PAC "6-Clicks" functional assessment scores predict acute care hospital discharge destination. Phys Ther 2014;94(9):1252–61.

Complications of Vascular Disease

Jesse Kiefer, MD, MSEd[a], Michael Mazzeffi, MD, MPH, MSc[b],*

KEYWORDS

- Vascular disease • Coronary disease • Hypertension • Stroke • Vasculitis

KEY POINTS

- Perioperative hypertension increases the odds of postoperative cardiovascular complications by approximately 35%. The 2017 American College of Cardiology/American Heart Association clinical practice guidelines for management of hypertension recommend delaying elective surgery when preoperative systolic blood pressure is greater than 180 mm Hg or diastolic blood pressure is greater than 110 mm Hg.
- American Heart Association guidelines recommend pharmacologic stress testing in cases where a patient has elevated predicted cardiovascular risk, poor, or unknown functional status, and the testing will impact clinical decision-making. Canadian guidelines recommend an approach based on the revised cardiac risk index and N-terminal-pro brain natriuretic peptide (BNP) or standard BNP testing.
- There is minimal evidence to guide the ideal timing of elective noncardiac surgery after a prior cerebrovascular accident (CVA). Expert recommendations suggest waiting at least 3 months, when possible, to reduce the risk of recurrent CVA and major adverse cardiac events.
- Surgical patients are at increased risk for venous thromboembolism, which is among the most preventable causes of death in hospitalized patients. The American College of Chest Physicians recommends that the overwhelming majority of patients should receive at a minimum mechanical prophylaxis.
- The pulmonary and renal systems are most commonly affected by inflammatory vascular diseases. Treatment is typically with glucocorticoids and immunosuppressive agents.

INTRODUCTION

Vascular disease is a major contributor to perioperative morbidity and mortality in noncardiac surgical patients. In this review, the authors discuss the complications of vascular disease and related implications for surgical patients. Specific diseases that are discussed include arterial hypertension, ischemic heart disease, cerebral vascular disease, venous thromboembolism (VTE), and inflammatory vasculitides.

---

[a] Department of Anesthesiology and Critical Care Medicine, University of Pennsylvania – Perelman School of Medicine, 3400 Spruce Street, Suite 680 Dulles Philadelphia, PA 19104, USA;
[b] Department of Anesthesiology, University of Virginia Health, PO Box 800710, Charlottesville, VA, USA
* Corresponding author.
E-mail address: syy4wa@hscmail.mcc.virginia.edu

Anesthesiology Clin 40 (2022) 587–604
https://doi.org/10.1016/j.anclin.2022.08.006
1932-2275/22/© 2022 Elsevier Inc. All rights reserved.

anesthesiology.theclinics.com

Abbreviations	
OR	odds ratio
PCI	percutaneous coronary intervention
IVIG	intravenous immunoglobulin
ICU	intensive care unit

ARTERIAL HYPERTENSION
Epidemiology and Pathophysiology

Arterial hypertension is the most common vascular disease in adults and most common preventable cause of death in the world. Approximately one-third of the world's population has hypertension with a higher prevalence in middle- and low-income countries.[1] The disease burden of arterial hypertension continues to grow in low-income countries, whereas small decreases have occurred in high-income countries during the last two decades.[1] Based on the 2020 International Society of Hypertension global hypertension guidelines, hypertension is diagnosed when systolic blood pressure is greater than 140 mm Hg and/or diastolic blood pressure is greater than 90 mm Hg in the office or clinic.[2] If ambulatory or home blood pressure monitoring is performed, slightly different cutoffs are used.[2] Grade 1 hypertension is when systolic blood pressure is between 140 and 159 mm Hg and/or diastolic blood pressure is between 90 and 99 mm Hg.[2] Grade 2 hypertension is when systolic blood pressure is $\geq$ 160 mm Hg and/or diastolic blood pressure is $\geq$ 100 mm Hg.[2]

The pathophysiology of arterial hypertension is complex with multiple medical causes. These include primary hyperaldosteronism, renovascular disease, chronic steroid use, pheochromocytoma, thyroid disease, chronic kidney disease, and drug-related hypertension. The initial evaluation for hypertension includes consideration of these conditions as well as screening for end-organ damage including kidney, cardiac, peripheral arterial, and cerebrovascular disease.

Essential hypertension is most common. Contributing factors include renin–angiotensin–aldosterone system dysfunction, oxidative stress, autonomic nervous system changes, endothelial cell dysfunction, and hypercoagulability.[3–5] Established risk factors for arterial hypertension include obesity, alcohol use, advanced age, family history of hypertension, insulin resistance, low high-density lipoprotein (HDL) levels, tobacco use, and high triglyceride levels.[6,7] In the typical patient with essential hypertension, the arterial tree stiffens, leading to increased systolic blood pressure, decreased diastolic blood pressure, and a widened pulse pressure.[8] Widened pulse pressure is a surrogate marker of the degree of vascular stiffness when there is no significant aortic insufficiency.[8]

Sequelae

Arterial hypertension leads to multiple sequelae over time including coronary artery disease, peripheral arterial disease, cerebrovascular disease, and renal microvascular disease. Poorly controlled hypertension also causes left ventricular hypertrophy, increased myocardial oxygen consumption, increased left-ventricular end diastolic pressure, and congestive heart failure. Approximately one-quarter of patients with arterial hypertension have coronary artery disease with almost half having at least two other comorbidities.[9,10] Arterial hypertension increases the relative risk for myocardial infarction in a dose-dependent manner. The relative risk for myocardial infarction in a patient with a systolic blood pressure of 140 to 159 mm Hg is 1.2, in a patient with a systolic blood pressure of 160 to 179 mm Hg is 1.3, and in a patient with a systolic blood pressure greater than 180 mm Hg is 1.8 compared with a normotensive patient.[11]

Uncontrolled arterial hypertension is a major risk factor for cerebrovascular disease with up to half of cerebrovascular accidents (CVAs) attributable to poorly controlled hypertension.[12,13] Arterial hypertension increases the risk for both ischemic and hemorrhagic stroke.[14] In patients with untreated arterial hypertension, the odds of hemorrhagic stroke are three-fold higher, and in patients with treated hypertension, the odds of hemorrhagic stroke are one-and-a-half-fold higher.[15]

Arterial hypertension contributes to over half the cases of end-stage renal disease (ESRD) with up to 2% of patients with severe arterial hypertension developing ESRD.[16] There is a clear relationship between the severity of arterial hypertension and the long-term risk of developing ESRD with odds ratios for ESRD varying from 2.6 for patients with Stage 1 hypertension to 4.2 for patients with systolic blood pressure greater than 210 mm Hg.[17]

Perioperative Risk

Perioperative hypertension significantly increases myocardial infarction risk after surgery. In a meta-analysis that included 30 studies (mostly observational), perioperative hypertension was found to increase the odds of postoperative cardiovascular complications by 35% (pooled OR = 1.35).[18] The incidence of postoperative cardiovascular complications in patients with uncontrolled hypertension (eg, systolic blood pressure >180 mm Hg) is close to 5%.[19] The risk for perioperative myocardial infarction in the general surgical population is around 0.4%.[20] Perioperative hypertension also increases the risk for postoperative bleeding, particularly in neurosurgical or ear, nose, and throat patients.[21]

The 2017 American College of Cardiology/American Heart Association clinical practice guidelines for management of hypertension recommend delaying elective surgery when preoperative systolic blood pressure is greater than 180 mm Hg or diastolic blood pressure is greater than 110 mm Hg.[22] Unfortunately, many patients who have surgery delayed because of poorly controlled hypertension return for surgery with a similar poorly controlled blood pressure.[19] Hence, it is unclear whether rescheduling surgery for medical optimization reduces perioperative cardiovascular or bleeding risk. We recommend an individualized approach based on medical comorbidities, level of surgical risk, insurance status, and socioeconomic factors when deciding whether or not to proceed with elective surgery in a severely hypertensive patient. If a patient has signs of new end-organ injury or hypertensive emergency (eg, new myocardial ischemia or a new neurologic deficit), elective surgery should be delayed. If these signs are absent, it may be reasonable to proceed with low-risk surgery when a patient's blood pressure is not well controlled.

Perioperative Management

There is considerable evidence that intraoperative hypotension increases risk for adverse postoperative outcomes, mainly acute kidney and myocardial injury, and risk is probably greater in chronically hypertensive patients.[23] Both a mean arterial pressure (MAP) less than 65 mm Hg and a relative decrease in blood pressure of greater than 30% from baseline are similarly predictive of acute myocardial injury.[24] There is high risk for organ injury when MAP is less than 65 mm Hg for greater than 20 minutes or MAP is less than 50 mm Hg for greater than 5 minutes.[25] What MAP should be targeted for an individual patient remains a difficult question because autoregulatory thresholds, comorbidities, and surgical factors differ between patients.[26] In a recent study testing "individualized" intraoperative blood pressure management, the investigators found that when systolic blood pressure 10% less than the baseline value was used as a vasopressor treatment trigger, compared with an absolute cutoff of 80 mm Hg, patients had less postoperative organ dysfunction.[27] In a recent expert consensus statement, the investigators recommended keeping MAP above 60 to 70 mm Hg and systolic blood pressure below 160 mm Hg during surgery in most noncardiac surgery patients.[28] These targets seem reasonable for most noncardiac surgery patients, although case-by-case decisions should be made for specific surgical procedures including neurosurgical procedures for intracranial hemorrhage and endoscopic sinus surgery.

CORONARY ARTERY DISEASE
Epidemiology and Pathophysiology

The prevalence of coronary artery disease is around 6% in adults in the United States.[29] Men have an approximately two-fold higher risk of ischemic heart disease than women.[29] The prevalence of prior myocardial infarction is around 3%, with men also having a two-fold higher risk than women. Although the prevalence of coronary artery disease has decreased over the last 30 years, it is less clear whether myocardial infarctions are decreasing. In fact, there has been a relative increase in the number of non-ST elevation myocardial infarctions diagnosed, perhaps because of improved diagnostic testing.[29] Approximately one-third of first myocardial infarctions are silent, and silent myocardial infarctions are more common in women and patients with diabetes mellitus.[30] Silent myocardial infarctions can be identified by the presence of Q waves on an electrocardiogram in the absence of myocardial infarction history.

Important risk factors for coronary artery disease include age, male sex, obesity, low HDL levels, elevated low-density lipoprotein levels, hypertension, tobacco use, diabetes mellitus, elevated plasma fibrinogen, and a family history of coronary artery disease.[31–33]

The pathophysiology of coronary artery disease is complex but is mainly related to the formation of atherosclerotic plaque. Atherosclerotic plaque forms when lipids deposit within the blood vessel wall.[34] Macrophages take residence in the subendothelial space, where they ingest oxidized and non-oxidized cholesterol leading to chronic inflammation.[34,35] "Foamy" macrophages release chemokines, cytokines, and reactive oxygen species and when they die, tissue factor is released leading to a procoagulant state.[34,35] Most acute coronary artery obstruction occurs when an atherosclerotic plaque ruptures, exposing a lipid-rich core, which leads to platelet adhesion and aggregation. If critical coronary artery obstruction occurs, it causes myocardial injury, and ultimately myocardial infarction if adequate blood flow cannot be restored.[34]

Type 1 myocardial infarction is diagnosed by elevated high-sensitivity troponin, signs and symptoms of ischemia, and evidence of coronary artery thrombosis on angiography.[36] Type 2 myocardial dysfunction is diagnosed by elevated high-sensitivity troponin, signs and symptoms of ischemia, and evidence of oxygen supply/demand mismatch unrelated to coronary artery thrombosis.[36] Other specific myocardial infarction types can occur from direct myocardial injury (eg, cardiac surgery).

Sequelae

Coronary artery disease predisposes patients to cardiac arrhythmias, myocardial infarction, chronic ischemic cardiomyopathy, and cardiac arrest. Perioperative ventricular arrhythmias (>30 ectopic ventricular beats per hour or ventricular tachycardia) occur in up to 40% of patients with coronary artery disease.[37] The incidence of perioperative myocardial infarction depends on the exact definition used, but in contemporary studies is around 5% with approximately three-quarters happening within

48 hours of surgery.[38] Most perioperative myocardial infarctions do not involve coronary artery thrombosis, but instead are due to a mismatch between oxygen supply and demand.[39]

Approximately 70% to 90% of congestive heart failure is caused by ischemic heart disease.[40] Both myocardial infarction and myocardial hibernation can lead to impaired diastolic and systolic function. It is estimated that up to 50% of patients with impaired systolic function and coronary artery disease have hibernating myocardium and revascularization can improve cardiac function in many cases.[41] For patients with New York Heart Association Class III or IV congestive heart failure, 5-year mortality is 50% and patients with a prolonged QRS duration have higher mortality near 70%.[42] Intraoperative cardiac arrest is a rare event occurring at a rate of approximately five events per 100,000 surgical cases.[43] Myocardial ischemia is a leading cause of intraoperative cardiac arrest.[43]

Perioperative Risk

In 2014, the American College of Cardiology updated its guideline on perioperative cardiovascular evaluation and management for patients having noncardiac surgery. For patients having elective surgery, the authors recommend using a validated cardiac risk assessment tool, such as the revised cardiac risk index (RCRI) or American College of Surgeons National Surgical Quality Improvement Program risk calculator, to evaluate an individual patient's risk for perioperative myocardial infarction.[44] The guidelines recommend pharmacologic stress testing in cases where a patient has elevated predicted cardiovascular risk, poor, or unknown functional status, and the testing will impact clinical decision-making.[44] The Canadian guidelines recommend a different approach, which is based on the RCRI as well as N-terminal (NT)-pro brain natriuretic peptide (BNP) or standard BNP testing. For patients who are age $\geq$ 65, have RCRI $\geq$ 1, or those with significant cardiovascular disease, NT-pro BNP or BNP testing should be performed. If levels are above a threshold (300 or 92 mg/L, respectively) postoperative troponin monitoring is warranted for 2 to 3 days along with postoperative electrocardiogram monitoring.[45]

Perioperative Management

Patients who have undergone recent angioplasty should wait 14 days until having elective noncardiac surgery.[44] Those with a bare-metal stent (BMS) should wait 30 days, and those with a drug-eluting stent (DES) should wait 12 months, when possible.[44] Recent data suggest that earlier surgery (eg, 3–6 months) may be safe after DES placement, but the competing risks of perioperative myocardial infarction and delaying surgery should be weighed for an individual patient.[46]

Other recommended interventions to reduce the risk of perioperative myocardial infarction include continuing beta blockers in patients with chronic use, starting beta blockers in patients with high cardiovascular risk (eg, 3 or more RCRI risk factors), continuing statins in patients with chronic use, starting statins in vascular surgery patients, continuing angiotensin-converting enzyme inhibitors and angiotensin receptor blockers in patients with chronic use, continuing dual antiplatelet therapy in patients with a recent BMS or DES (4–6 weeks) and low bleeding risk, and continuing aspirin after a BMS or DES whenever feasible.[44]

There is no strong evidence to suggest that performing surgery under monitored anesthesia care or regional anesthesia reduces perioperative myocardial infarction.[44] Similarly, there is no strong evidence to support the use of total intravenous anesthesia compared with volatile anesthesia to reduce perioperative myocardial infarction.[44] Revascularization before elective noncardiac surgery with PCI or coronary artery bypass grafting may be indicated for select surgical procedures and generally is reserved for patients with left main coronary artery disease and patients with acute coronary syndromes.[44] There are no randomized controlled trials demonstrating that revascularization reduces perioperative myocardial infarction risk and the largest trial to date found no benefit in terms of reducing major adverse cardiovascular events.[47]

CEREBROVASCULAR DISEASE
Epidemiology and Pathophysiology

The prevalence of CVA is 3% in adults in the United States and there are 800,000 new CVAs pear year.[48] These numbers translate to a CVA incidence of approximately 200 events per 100,000 persons.[48] Ischemic CVA (87% of all events) is nine-fold more common than hemorrhagic CVA (10% of all events) with subarachnoid hemorrhage being an uncommon cause of CVA (3% of all events).[48]

Most ischemic CVAs are caused by vascular thrombosis or thromboembolism. Approximately one-quarter of ischemic CVAs are from large vessel occlusion, one-quarter are from small vessel thrombosis, one-quarter are from thromboembolism, and the final quarter are from an unknown etiology.[49]

Sequelae

The symptoms of CVA depend on its size and territory. Sequelae range from being largely asymptomatic, to being hemiplegic, or even comatose. Patients with a prior CVA may present for surgery with impaired functional status, impaired nutritional status, altered airway reflexes and swallowing, and existent deep venous thrombosis from immobility. Muscle contractures are also present in many patients with motor CVAs and can make positioning for surgery challenging in some cases.

Perioperative Risk

Patients with a prior CVA are at increased risk for multiple adverse perioperative events including aspiration from impaired airway reflexes, postoperative respiratory failure and reintubation from poor cough, recurrent CVA, and cardiovascular complications, including myocardial infarction. There is minimal evidence to guide the ideal timing of elective noncardiac surgery after a prior CVA. Expert recommendations suggest waiting at least 3 months, when possible, to reduce the risk of recurrent CVA and major adverse cardiac events.[50–52] This recommendation is supported by a recent observational study of over 5.8 million patients, which found that the risk for recurrent CVA leveled off 90-days after a prior ischemic CVA.[53] Waiting for 90-days allows time for a patient's neurological and hemodynamic status to stabilize and cerebral autoregulation to return to normal.[51] In patients with hemorrhagic CVA, delaying surgery for several months may also reduce the risk of rebleeding.

The risk for perioperative CVA in patients having noncardiac, non-neurologic surgery is low (0.2–0.7%) but is two-fold higher in patients with a prior CVA.[54–56] Over half of perioperative events occur within 24 hours of surgery.[57] Intraoperative hypotension is inconsistently associated with perioperative CVA in prior studies, and the association is mainly with long durations of hypotension (eg, >20 minutes).[54,56,58] Hemorrhagic CVA risk is increased in patients with uncontrolled hypertension, and elective surgery should be postponed in patients with hypertensive urgency or emergency.

Perioperative Management

For patients with a prior ischemic CVA, blood pressure should be kept within 20% of its baseline value and MAP should be kept above 70 mm Hg.[52] Antiplatelet drugs should be started as soon as feasible, and in highrisk patients with atrial fibrillation, systemic anticoagulation should be restarted when bleeding risk is low (eg, after 24 to 48 hours).[52] For patients with prior hemorrhagic CVA, severe hypertension should be avoided and ideally systolic blood pressure should be kept below 180 mm Hg during the perioperative period.[59] In surgical patients with new symptoms suggestive of CVA and large vessel occlusion, urgent computed tomography angiography and perfusion imaging should be performed. Select patients are eligible for thrombectomy up to 24 hours after symptom onset.[57]

VENOUS THROMBOEMBOLIC DISEASES
Epidemiology and Pathophysiology

VTE includes both deep vein thrombosis and pulmonary embolism. Perioperative VTE is among the most preventable causes of death in hospitalized patients, and surgical patients are at increased risk.[60] Although there is uncertainty about VTEs exact incidence, it may affect up 25% of surgical patients.[61] In a thoughtful review, Gordon and colleagues[60] noted that VTE morbidity has not changed considerably in the last 20 years.

The mechanisms causing VTE are not completely understood, although there are a number of critical events that contribute including venous stasis, venous valve hypoxia, endothelial dysfunction, tissue factor activation, and platelet and leukocyte activation causing thrombus propagation.[60]

Sequelae

Deep vein thrombosis can cause post-thrombotic syndrome leading to chronic limb swelling, chronic pain, skin ulceration, and poor wound healing.[62] Acute pulmonary embolism causes hypoxemia, increased pulmonary vascular resistance, and right ventricular dysfunction. Chronic pulmonary thromboembolic disease causes chronic pulmonary hypertension, chronic right ventricular dysfunction, and in severe cases, right ventricular failure with cardiac cirrhosis and renal failure.

Perioperative Risk

There are multiple VTE risk factors including surgery type, surgery length, age, body mass index, VTE history, renal disease, immobility, oncologic history, and postoperative coagulopathy. The Caprini score provides guidance on VTE risk (**Table 1**). A large recent meta-analysis supported the use of the Caprini score in the perioperative setting, noting a benefit of chemoprophylaxis in surgical patients with a Caprini score ≥7.[63] Patients with the Caprini scores ≤6 did not benefit from chemoprophylaxis in the meta-analysis.[63] The same study identified no association between the Caprini score and major bleeding.[63] In a larger and more recent meta-analysis, McAlpine and colleagues[64] found a nonsignificant decrease in VTE and a nonsignificant increase in bleeding when thromboprophylaxis was initiated preoperatively compared with postoperatively. These findings highlight remaining uncertainty in how to best provide VTE prophylaxis during the perioperative period.

Perioperative Management

Multiple medical organizations including the American College of Surgeons, the American College of Chest Physicians (ACCP), and the Joint Commission have highlighted the importance of perioperative VTE risk assessment and prophylaxis. A large multinational study found that at-risk surgical patients received VTE prophylaxis only 60% of the time, demonstrating an opportunity for improvement.[65]

The ACCP published a clinical practice guideline for VTE prevention in nonorthopedic surgical patients in 2012, which was separated according to surgical subspecialty.

Table 1
Summary of Caprini score

1 Point	2 Points	3 Points	5 Points	1 Point (Women Only)

• Age 41–60 y
• Minor surgery
• Prior major surgery (<1 mo)
• Varicose veins
• Inflammatory bowel disease
• Swollen legs (current)
• Obesity (body mass index [BMI] >25 kg/m²)
• Acute myocardial infarction (<1 mo)
• Congestive heart failure
• Sepsis (<1 mo)
• Abnormal pulmonary function
• Current bed rest
	• Age 60–74 y
	• Arthroscopic surgery
	• Malignancy (present or previous)
	• Major surgery (>45 min)
	• Laparoscopic surgery (>45 min)
	• Bedbound (>72 h)
	• Immobilizing plaster cast (<1 mo)
	• Central venous access
		• Age > 75 y
		• History of VTE
		• Family history of VTE
		• Factor V Leiden
		• Prothrombin gene mutation
		• Elevated homocysteinemia
		• Lupus anticoagulant
		• Anticardiolipin antibodies
		• Heparin-induced thrombocytopenia
		• Other congenital/ acquired thrombophilia
			• Elective major lower extremity arthroplasty
			• Hip, pelvis, or leg fracture (<1 mo)
			• Stroke (<1 mo)
			• Multiple trauma (<1 mo)
			• Acute spinal cord injury (<1 mo)
				• Oral contraceptive use
				• Hormone replacement therapy
				• Pregnancy, postpartum
				• History of:
				  ○ Unexplained stillborn infant
				  ○ Recurrent spontaneous abortions (>3)
				  ○ Premature birth with toxemia
				  ○ Growth-restricted infant

Interpretation of VTE risk and recommended prophylaxis. Patients with a score of 0 are "very low" risk for VTE with an incidence of 0.5% and do not warrant mechanical or pharmacologic prophylaxis. Patients with a score of 1–2 are "low" risk for VTE with an incidence of 1.5% and warrant mechanical prophylaxis. Patients with a score of 3–4 are "moderate" risk for VTE with an incidence of 3.0% and warrant pharmacologic ± mechanical prophylaxis. Patients with a score of 5+ are "high" risk for VTE with an incidence of 6.0% and warrant mechanical and pharmacologic prophylaxis.

The ACCP stratified VTE risk using the Caprini score (see **Table 1**). Although there are subspecialty specific recommendations, the guideline generally recommended the following: no prophylaxis in very low-risk patients; mechanical prophylaxis in low-risk patients; chemical prophylaxis or mechanical prophylaxis in moderate-risk patients depending on bleeding risk; and chemical prophylaxis and mechanical prophylaxis in high-risk patients depending on bleeding risk.[66] Mechanical prophylaxis includes intermittent pneumatic compression, graduated compression stockings, and venous foot pumps, all of which enhance blood flow in the deep veins of the lower extremities. Mechanical prophylaxis is preferred over no prophylaxis when a contraindication for chemical prophylaxis exists.[66] The exception for mechanical prophylaxis is in patients with acute deep vein thrombosis, where the ACCP guideline recommends against its use to prevent post-thrombotic syndrome (Grade 2B).[67]

There is debate surrounding the additional benefit of mechanical prophylaxis in patients who receive chemical prophylaxis. A large randomized controlled trial found that in critically ill patients, the addition of mechanical prophylaxis did not result in a significantly lower VTE incidence when compared with chemical prophylaxis alone.[68] A more recent meta-analysis found that dual mechanical and chemical prophylaxis reduced the incidence of both pulmonary embolism and deep vein thrombosis when compared with mechanical prophylaxis alone and reduced the incidence of both pulmonary embolism and deep vein thrombosis when compared with chemical prophylaxis alone.[69]

SYSTEMIC INFLAMMATORY VASCULAR DISEASES
General Classification and Pathophysiology

Systemic inflammatory vascular diseases, more commonly referred to as vasculitides, are a spectrum of multisystem disorders characterized by blood vessel inflammation, causing tissue or organ damage. Inflammation of blood vessels is a shared feature, but specific classification is challenging, as there is overlap along the disease spectrum.[70] The current nomenclature for vasculitides comes from the 2012 Chapel Hill Consensus Conference (CHCC2012), which was composed of an international, multidisciplinary group of experts. Initial categorization is based on the predominant vessel type that is involved—large vessel, medium vessel, or small vessel (**Table 2**). Final categorization also considers structural and functional attributes.[70,71] Large vessels are the aorta, its major branches, and their corresponding veins. Medium vessels are the main visceral arteries, veins, and their initial branches. Small vessels are intraparenchymal arteries, arterioles, capillaries, venules, and veins.

Large-Vessel Vasculitis

Takayasu arteritis (TAK) and Giant cell arteritis (GCA) are the most common large-vessel vasculitides, both affecting the aorta and its major branches. GCA has a preference for branches of the carotid and vertebral arteries (previously referred to as temporal arteritis).[70,72] TAK and GCA are both characterized by granulomatous inflammation of the blood vessel wall with a dysfunctional immune response to injury, which ultimately threatens perfusion.[73] TAK was initially described in Japan and affects Asians more frequently than Europeans, 6 to 71 per million compared with 1 to 2 per million, respectively.[71,74] Comparatively, GCA predominantly affects Europeans, specifically Northern Europeans.[74,75] Watts and colleagues[71,74] reported an incidence for GCA of 14 to 27 per million for Northern Europeans. The initial 1990 American College of Rheumatology classification criteria included age of less than 40 for TAK and greater than 50 for GCA, which has recently been called into

Table 2
Summary of vasculitides

CHCC2012 Category	Disease	Typical Population	Notable Vessels Effected	Possible Systemic Findings
Large vessel	Takayasu arteritis	Asian descent Female > male <40–50 y of age	Aorta	Aortic regurgitation Angina Carotidynia Hypertension limb claudication Reduced/absent pulses
	Giant cell arteritis (temporal arteritis)	European descent Female > male >50 y of age	Aorta Carotid artery and branches Temporal artery	Cerebral vascular accident Headache Jaw claudication Neck pain Visual disturbances
Medium vessel	Polyarteritis nodosa	40–60 y of age Male > female	Renal and interlobar arteries Coronary arteries	Heart failure Gastrointestinal dysfunction Renal dysfunction/failure Peripheral ischemia Peripheral neuropathy
	Kawasaki disease (mucocutaneous lymph node syndrome)	Asian descent <5 year old	Coronary arteries	Cervical lymphadenopathy Heart failure Myocardial ischemia Nonexudative conjunctivitis Oropharyngeal mucosal erythema Truncal rash
Small vessel: Antineutrophil cytoplasmic antibody (ANCA)-associated vasculitis	Microscopic polyangiitis	European descent	—	Cutaneous purpura Glomerulonephritis and renal failure Pulmonary hemorrhage
	Granulomatosis with polyangiitis (Wegener's)	European descent 40–60 y of age	—	ENT findings otitis, rhinitis, and sinusitis Glomerulonephritis and renal failure

Category	Disease	Epidemiology/Association	Vessel involved	Clinical features
Small vessel: Immune complex-mediated	Eosinophilic granulomatosis with polyangiitis (Churg–Strauss)	European descent	—	Pulmonary hemorrhage, hypertension, and fibrosis; Allergic asthma attacks; Allergic rhinitis/sinusitis; Glomerulonephritis; Mononeuritis/polyneuropathy
	Anti-glomerular basement membrane disease (Goodpasture's syndrome)	—	Glomerular capillaries; Pulmonary capillaries	Glomerulonephritis with necrosis and crescents; Pulmonary hemorrhage
	Cryoglobulinaemic vasculitis	70–90% association with hepatitis C infection	—	Acrocyanosis; Cutaneous purpura with ulceration/necrosis; Polyneuropathy; Raynaud's phenomenon; Arthritis/arthralgia
	IgA vasculitis (Henoch–Schonlein)	<10 y of age; Female > male	—	Colicky abdominal pain; Cutaneous erythematous macules/urticaria progressing to palpable purpura; Nephritis progressing to nephritic syndrome
	Hypocomplementaemic urticarial vasculitis (anti-C1q vasculitis)	Up to 90% association with bacterial or viral infection	—	Urticaria
Variable vessel	Behcet's disease	Mediterranean/Middle Eastern/East Asian descent; 20–40 y of age	—	Arterial and venous thrombosis; Arthritis; Cutaneous lesions; Gastrointestinal findings; Ocular disease; Recurrent genital and oral ulcers
	Cogan's syndrome	Rare <500 cases published; 20–50 y of age	Aorta (10% of cases)	Arteritis; Ocular lesions: keratitis, uveitis, and episcleritis; Inner ear disease: sensorineural hearing loss, and vestibular dysfunction

question.[74] However, Li and colleagues[75] demonstrated in a large meta-analysis that GCA is the most common systemic vasculitis in adults aged greater than 50 years. Both TAK and GCA have a predilection for affecting females with percent of cases being 61% to 91% and 67% to 79%, respectively.[76]

Generalized symptoms of inflammation are often preset in both TAK and GCA, including arthralgia, fatigue, fevers, myalgia, sweats, and weight loss.[73] TAK is more commonly associated with abdominal pain, aortic regurgitation, carotidynia, chest pain, dyspnea, hypertension, lightheadedness, limb claudication, and reduced pulses.[72,73] GCA is more commonly associated with cough, headache, jaw claudication, neck pain, scalp tenderness, visual disturbances, and tender/thickened temporal arteries.[73,76] Comparatively, GCA also carries a higher stroke risk with reports as high as 7%.[76] There is limited information surrounding the perioperative setting. Patient management focuses predominantly on managing symptoms and potential sequelae including end-organ dysfunction, hypertension, and large vessel stenosis.[72]

The mainstay of treatment of both TAK and GCA is glucocorticoids, often at doses which can cause adrenal suppression. Careful preoperative medication review is paramount, as supplemental glucocorticoid administration is frequently required to maintain adequate levels during stress.[72,73,76] Some patients with severe disease require additional treatment including methotrexate, tocilizumab, and antiplatelet drugs, whose continuation during the perioperative period must be carefully considered.

Medium-Vessel Vasculitis

Polyarteritis nodosa (PAN) and Kawasaki disease (KD) are the most common medium-vessel vasculitides, affecting the visceral arteries and their associated branches.[70,76] Both PAN and KD have a more acute onset of inflammation and are more predisposed to necrotizing lesions compared with large-vessel vasculitides.[76] PAN and KD are differentiated by age, ethnic background, symptoms, and the specific vessels affected.

PAN is rare with an incidence of 1 to 8 per million, is more common in men, and typically affects patients 40 to 60 years of age.[71,74,76] Most recently, PAN has been differentiated from the antineutrophil cytoplasmic-associated vasculitides (AAV). PAN is a systemic illness that causes fevers, peripheral ischemia/neuropathy, and multiorgan system dysfunction including cardiovascular, gastrointestinal, neurologic, and renal failure. The most common early symptom is peripheral neuropathy.[76] Renal symptoms are present in 26% to 44% of patients, which include hematuria, moderate proteinuria, slowly progressive renal failure, and hypertension. Renal injury is thought to be secondary to aneurysm formation, infarction, and/or hematoma.[76] Cardiovascular symptoms are present in up to 25% of patients, which include predominantly left-sided heart failure and pericarditis.[76] Treatment of PAN is similar to other vasculitides with glucocorticoids and immunomodulators. Even with treatment, outcomes remain relatively poor with 5-year survival of only 59% to 67%.[71,76]

As with other vasculitides, perioperative management focuses on symptom management and appropriate medication continuation and discontinuation. Of note, patients often require surgery for gastrointestinal complications of PAN, which is associated with high mortality.[71]

KD predominantly affects infants and children under the age of 5 (up to 85% patients) and is often self-limited with many patients completely recovering.[74] The highest incidence of KD is among Asians with reports of 60 to 300 cases per 100,000 children less than 5 year old.[71,74] The overall incidence in the United States is 20 cases per 100,000 children aged less than 5 year old.[77]

There is a notable seasonality, temporal, and spatial clustering of KD with peaks in winter, spring, and mid-summer.[74] Symptoms of KD include cervical lymphadenopathy, fever, nonexudative conjunctivitis, oropharyngeal mucosal ery-thema "strawberry tongue," and truncal rash. Coronary arteries are affected in 20% with findings of aneurysm, thrombosis, or coronary dissection that can progress to heart failure, infarction, and/or sudden death.[76] The first-line treatment following diag-nosis of KD is IVIG therapy, which has been shown to reduce progression to coronary involvement. For KD patients who have coronary artery involvement, perioperative risks include aneurysm rupture, thrombosis, and myocardial ischemia.[76]

Small-Vessel Vasculitis

Small-vessel vasculitides (SVV) predominately affect small intraparenchymal arteries, arterioles, capillaries, and venules. There are two main categories for SVV differenti-ated by deposition of immunoglobin in the vessel wall for immune complex mediated and paucity of immunoglobin deposits for antineutrophil cytoplasmic antibody (ANCA)-associated vasculitis.[70] SVVs have an incidence of 10 to 30 cases per million among the general population, and when compared with other systemic autoimmune diseases are associated with higher rates of mechanical ventilation, renal replacement therapy, and ICU mortality.[74,78]

Immune complex-mediated SVV includes anti-glomerular basement membrane (anti-GBM) disease, cryoglobulinaemic vasculitis, IgA vasculitis, and hypocomple-mentaemic urticarial vasculitis.[70] Of these, the most relevant in the perioperative setting is anti-GBM disease previously known as Goodpasture's syndrome, which af-fects the glomerular capillaries causing renal failure and pulmonary capillaries causing alveolar hemorrhage.[70,74] Treatment of anti-GBM disease includes therapeutic plasma exchange, cyclophosphamide, and corticosteroids. These treatments together remove and prevent the continued formation of autoantibodies.[79] The degree of renal injury at presentation is predictive of progression to ESRD. Severe cases with ESRD may present for renal transplantation or arteriovenous fistula creation. Sus-tained seronegativity is important for the prevention of disease recrudescence following transplant.[79]

The ANCA-associated SVVs include granulomatosis with polyangiitis (GPA), micro-scopic polyangiitis (MPA), and eosinophilic GPA (EGPA).[70] The combined incidence is approximately 20 per million in Europeans.[71] GPA and MPA are clinically difficult to differentiate given many overlapping features.[80] GPA, previously named Wegener's disease, includes necrotizing granulomatous inflammation of the upper and lower res-piratory tract, necrotizing glomerulonephritis, pulmonary hemorrhage, and ocular vasculitis.[81] MPA includes necrotizing capillaritis of lungs and kidney leading to diffi-culty breathing and reduced kidney function or failure.[81] As with other vasculitides, the first-line treatment of these diseases is glucocorticoids. For more severe cases, treatment includes cyclophosphamide, methotrexate, or rituximab.[80,81]

CLINICS CARE POINTS

- Patients who have undergone recent angioplasty should wait 14 days until having elective noncardiac surgery. Those with a bare-metal stent (BMS) should wait 30 days, and those with a drug-eluting stent (DES) should wait 12 months, when possible. Recent data suggest that earlier surgery (eg, 3–6 months) may be safe after DES placement.

- For patients with a prior ischemic CVA, blood pressure should be kept within 20% of its baseline value and MAP should be kept above 70 mm Hg.

- After a prior ischemic stroke, experts recommend waiting for at least 3 months for elective surgery to reduce the risk of recurrent CVA and major adverse cardiac events.

- Patients with a Caprini score of 0 are "very low" risk for VTE with an incidence of 0.5% and do not warrant mechanical or pharmacologic prophylaxis. Patients with a score of 1–2 are "low" risk for VTE with an incidence of 1.5% and warrant mechanical prophylaxis. Patients with a score of 3–4 are "moderate" risk for VTE with an incidence of 3.0% and warrant pharmacologic ± mechanical prophylaxis. Patients with a score of 5+ are "high" risk for VTE with an incidence of 6.0% and warrant mechanical and pharmacologic prophylaxis.

DISCLOSURE

M. Mazzeffi has previously received consulting fees from Hemosonics and Octapharma.

REFERENCES

1. Mills KT, Bundy JD, Kelly TN, et al. Global disparities of hypertension prevalence and control: a systematic analysis of population-based studies from 90 countries. Circulation 2016;134(6):441–50.
2. Unger T, Borghi C, Charchar F, et al. 2020 International Society of Hypertension global hypertension practice guidelines. J Hypertens 2020;38(6):982–1004.
3. Beevers G, Lip GY, O'Brien E. ABC of hypertension: the pathophysiology of hypertension. BMJ 2001;322(7291):912–6.
4. Alexander RW. Theodore Cooper Memorial Lecture. Hypertension and the pathogenesis of atherosclerosis. Oxidative stress and the mediation of arterial inflammatory response: a new perspective. Hypertension 1995;25(2):155–61.
5. Wilkinson IB, McEniery CM, Cockcroft JR. Arteriosclerosis and atherosclerosis: guilty by association. Hypertension 2009;54(6):1213–5.
6. Wang W, Lee ET, Fabsitz RR, et al. A longitudinal study of hypertension risk factors and their relation to cardiovascular disease: the Strong Heart Study. Hypertension 2006;47(3):403–9.
7. van Oort S, Beulens JWJ, van Ballegooijen AJ, et al. Association of cardiovascular risk factors and lifestyle behaviors with hypertension: a mendelian randomization study. Hypertension 2020;76(6):1971–9.
8. Steppan J, Barodka V, Berkowitz DE, et al. Vascular stiffness and increased pulse pressure in the aging cardiovascular system. Cardiol Res Pract 2011;2011: 263585.
9. Liu J, Ma J, Wang J, et al. Comorbidity analysis according to sex and age in hypertension patients in China. Int J Med Sci 2016;13(2):99–107.
10. Noh J, Kim HC, Shin A, et al. Prevalence of comorbidity among people with hypertension: the korea national health and nutrition examination survey 2007-2013. Korean Circ J 2016;46(5):672–80.
11. Kaplan RC, Psaty BM, Heckbert SR, et al. Blood pressure level and incidence of myocardial infarction among patients treated for hypertension. Am J Public Health 1999;89(9):1414–7.
12. Li C, Engstrom G, Hedblad B, et al. Blood pressure control and risk of stroke: a population-based prospective cohort study. Stroke 2005;36(4):725–30.
13. Gaciong Z, Sinski M, Lewandowski J. Blood pressure control and primary prevention of stroke: summary of the recent clinical trial data and meta-analyses. Curr Hypertens Rep 2013;15(6):559–74.
14. Hagg-Holmberg S, Dahlstrom EH, Forsblom CM, et al. The role of blood pressure in risk of ischemic and hemorrhagic stroke in type 1 diabetes. Cardiovasc Diabetol 2019;18(1):88.

15. Woo D, Haverbusch M, Sekar P, et al. Effect of untreated hypertension on hemorrhagic stroke. Stroke 2004;35(7):1703–8.
16. Tozawa M, Iseki K, Iseki C, et al. Blood pressure predicts risk of developing end-stage renal disease in men and women. Hypertension 2003;41(6):1341–5.
17. Hsu CY, McCulloch CE, Darbinian J, et al. Elevated blood pressure and risk of end-stage renal disease in subjects without baseline kidney disease. Arch Intern Med 2005;165(8):923–8.
18. Howell SJ, Sear JW, Foex P. Hypertension, hypertensive heart disease and perioperative cardiac risk. Br J Anaesth 2004;92(4):570–83.
19. Wax DB, Porter SB, Lin HM, et al. Association of preanesthesia hypertension with adverse outcomes. J Cardiothorac Vasc Anesth 2010;24(6):927–30.
20. Wilcox T, Smilowitz NR, Xia Y, et al. Cardiovascular Risk factors and perioperative myocardial infarction after noncardiac surgery. Can J Cardiol 2021;37(2):224–31.
21. Basali A, Mascha EJ, Kalfas I, et al. Relation between perioperative hypertension and intracranial hemorrhage after craniotomy. Anesthesiology 2000;93(1):48–54.
22. Whelton PK, Carey RM, Aronow WS, et al. 2017 ACC/AHA/AAPA/ABC/ACPM/AGS/APhA/ASH/ASPC/NMA/PCNA guideline for the prevention, detection, evaluation, and management of high blood pressure in adults: executive summary: a report of the american college of cardiology/american heart association task force on clinical practice guidelines. Circulation 2018;138(17):e426–83.
23. Walsh M, Devereaux PJ, Garg AX, et al. Relationship between intraoperative mean arterial pressure and clinical outcomes after noncardiac surgery: toward an empirical definition of hypotension. Anesthesiology 2013;119(3):507–15.
24. Salmasi V, Maheshwari K, Yang D, et al. Relationship between intraoperative hypotension, defined by either reduction from baseline or absolute thresholds, and acute kidney and myocardial injury after noncardiac surgery: a retrospective cohort analysis. Anesthesiology 2017;126(1):47–65.
25. Wesselink EM, Kappen TH, Torn HM, et al. Intraoperative hypotension and the risk of postoperative adverse outcomes: a systematic review. Br J Anaesth 2018;121(4):706–21.
26. Joshi B, Ono M, Brown C, et al. Predicting the limits of cerebral autoregulation during cardiopulmonary bypass. Anesth Analg 2012;114(3):503–10.
27. Futier E, Lefrant JY, Guinot PG, et al. Effect of individualized vs standard blood pressure management strategies on postoperative organ dysfunction among high-risk patients undergoing major surgery: a randomized clinical trial. JAMA 2017;318(14):1346–57.
28. Sessler DI, Bloomstone JA, Aronson S, et al. Perioperative Quality Initiative consensus statement on intraoperative blood pressure, risk and outcomes for elective surgery. Br J Anaesth 2019;122(5):563–74.
29. Writing Group M, Mozaffarian D, Benjamin EJ, et al. Executive summary: heart disease and stroke statistics–2016 update: a report from the american heart association. Circulation 2016;133(4):447–54.
30. Sanchis-Gomar F, Perez-Quilis C, Leischik R, et al. Epidemiology of coronary heart disease and acute coronary syndrome. Ann Transl Med 2016;4(13):256.
31. Wilson PW. Established risk factors and coronary artery disease: the Framingham Study. Am J Hypertens 1994;7(7 Pt 2):7S–12S.
32. Myers RH, Kiely DK, Cupples LA, et al. Parental history is an independent risk factor for coronary artery disease: the Framingham Study. Am Heart J 1990; 120(4):963–9.
33. Hajar R. Risk factors for coronary artery disease: historical perspectives. Heart Views 2017;18(3):109–14.

34. Bergheanu SC, Bodde MC, Jukema JW. Pathophysiology and treatment of atherosclerosis : current view and future perspective on lipoprotein modification treatment. Neth Heart J 2017;25(4):231–42.

35. Moore KJ, Sheedy FJ, Fisher EA. Macrophages in atherosclerosis: a dynamic balance. Nat Rev Immunol 2013;13(10):709–21.

36. Thygesen K, Alpert JS, Jaffe AS, et al. Fourth universal definition of myocardial infarction (2018). Circulation 2018;138(20):e618–51.

37. O'Kelly B, Browner WS, Massie B, et al. Ventricular arrhythmias in patients undergoing noncardiac surgery. The Study of Perioperative Ischemia Research Group. JAMA 1992;268(2):217–21.

38. Devereaux PJ, Xavier D, Pogue J, et al. Characteristics and short-term prognosis of perioperative myocardial infarction in patients undergoing noncardiac surgery: a cohort study. Ann Intern Med 2011;154(8):523–8.

39. Sheth T, Natarajan MK, Hsieh V, et al. Incidence of thrombosis in perioperative and non-operative myocardial infarction. Br J Anaesth 2018;120(4):725–33.

40. Cleland JG, McGowan J. Heart failure due to ischaemic heart disease: epidemiology, pathophysiology and progression. J Cardiovasc Pharmacol 1999;33(Suppl 3):S17–29.

41. Di Carli MF, Davidson M, Little R, et al. Value of metabolic imaging with positron emission tomography for evaluating prognosis in patients with coronary artery disease and left ventricular dysfunction. Am J Cardiol 1994;73(8):527–33.

42. Braunschweig F, Linde C, Benson L, et al. New York Heart Association functional class, QRS duration, and survival in heart failure with reduced ejection fraction: implications for cardiac resynchronization therapy. Eur J Heart Fail 2017;19(3):366–76.

43. Moitra VK, Einav S, Thies KC, et al. Cardiac arrest in the operating room: resuscitation and management for the anesthesiologist: part 1. Anesth Analg 2018;126(3):876–88.

44. Fleisher LA, Fleischmann KE, Auerbach AD, et al. 2014 ACC/AHA guideline on perioperative cardiovascular evaluation and management of patients undergoing noncardiac surgery: a report of the American College of Cardiology/American Heart Association Task Force on practice guidelines. J Am Coll Cardiol 2014;64(22):e77–137.

45. Duceppe E, Parlow J, MacDonald P, et al. Canadian cardiovascular society guidelines on perioperative cardiac risk assessment and management for patients who undergo noncardiac surgery. Can J Cardiol 2017;33(1):17–32.

46. Smilowitz NR, Berger JS. Perioperative cardiovascular risk assessment and management for noncardiac surgery: a review. JAMA 2020;324(3):279–90.

47. McFalls EO, Ward HB, Moritz TE, et al. Coronary-artery revascularization before elective major vascular surgery. N Engl J Med 2004;351(27):2795–804.

48. Saini V, Guada L, Yavagal DR. Global epidemiology of stroke and access to acute ischemic stroke interventions. Neurology 2021;97(20 Suppl 2):S6–16.

49. Ornello R, Degan D, Tiseo C, et al. Distribution and temporal trends from 1993 to 2015 of ischemic stroke subtypes: a systematic review and meta-analysis. Stroke 2018;49(4):814–9.

50. Jorgensen ME, Torp-Pedersen C, Gislason GH, et al. Time elapsed after ischemic stroke and risk of adverse cardiovascular events and mortality following elective noncardiac surgery. JAMA 2014;312(3):269–77.

51. Mehdi Z, Birns J, Partridge J, et al. Perioperative management of adult patients with a history of stroke or transient ischaemic attack undergoing elective noncardiac surgery. Clin Med (Lond) 2016;16(6):535–40.

52. Ng JL, Chan MT, Gelb AW. Perioperative stroke in noncardiac, nonneurosurgical surgery. Anesthesiology 2011;115(4):879–90.
53. Glance LG, Benesch CG, Holloway RG, et al. Association of time elapsed since ischemic stroke with risk of recurrent stroke in older patients undergoing elective nonneurologic, noncardiac surgery. JAMA Surg 2022;157(8):e222236.
54. Mazzeffi M, Chow JH, Anders M, et al. Intraoperative hypotension and perioperative acute ischemic stroke in patients having major elective non-cardiovascular non-neurological surgery. J Anesth 2021;35(2):246–53.
55. Bateman BT, Schumacher HC, Wang S, et al. Perioperative acute ischemic stroke in noncardiac and nonvascular surgery: incidence, risk factors, and outcomes. Anesthesiology 2009;110(2):231–8.
56. Wongtangman K, Wachtendorf LJ, Blank M, et al. Effect of intraoperative arterial hypotension on the risk of perioperative stroke after noncardiac surgery: a retrospective multicenter cohort study. Anesth Analg 2021;133(4):1000–8.
57. Benesch C, Glance LG, Derdeyn CP, et al. Perioperative neurological evaluation and management to lower the risk of acute stroke in patients undergoing noncardiac, nonneurological surgery: a scientific statement from the american heart association/american stroke association. Circulation 2021;143(19):e923–46.
58. Bijker JB, Persoon S, Peelen LM, et al. Intraoperative hypotension and perioperative ischemic stroke after general surgery: a nested case-control study. Anesthesiology 2012;116(3):658–64.
59. Rabinstein AA. Optimal blood pressure after intracerebral hemorrhage: still a moving target. Stroke 2018;49(2):275–6.
60. Gordon RJ, Lombard FW. Perioperative venous thromboembolism: a review. Anesth Analg 2017;125(2):403–12.
61. Buesing KL, Mullapudi B, Flowers KA. Deep venous thrombosis and venous thromboembolism prophylaxis. Surg Clin North Am 2015;95(2):285–300.
62. Kahn SR. The post-thrombotic syndrome. Hematol Am Soc Hematol Educ Program 2016;2016(1):413–8.
63. Pannucci CJ, Swistun L, MacDonald JK, et al. Individualized venous thromboembolism risk stratification using the 2005 caprini score to identify the benefits and harms of chemoprophylaxis in surgical patients: a meta-analysis. Ann Surg 2017; 265(6):1094–103.
64. McAlpine K, Breau RH, Werlang P, et al. Timing of perioperative pharmacologic thromboprophylaxis initiation and its effect on venous thromboembolism and bleeding outcomes: a systematic review and meta-analysis. J Am Coll Surg 2021;233(5):619–31.e614.
65. Cohen AT, Tapson VF, Bergmann JF, et al. Venous thromboembolism risk and prophylaxis in the acute hospital care setting (ENDORSE study): a multinational cross-sectional study. Lancet 2008;371(9610):387–94.
66. Gould MK, Garcia DA, Wren SM, et al. Prevention of VTE in nonorthopedic surgical patients: antithrombotic therapy and prevention of thrombosis, 9th ed: american college of chest physicians evidence-based clinical practice guidelines. Chest 2012;141(2 Suppl):e227S–77S.
67. Stevens SM, Woller SC, Kreuziger LB, et al. Antithrombotic therapy for VTE disease: second update of the chest guideline and expert panel report. Chest 2021;160(6):e545–608.
68. Arabi YM, Al-Hameed F, Burns KEA, et al. Adjunctive intermittent pneumatic compression for venous thromboprophylaxis. N Engl J Med 2019;380(14): 1305–15.

69. Kakkos S, Kirkilesis G, Caprini JA, et al. Combined intermittent pneumatic leg compression and pharmacological prophylaxis for prevention of venous thromboembolism. Cochrane Database Syst Rev 2022;1:CD005258.

70. Jennette JC, Falk RJ, Bacon PA, et al. 2012 revised international chapel hill consensus conference nomenclature of vasculitides. Arthritis Rheum 2013; 65(1):1–11.

71. Watts RA, Robson J. Introduction, epidemiology and classification of vasculitis. Best Pract Res Clin Rheumatol 2018;32(1):3–20.

72. Yoshida M, Yamamoto T, Shiiba S, et al. Anesthetic management of a patient with takayasu arteritis. Anesth Prog 2016;63(1):31–3.

73. Pugh D, Karabayas M, Basu N, et al. Large-vessel vasculitis. Nat Rev Dis Primers 2022;7(1):93.

74. Watts RA, Hatemi G, Burns JC, et al. Global epidemiology of vasculitis. Nat Rev Rheumatol 2022;18(1):22–34.

75. Li KJ, Semenov D, Turk M, et al. A meta-analysis of the epidemiology of giant cell arteritis across time and space. Arthritis Res Ther 2021;23(1):82.

76. Saadoun D, Vautier M, Cacoub P. Medium- and large-vessel vasculitis. Circulation 2021;143(3):267–82.

77. Maddox RA, Person MK, Kennedy JL, et al. Kawasaki disease and kawasaki disease shock syndrome hospitalization rates in the United States, 2006-2018. Pediatr Infect Dis J 2021;40(4):284–8.

78. Włudarczyk A, Polok K, Górka J, et al. Patients with small-vessel vasculitides have the highest mortality among systemic autoimmune diseases patients treated in intensive care unit: a retrospective study with 5-year follow-up. J Crit Care 2018;48:166–71.

79. McAdoo SP, Pusey CD. Anti-glomerular basement membrane disease. Clin J Am Soc Nephrol 2017;12(7):1162–72.

80. Geetha D, Jefferson JA. ANCA-associated vasculitis: core curriculum 2020. Am J Kidney Dis 2020;75(1):124–37.

81. Lopalco G, Rigante D, Venerito V, et al. Management of small vessel vasculitides. Curr Rheumatol Rep 2016;18(6):36.

Patient Blood Management in Vascular Surgery

Richard Gyi, DO[a], Brian C. Cho, MD[a,b], Nadia B. Hensley, MD[b,*]

KEYWORDS

- Patient blood management • Vascular surgery • Bleeding management • Anemia
- Blood transfusion • Antiplatelet agents • Coagulopathy

KEY POINTS

- Vascular surgery is one of the highest utilizers of allogeneic blood components, making it second only to cardiac surgery in the allocation of the nation's blood supply.
- Studies have shown a positive correlation between preoperative anemia in vascular surgical patients and two times increased likelihood of 30-day mortality. Given the increased risk, identification and appropriate treatment of preoperative anemia should be prioritized in this high-risk surgical population.
- Surgery-specific risk factors of increased blood loss are related to the anatomical location of the surgical site, vascularity of the involved organ or tissue, and surgical approach such as open versus minimally invasive methods.
- In general, a restrictive transfusion threshold, defined as 7-8 g/dL, has been shown to reduce transfusion exposure with no increase in mortality, myocardial events, or cerebrovascular events for the vascular surgery population. Antifibrinolytics have demonstrated reduced bleeding and transfusions in patients undergoing vascular surgery.
- Hypothermia has been known to impair platelet function and coagulation cascade. Even mild intraoperative hypothermia at a core temperature of 35 C is associated with 16% increased blood loss and 22% increased risk of transfusion. Avoiding hypothermia after aortic cross-clamp removal is important to preventing coagulopathy.

INTRODUCTION

Patient blood management (PBM) is an evidence-based, multidisciplinary approach aimed at appropriately allocating blood products to patients requiring transfusion while simultaneously minimizing inappropriate transfusions. The 3 pillars of patient blood management are optimizing erythropoiesis, minimizing blood loss, and optimizing physiological reserve of anemia. Benefits seen from PBM include limiting hospital costs and mitigating harm from numerous risks of transfusion.[1]

---

[a] Department of Anesthesiology, Johns Hopkins Hospital, 1800 Orleans Avenue, Zayed Tower 6212, Baltimore, MD 21287, USA; [b] Division of Cardiothoracic Anesthesiology, Johns Hopkins University School of Medicine, 1800 Orleans Avenue, Zayed Tower 6212, Baltimore, MD 21287, USA
* Corresponding author.
E-mail address: nhensle2@jhmi.edu

Anesthesiology Clin 40 (2022) 605–625
https://doi.org/10.1016/j.anclin.2022.08.007
anesthesiology.theclinics.com
1932-2275/22/© 2022 Elsevier Inc. All rights reserved.

Vascular surgery is one of the highest utilizers of allogeneic blood components, making it second only to cardiac surgery in the allocation of the nation's blood supply. This may be due to the high risk of blood loss often associated with vascular surgical interventions, as well as the comorbidities of the patient population and medications such as anticoagulants or platelet inhibitors. Furthermore, both anemia and blood transfusion have been found to be independently associated with poor outcomes such as postoperative myocardial infarction, worse survival, and longer length of stay after vascular surgeries.[1–3]

Given this predisposition, it is important for vascular surgical patients to have preoperative, intraoperative, and postoperative blood management optimization. It is vital that there is support for the implementation of a PBM program from all facets of the medical system as it requires significant time, education, and financial support. However, with the ever-present blood supply challenges and the growing literature on the morbidities associated with transfusion, PBM programs are becoming a centerpiece in individualized patient care.[4,5]

Preoperative Patient Blood Management for Vascular Surgery

The implementation of an effective PBM program begins in the preoperative period. This includes evaluating and treating anemia, assessing the bleeding risks associated with the procedure, managing medications such as antiplatelet agents, anticoagulants, and direct oral anticoagulants, considering preoperative autologous blood donation, and anemia tolerance. Other important considerations include implementing a maximum surgical blood order schedule, which is ordering only amount of blood products necessary for procedure, and using minimally invasive surgical techniques.

Evaluation and treatment of preoperative anemia

Preoperative anemia is common in the vascular surgical patient population. In hospitalized patients 65 and older, the prevalence of anemia is 24 to 40%.[2] Studies have shown a positive correlation between preoperative anemia in vascular surgical patients and two times increased likelihood of 30-day mortality. Given the increased risk, identification and appropriate treatment of preoperative anemia should be prioritized in this high-risk surgical population.

Preoperative anemia in this population is most often secondary to iron deficiency anemia and anemia of chronic disease. The workup, diagnosis, and appropriate treatment of anemia takes time, often taking up to 30 days to achieve optimal effect. Patient should have lab work to determine the cause of anemia which can help direct treatment options. Lab tests frequently used to inform treatment plans include ferritin and transferrin (for iron deficiency), endogenous erythropoietin, holotranscobalamine (for possible B12 treatment), and folic acid. Treatments such as iron infusions, oral iron supplements, vitamin B12, folic acid, and erythropoietin may be used to optimize erythropoiesis and correct preoperative anemia.[4]

Intravenous iron infusion. The use of intravenous iron therapy can be a feasible method to treat preoperative anemia. The CAVIAR study was an observational study out of the United Kingdom which compared cardiac and vascular surgical patients without anemia, patients with anemia who received no preoperative treatment, and patients with anemia who received preoperative intravenous iron. The study concluded that patients with anemia who received intravenous iron preoperatively had a higher postoperative hemoglobin level than those without preoperative intravenous iron treatment. These findings were furthermore reinforced with the PREVENTT trial.[6] Although the PREVENTT trial showed no difference in the primary outcome of transfusions between those treated with IV iron, there was significantly higher hemoglobin at 8 weeks [mean difference (MD) 10.7 g/dL, (95%CI 7.3, 3.6–11.1)], and at 6-month follow-up (MD 7.3, 3.6–11.1).

One of the major limitations of preoperative intravenous iron is the establishment of programs that identify preoperative anemia early enough for intervention as it usually takes 30 days to improve hemoglobin levels.[6] The timeline for this is a matter of debate; however, as one study showed that the initiation of erythropoiesis-stimulating agents and intravenous iron even as short as 2 days prior to surgery can reduce RBC transfusion requirement.[7] Additionally, the efficacy of preoperative iron still requires further study in larger randomized controlled trials. The small increase in hemoglobin levels has yet to show a definitive beneficial relationship with postoperative outcomes.[3,4]

Erythropoietin use. Erythropoietin's role in treating anemia in vascular surgery patients has not been defined. However, extrapolating from studies of cardiac surgical patients and elective orthopedic patients, erythropoietin may have a role in treating anemia preoperatively in vascular surgical patients. In a recent meta-analysis, erythropoietin administration preoperatively showed a decrease in perioperative allogenic blood transfusions in the intraoperative period, postoperative period, and the entire hospital stay. Although many of the studies included in the meta-analysis did not include quantitative hemoglobin levels, in those that did, there was a significant increase in preoperative and postoperative hemoglobin levels in those treated with erythropoietin as compared to placebo.[5] In this meta-analysis, among cardiac and orthopedic surgery patients, erythropoietin treatment was not associated with increased risks of thromboembolic events or other significant known side effects. Further study of preoperative erythropoietin in vascular surgery patients is needed.

Assessment of bleeding risk

The bleeding risk of a patient is a combination of surgery-specific risk factors and patient-related risk factors. Surgery-specific risk factors of increased blood loss are related to the anatomical location of the surgical site, vascularity of the involved organ or tissue, and surgical approach such as open versus minimally invasive methods.[8] Surgeries with highest bleeding risks are cardiac surgeries, followed by vascular surgeries.

Common patient-related risk factors for increased bleeding include the use of antiplatelet or anticoagulant agents, family and personal history of significant bleeding, platelet or clotting abnormalities.[8] For patients with a positive bleeding history, further testing and referral to hematology can be helpful in developing an individualized strategy in perioperative hemostasis. There are few existing scoring systems for bleeding risk stratification but none are validated in large prospective studies for general surgeries.[8] One scoring system, ACTA PORT score, has been validated to predict the risk of blood transfusion for adult cardiac surgery, and it considers age, sex, body surface area, preoperative hemoglobin, creatinine, type of cardiac operation, and EURO-SCORE, a marker for mortality used in Europe.[9] Though validated for cardiac surgeries, it is not yet applicable to other types of surgeries. A detailed history, lab work, and hematology consult, if indicated, are steps to identify patient-related risk factors that can be optimized prior to surgery.

The use of antiplatelet or anticoagulant agents is frequently encountered in patients undergoing vascular surgeries, as patients in this cohort often share similar cardiovascular risk factors such as coronary artery disease, peripheral vascular disease, or thromboembolic events. Perioperative management of antiplatelet therapy and anticoagulants is a fine balance between bleeding risk and major cardiovascular and thrombotic risk, often requiring delicate multidisciplinary risk-benefit discussions between surgeons, hematologists, cardiologists, anesthesiologists, and patients.

Antiplatelet agents. Patients with coronary artery disease requiring stent placement are placed on dual antiplatelet therapy with aspirin and clopidogrel or other P2Y12 receptor antagonists, such as ticagrelor and prasugrel, for 4 weeks for bare metal stents (BMS) and for 1 year for drug-eluting stents (DES), and aspirin is a life-long therapy for patients with coronary artery disease.[10] The impact of continuation or discontinuation of antiplatelet therapy on the risk of bleeding and cardiovascular events has been studied, but no strong evidence so far has provided guidance on the preoperative management of antiplatelet therapy.[8,10–13] Some studies concluded that the risk of a cardiovascular event with the discontinuation of antiplatelet agent is higher than the risk of surgical bleeding with continuation, except for neurosurgery, closed eye surgery, or surgeries with high bleeding risks,[8,10,12] so antiplatelet agents should be continued if the risk of not having the vascular surgery prior to 6 months after DES outweighs the risk of bleeding. Other studies concluded that short-term discontinuation of antiplatelet agents confers no increased risk in thrombotic events and bleeding risk is lessened, thus antiplatelet agents should be held preoperatively.[13] Recommendations currently are that aspirin should not be continued for most procedures; clopidogrel, ticagrelor, or prasugrel can be stopped 5–7 days prior for vital surgeries with high bleeding risk that cannot be postponed until the discontinuation of P2Y12 inhibitors or 6 months after a DES.[10,14] In emergent surgeries with significant bleeding risk, the antiplatelet effect can be reversed with allogeneic platelet transfusions, which will be discussed further in a later section.[15]

Anticoagulant agents

Warfarin and bridging therapy with heparin Warfarin is a vitamin K antagonist that blocks the function of the vitamin K epoxide reductase complex in the liver, leading to a decrease in the reduced form of vitamin K which normally acts as a cofactor for vitamin K-dependent coagulation factors.[16] Warfarin has a long half-life of 36 hours and needs to be stopped 5 days prior to elective surgery to ensure adequate normalization of coagulation function. An INR should be checked the day prior to surgery to allow time for reversal with vitamin K or phytomenadione if INR >1.5 and again on the day of surgery.[14] If warfarin is held preoperatively, some patients at high risk of thromboembolic events may require bridging with treatment dose heparin or low molecular weight heparin (LMWH).[14]

When assessing the risk and need for bridging therapy, patients taking warfarin for stroke prevention due to atrial fibrillation, secondary prevention of venous thromboembolism (VTE), or mechanical heart valves need to be considered separately.[14] Unfortunately, the current recommendations are largely based on expert opinion and not yet supported by clear evidence.[17]

The risk stratification for stroke in patients with atrial fibrillation is based on CHA2DS2-VASc scores that are calculated from the history of congestive heart failure, hypertension, age, diabetes, stroke, vascular disease, and sex category, with a 0–4 score being low risk, 5–6 being moderate risk, and >7 as high risk.[17,18] Guidelines have suggested considering bridging therapy for those with stroke in the past 3 months or multiple risk factors, in other words, those with moderate to high risk as assessed by CHA2DS2-VASc score.[18]

For patients taking warfarin for a recent venous thromboembolic event, they are considered high risk if the VTE occurred within the past 3 months, moderate risk if the VTE occurred in the past 3–12 months, and low risk if it occurred more than

1 year ago.[14,18,19] Bridging therapy should be considered for those with high risk for VTE, or those who had VTE within the last 3 months.[14]

For patients taking warfarin for mechanical heart valves, the thrombotic risk is considered high, and bridging therapy is recommended for all types of mechanical valves except for bi-leaflet aortic valves and for any patients with prothrombotic risk factors such as atrial fibrillation, congestive heart failure, hypertension, diabetes, prior stroke, and age>75 years.[14,18]

In emergent surgeries with significant bleeding risk, 4-factor prothrombin complex concentrate (4F PCC) should be administered to provide rapid reversal of the anticoagulant effect of warfarin as well as intravenous vitamin K for the sustained effect of reversal.[15]

Direct oral anticoagulants The direct oral anticoagulants are becoming more widely used for stroke risk reduction in patients with nonvalvular atrial fibrillation and treatment of deep vein thrombosis and pulmonary embolism.[19] The common DOACs include dabigatran, a direct thrombin/factor IIa inhibitor, and 3 selective factor Xa inhibitors: rivaroxaban, apixaban, and edoxaban. Compared to warfarin, all the DOACs have faster onset, similar shorter half-lives of 10–12 hrs, more predictable pharmacokinetics and pharmacodynamics.[18,20] While DOACs are more predictable than warfarin, each DOAC has a slightly different elimination mechanism. All DOACs' half-lives are subject to renal function to varying degrees, and apixaban and rivaroxaban are also dependent on liver function.[20] These are important properties to consider for the perioperative management of DOACs.

In general, due to their predictable properties, all DOACs can be stopped 48 hours before most surgeries in the presence of normal hepatic and renal function.[8] The DOACs act similarly to LMWHs in terms of these predictable pharmacokinetic properties, so bridging therapy is often not recommended when suspending DOACs perioperatively.[18,21,22] However, for patients with impaired renal function, there is no published data or established protocols for the discontinuation of individual DOACs, and the wide variability of recommendations are largely based on manufacturers' advice and expert opinions.[14,18,20] The range of time recommended for stopping DOACs prior to surgery range from 24 hrs to 96 hrs preoperatively, depending on renal function and bleeding risk of the surgery.[8,14]

Currently, no laboratory studies are recommended for routine measures of return to normal coagulation or quantification of DOAC levels after discontinuation.[14,18] In rare incidents when DOAC level needs to be measured, drug-specific anti-Xa trough levels for apixaban, rivaroxaban, and edoxaban, and diluted thrombin time for dabigatran can be helpful if they are available.[18,20] Routine coagulation tests such as PT and aPTT should not be used to judge anticoagulation with DOACs as the sensitivity of these tests is dependent on the different laboratory reagents used, and normal values of PT and PTT cannot exclude anticoagulation in patients on DOACs.[20] Due to the challenge in measuring the anticoagulation effect of DOACs, the administration of tranexamic acid should be considered in patients undergoing urgent surgery with high bleeding risks where residual levels of DOACs are suspected.[8] Nonspecific reversal of DOACs' anticoagulant effect has also been achieved by prothrombin complex concentrate (PCCs) prior to the advent of two new specific reversal agents approved in the United States: idarucizumab for dabigatran reversal and andexanet alfa for apixaban and rivaroxaban reversal.[23]

Other preoperative planning
Preoperative autologous blood donation. Preoperative autologous donation first gained interest as a result of the AIDS epidemic in the 1980s. This was in response

to the fear of blood-born pathogen transmission with viruses such as hepatitis through allogenic transfusion. The goal of preoperative autologous blood donation is to decrease allogenic transmission and stimulate erythropoiesis. A meta-analysis of 6 randomized studies with vascular surgical patients included in the cohort concluded that preoperative autologous donation does reduce the exposure to allogenic blood, however, patients who predonated were also predisposed to receive any type of transfusion (autologous or allogenic).[24] This poses the question of whether patients truly benefit from preoperative donation, given the inherent risks of transfusion of the wrong unit of autologous blood secondary to administrative errors, the patient tolerance to autologous donation preoperatively and relative safety of allogenic transfusion in the modern error of blood banking technology.

The meta-analysis and randomized controlled trials looking at preoperative autologous donation were based on transfusion triggers of 10 g/dL, as compared to current evidence that lower transfusion triggers may be more beneficial. Therefore, although preoperative autologous donation may cause an increase in total transfusion rates, the data may need to be reassessed with modern transfusion triggers.[6]

Practitioners should continue to keep in mind that patients with vascular pathology undergoing vascular surgery may have additional comorbidities, such as coronary artery disease, that place them at higher risk of adverse events with preoperative autologous donation. Patient selection is key.

Transfusion threshold: anemia tolerance. Historically, blood transfusion was used to maintain blood hemoglobin concentration above 10 g/dL and hematocrit above 30%. There has been an emphasis in recent years to reduce blood transfusion and lower the blood transfusion threshold to conserve scarce resources and minimize exposure to allogeneic blood and its associated adverse effects. While it is widely agreed that perioperative anemia should be addressed, despite the multitude of studies, there is still no agreement on a clear transfusion threshold for patients undergoing general surgeries and likewise, for patients with cardiovascular risk factors undergoing vascular surgeries. Traditionally, the restrictive transfusion threshold uses the hemoglobin concentration of 7.0–8.0 g/dL as the transfusion trigger, and the liberal approach uses the hemoglobin concentration of 9.0–10.0 g/dL. The restrictive transfusion strategy has been shown to reduce the exposure to RBC transfusion by 41% across a broad range of surgical patients,[25,26] but no difference in mortality or cardiac events, myocardial infarction, stroke, thromboembolism, or infection were observed between patients assigned to a restrictive or liberal transfusion approach.[25,27–29]

However, the data are less certain in terms of the safety of restrictive transfusion thresholds for subgroups of patients with cardiovascular disease undergoing high risk surgeries such as cardiac or vascular procedures.[25–29] There seems to be no difference in mortality between patients who received restrictive transfusion strategy compared to those who were managed with liberal transfusion strategy, but there seems to be an increased risk of secondary outcomes of cardiovascular events in the restrictive approach.[25–29] A context-specific meta-analysis examined outcomes in patients with cardiovascular disease undergoing cardiac or vascular procedures and elderly patients with varying cardiovascular disease undergoing orthopedic surgeries separate from other patients' populations and surgeries.[27] In this risk-stratified meta-analysis, the restrictive transfusion threshold strategy was found to have a mildly elevated risk of composite outcomes of mortality and events related to inadequate oxygen delivery, such myocardial infarction, arrhythmia, angina, stroke, transient ischemic attack, acute kidney injury, and mesenteric ischemia.[27] In another meta-analysis specifically examining patients with cardiovascular disease undergoing noncardiac surgeries, mortality is not statistically different, but the risk of acute coronary syndrome is increased in the patients managed with restrictive transfusion strategy compared to liberal transfusion approach, defined as a hemoglobin concentration threshold of > 8.0 g/dL.[28]

In a retrospective database study examining patients with preoperative anemia undergoing elective endovascular aortic repair (EVAR), red cell transfusion was associated with increased risk of death and complications, suggesting that the restrictive approach of blood transfusion combined with preoperative management of anemia may be safer in this specific patient population and procedure.[30] However, with many observational studies analyzing outcomes with different hemoglobin triggers, confounding by indication is a significant limitation.

Maximum surgical blood order schedule. Maximum surgical blood ordering schedule (MSBOS) is a list of the recommended number of units of blood to be cross-matched for elective surgeries. Friedman and colleagues[31] first created the concept of MSBOS in 1976 by compiling the mean number of units crossmatched and transfused for elective surgeries from the University of Michigan over a 3-month period. He noted that, for example, while elective cholecystectomies were commonly crossmatched for 2 units of RBCs, the average number required intraoperatively was only 0.5 unit. The first MSBOS reduced the blood unit expiration rate from 6.5% to 4.5%. Friedman and colleagues's[31] MSBOS suggested surgical blood orders and type and screen recommendations for 63 common elective surgical procedures. An evolution in surgical techniques such as laparoscopic and minimally invasive procedures and other patient blood management strategies have naturally led to changes in the MSBOS. Additionally, inter-institutional practice variations also require institution-specific adjustments to the MSBOS.[8,32] Frank and colleagues[32] in 2013 described methods to create up-to-date, institution-specific, data-driven MSBOS to guide preoperative blood ordering. Following their described method of data-driven, institution-specific MSBOS, there was an effective reduction in unnecessary type and screen samples and cross-matched blood ordered preoperatively.[32,33]

As MSBOS only considers the nature of the surgery at a specific institution, there are several limitations of MSBOS that still require joint clinical decisions between surgeons and anesthesiologists for individual cases. For example, MSBOS does not consider specific preoperative patient considerations such as anemia or cardiovascular risk factors[34]; intraoperative estimation of blood loss may not be accurate, and restrictive transfusion thresholds in the setting of acute blood loss are unreasonable. Hence, intraoperative transfusion requirement often relies on the anesthesiologist's and surgeon's clinical judgment despite the average transfusion requirements for any particular case.[34]

On many MSBOS, vascular surgeries, especially aortic repairs and major artery repairs, often have the 2nd highest recommended numbers of cross-matched blood to prepare for preoperatively, only second to cardiac surgeries.[34] With advances in endovascular approaches, the transfusion requirement for elective aortic repairs have decreased significantly.[35]

Minimally invasive surgery: thoracic endovascular aortic repair or endovascular aortic repair. The advances made in minimally invasive surgical techniques in the past few decades such as with laparoscopic, robotic, and endovascular methods as opposed to open approaches have decreased blood loss and transfusion requirements across all surgical fields.[8,31] In vascular surgery, the endovascular approaches have been performed in not only peripheral arterial repair[32] but also have become a significant contributor in aortic repair.[34–37] While patients with peripheral arterial injuries resulting in free hemorrhage or significant blood loss may still be best served with open repair, endovascular therapy can provide some advantage in cases of challenging anatomy and can lead to less blood transfusion requirement and less physiologic derangement.[32,33] Open thoracic or abdominal aortic repairs often have high risk of bleeding and requirement for blood transfusions. Compared to open repairs, patients who received the endovascular approach with thoracic endovascular aortic repair (TEVAR) or abdominal endovascular aortic repair (EVAR) have a significantly reduced risk of bleeding and perioperative transfusion.[34–36]

Advantages of endovascular approaches include shorter length of hospital stay, improved short-term mortality, and decreased surgical time. Some studies have demonstrated worse long-term survival, higher rates of postoperative ischemia, reintervention, and costs with endovascular approaches. Yet, perioperative bleeding and transfusions have been consistently reported to be less in TEVARs and EVARS compared to open aortic repair.[34–36]

Intraoperative Methods

Cell salvage

Cell salvage, or auto-transfusion, is the collection of blood from the operative field or wound site and reinfusion of the washed autologous red cells back into the patient.[38,39] It is an important part of patient blood management that helps limit the need for allogeneic red cell transfusion and associated risks of alloimmunization and infection. It is used in multiple surgical disciplines including cardiac, vascular, orthopedic, obstetrics, trauma, transplant, and cancer surgeries.

The concept of cell salvage and autotransfusion has been described since 1874 by Highmore when he proposed collecting the hemorrhaged blood from an obstetric patient and reinfusing it back into the patient.[40] However, it was not until the 1970s when the technology of "cell-saver" was developed to concentrate and wash the salvaged blood before it was readministered.[39] With the advances in filtration and washing technology, intraoperative cell salvage can provide high-quality blood products for autotransfusion.[39] The method of filtration allows the separation of RBCs from the surgical field debris. Centrifugal washing allows the separation of RBCs from anticoagulants, resulting in concentrated RBCs suspended in saline, without plasma and platelets, with a hematocrit of 55–70%.[41]

Compared to banked blood, the RBCs from cell salvage have not been subjected to the adverse effects of storage and thus have a few advantages[41]: (1) salvaged RBCs have a normal level of 2,3-diphosphoglucerate (2,3-DPG), whereas stored blood cells have almost completely depleted 2,3-DPG levels after 3 weeks, leading to a left shift in the hemoglobin-oxygen dissociation curve and less oxygen delivery at the tissue level[42]; (2) salvaged RBCs have normal cell membrane deformability that allows them to change shape and flow through small capillaries for optimal oxygen delivery[43,44]; (3) salvaged RBCs do not contain citrate as in stored blood, which can cause profound hypotension, decreased cardiac contractility, and vasoplegia due to calcium chelation.[41]

Studies have shown the overall effectiveness of cell salvage in reducing exposure to allogeneic blood transfusion across different types of surgery, vascular surgery included. A recent Cochrane review of 75 randomized controlled trials showed that the use of cell salvage is efficacious in reducing allogeneic RBC transfusion in elective cardiac and orthopedic surgeries and did not adversely impact clinical outcomes.[45] A 2016 meta-analysis of 47 RCTs also showed that cell salvage reduced the rate of allogeneic RBC transfusion, reduced the risk of infection, length of stay, with no increased risk of mortality. These findings remained statistically significant in the subgroup of 6 vascular surgery trials included in the meta-analysis.[38,45–49]

Cell salvage is also more cost-effective compared to allogeneic blood transfusion. While a full setup of cell salvage costs on average $120,[50] the total cost of acquisition of 1 unit of PRBC from donor, storage, and delivery to the recipient is approximately $800.[51] Therefore, the most suitable cases for cell salvage are the cases with large blood loss, including cardiac surgeries, major vascular surgeries,[45–49,52,53] heart, lung, and liver transplant surgeries, and major orthopedic and spine surgeries.[41,53,54]

Like banked blood cells, cell salvage does not contain any clotting factors and platelets, thus reinfusion of large amounts of cell salvage should be accompanied by plasma and platelet transfusion to achieve a balanced transfusion ratio. Cases of coagulopathy have been reported in cases that used large volumes of cell salvage without the coadministration of plasma, cryoprecipitate, or platelets.[55,56]

In cases of malignancy or grossly contaminated surgical fields, infection and metastasis were traditionally considered contraindications for cell salvage, but there is now increasing evidence to support its use in these settings as well.[8] Studies have not identified the association between the use of cell saver and increased risk of metastasis during cancer surgery, and leukocyte depletion filters remove 99% of bacterial contamination in the blood.[8] However, small metal fragments will not be removed with any currently available filter, so cell salvage should be avoided in surgeries involving revision of metalwork.[8]

Acute normovolemic hemodilution

Acute normovolemic hemodilution (ANH) has primarily been studied in cardiac surgery. The goal of ANH is to remove whole blood from patients with subsequent hemodilution with colloid or crystalloid in effort to limit the red cell mass lost. This is particularly useful in procedures with large anticipated blood loss. After the procedure is complete and the risk of further blood loss is low, the removed whole blood is reinfused back to the patient. The preservation of coagulation factors in the removed whole blood is an added benefit to the goal of limiting allogenic exposure.

While ANH has been well studied in cardiac surgery, its utility in vascular surgery has not been studied as extensively. A subset of vascular patients that may benefit from ANH is open vascular surgical patients, due to the anticipated high-volume blood loss. Studies have shown that in abdominal aortic aneurysms, the use of ANH overall lessened rates of intraoperative and whole hospital transfusions, as well as contributed to higher platelet counts and evidence of less coagulopathy postoperatively.[26] Although the sample sizes of these studies are limited, they provide the framework for applying ANH to vascular surgery patients.

Antifibrinolytics: tranexamic acid and aminocaproic acid

The 2 main antifibrinolytic agents are synthetic lysine analogs, tranexamic acid (TXA), and epsilon aminocaproic acid. TXA has been widely established to reduce bleeding and transfusion requirements for multiple surgical fields ranging from cardiac, orthopedic, spine, abdominal, trauma, plastic, and obstetrics surgeries and even epistaxis and upper gastrointestinal bleeds, without increased complications in thrombotic adverse effects.[57–64] Seizure has been reported in cardiac surgery cases of high dose tranexamic acid administration in patients with chronic kidney disease.[65,66]

Primary literature specific to the use of TXA and aminocaproic acid in vascular surgery, however, is lacking. A study reported that both aminocaproic acid and tranexamic acids are equally effective in reducing perioperative blood loss and transfusion requirements in patients undergoing thoracic aortic surgery with different adverse effect profiles. Renal injury was observed with aminocaproic acid, and higher incidence of seizure was seen with TXA.[67] Another study with TXA reported no difference in intraoperative blood loss and transfusion in open abdominal aortic aneurysm repair, but it reduced postoperative bleeding without increasing complications.[68]

DDAVP/desmopressin

Desmopressin (DDAVP) is a synthetic analog of vasopressin, or antidiuretic hormone. It has been used to treat hemophilia A and von Willebrand disease by transiently increasing the plasma levels of factor VIII and von Willebrand factor. It can be given subcutaneously or intravenously at a dose of 0.3 μg/kg.[8] Rare but possible adverse effects of desmopressin are the risk of thrombosis, hyponatremia, seizures, and hypotension.[8] Guidelines recommend the administration of desmopressin to patients with platelet dysfunction secondary to medication, uremia, or cardiopulmonary bypass,[8,69–71] but the evidence for such recommendation is weak. Most evidence for 1-deamino-8-D-arginine vasopressin (DDAVP) was obtained from cardiac surgeries where DDAVP was administered after cardiopulmonary bypass, and the resulting reduction in blood loss and red cell transfusion was statistically significant, but small. No difference in blood transfusion was observed in other surgeries such as orthopedic, vascular, or hepatic surgeries.[72] Further examination of the evidence for desmopressin in patients with platelet dysfunction either due to antiplatelet agents or cardiopulmonary bypass showed that patients treated with DDAVP had less blood loss, required less transfusion, and had a lower risk of reoperation due to bleeding. Yet, the quality of evidence was again low to moderate due to the small sample size.[73]

Factor concentrates

Correction of coagulopathy is important to achieve hemostasis and limit transfusions. Coagulopathy can exist preoperatively due to home medications or pre-existing condition or can develop perioperatively for multiple reasons such as excessive RBC transfusions. The correction of coagulopathy has often been treated by infusion of plasma or cryoprecipitate, which has several disadvantages such as infectious risks associated with blood component transfusion, adverse transfusion reactions, and allergic transfusion reactions. In certain cases, factor concentrates may be a good alternative to plasma or cryoprecipitate due to these risks.

Prothrombin complex concentrates. Prothrombin complex concentrates are the concentrated, virus-inactivated, pooled extracts from donated human plasma after the removal of antithrombin and factor XI. PCCs have a final clotting factor concentration 25 times higher than that of one unit of plasma. There are either three-factor formulations with factors II, IX, and X or 4-factor formulations with factors II, VII, IX, and X. It is approved for urgent reversal of warfarin.[15,74] While both FFP and PCCs are used to rapidly reverse the anticoagulation effect of warfarin, the four-factor PCC containing factor VII has been shown in recent studies to be at least noninferior or superior to FFP in warfarin reversal.[75–79] In addition, PCCs have also been used for nonspecific reversal of direct oral anticoagulants (DOACs) in emergent situations with increased bleeding risk.[23]

Recombinant activated factor VII (NovoSeven or rFVIIa). For perioperative bleeding patients without hemophilia, the rFVIIa should be considered a last resort treatment of life-threatening bleeding that cannot be controlled by any other pharmacological, surgical or interventional radiological means. Due to the lack of mortality benefit, weak evidence for reducing blood loss and transfusion requirement, and evidence for increased risk of arterial thromboembolic events recombinant activated factor VII should be used cautiously.[15,80,81]

Fibrinogen concentrate. Fibrinogen is an important part of hemostasis, and fibrinogen deficiency can develop from consumptive or dilutional coagulopathy during massive transfusion. Hypofibrinogenemia is a risk factor for hemorrhage and often develops before any other markers of hematologic deficiencies manifest. Fibrinogen concentrate is currently only approved for the prevention and treatment of bleeding in the rare fibrinogen congenital deficiency, but it has been used in other, off-label circumstances and found to be effective in reducing perioperative bleeding and transfusion requirement in patients in acquired hypofibrinogenemia[82–84(p)]. Compared to FFP, fibrinogen concentrate was associated with better outcomes such as decreased blood loss, decreased transfusion requirement, shorter length of stay, and better survival in patients in perioperative or massive trauma setting.[85] The benefit of reduced blood transfusion has been demonstrated without an increase in thrombotic events or mortality,[86] and the same benefit has been demonstrated in major vascular surgery such as thoraco-abdominal aortic aneurysm repair.[87]

Point of care tests for blood management during vascular surgeries
Activated clotting time and anti-factor Xa assay. During cardiac and vascular surgeries, safe and adequate anticoagulation is crucial for cardiopulmonary bypass, vascular bypass, and patency of vascular grafts. Anticoagulation is most often achieved with unfractionated heparin and monitored real-time with a point-of-care test, activated clotting time (ACT), to avoid inadequate or overdose of heparin, to decrease bleeding or avoid thrombotic events.[88,89] Different technologies of ACT measurements have been used, contributing to inter-institutional variations in target ACTs and necessary heparin dose in cardiac and vascular surgeries. Anti-factor Xa assay has emerged as a possibly superior means to measure anticoagulation, with better association with periprocedural bleeding although it takes considerable time for results.[88–91]

Thromboelastography and rotational thromboelastometry. In the management of severe acute bleeding, the 2 most commonly used point-of-care viscoelastic hemostatic assays are thromboelastography (TEG) and rotational thromboelastometry (ROTEM) due to their fast results in a few minutes are crucial for providing real-time information for making timely clinical decisions in life-threatening hemorrhage situations.[8] In TEG and ROTEM, a rotating pin connected to an electrode measures the strength of a clot formed from patients' whole blood, and the physical properties of the clot are measured and converted to electrical signals to generate the different parameters of clot formation.[8] TEG and ROTEM have been useful in the management of bleeding in cardiac, liver, obstetric, and trauma surgeries.[8,92–95] Compared to transfusion strategies guided by other methods, TEG or ROTEM have been found to reduce overall mortality and decrease red cell, FFP, and platelet transfusions.[96] Most studies on TEG or ROTEM are in cardiac surgery patients. In vascular surgery, TEG or ROTEM has been used in small studies, but no robust data have provided clear evidence of the efficacy of TEG or ROTEM to affect specific outcomes. For instance, TEG has been used to uncover resistance to antiplatelet therapy after carotid artery stenting in some patients with cerebrovascular disease. It has been used to predict hypercoagulability and thromboembolic events among various patient populations. Finally, TEG can be used in perioperative settings to predict hemorrhage and transfusion requirements in major vascular surgeries.[97]

Platelet function monitoring. As many vascular surgery patients may require antiplatelet agents, specific monitoring of the platelet function can be helpful in not only managing perioperative bleeding but also in dosing antiplatelet agents to decrease thrombotic risk. The need for monitoring of platelet function is also driven by the variable responses individual patients have with P2Y12 receptor inhibitors.[98] The gold standard to measure platelet function is light transmission aggregometry (LTA).[98] However, LTA is time-consuming, laborious, and not standardized, so a number of point-of-care (POCTs) tests for platelet function have become available in recent years.[98] Not one platelet function test has been shown to be superior to another in a large meta-analysis, and the data on their generalizability and accuracy are limited.[99] In one study, when a platelet function point-of-care test is used in combination with TEG or ROTEM to guide transfusion, there was a greater reduction in red cell transfusion but increased transfusion of platelets.[99] Clinical correlation between bleeding or hematomas and the degree of platelet function inhibition measured on POCTs, has been observed in a study on carotid endarterectomy patients.[100]

Permissive hypotension. The ultimate goal of resuscitation is to restore adequate tissue oxygenation, and thus the normotensive resuscitation strategy is intuitive in targeting a normal systolic blood pressure above 100 mm Hg. However, return to normal blood pressure after hypoperfusion can reverse vasoconstriction, dislodge blood clots, and increase surgical bleeding. If a large volume of resuscitation is required to achieve normotension, concerns for coagulopathy arise. The strategy of permissive hypotension, or hypotensive resuscitation, therefore, targets a SBP lower than 100 mm Hg, with the goal of reducing bleeding in the surgical field and overall blood loss.[15]

Permissive hypotension is balanced with the goal of maintaining tissue perfusion and oxygenation, so it should be carefully considered in patients with coronary artery disease or cerebrovascular disease. Patient selection for permissive hypotension is important, and signs of organ hypoperfusion must be monitored when the strategy is selected.[101]

While permissive hypotension of varying ranges has been studied across different surgical specialties such as orthopedic, oral and maxillofacial, and trauma surgeries with varying results, and the reduction in blood loss has been found to be associated with the strategy, strong evidence is lacking and these studies did not evaluate harm.[101–103] Only orthopedic surgery studies have observed a reduction in blood transfusion with permissive hypotension strategy.[102] Survival benefit is observed in the permissive hypotension group in trauma surgery,[103] when the SBP ranges 50–70 mm Hg and mean arterial pressure (MAP) 50–65 mm Hg, compared to the normotensive group of SBP 70–100 mm Hg or MAP>65 mm Hg. In TEVAR and EVAR cases, however, hypotension in a such extreme range can be associated with higher risk of spinal cord ischemia and should be avoided.[104]

In studies examining ruptured abdominal aortic aneurysm repair (rAAA), there is endorsement of the practice of permissive hypotension by multiple guidelines, but no randomized controlled trial has been conducted to support the recommendations.[105] A small case series observed a survival benefit with permissive hypotension of SBP 50–70 mm Hg and restrictive fluid restriction.[106] In 2018, the society of vascular surgery guideline recommended restricting aggressive volume infusion and implementing permissive hypotension of SBP 70–90 mm Hg in patients with rAAA.[107] The best evidence to date to guide the range of permissive hypotension in rAAA perhaps is based on the observation data from the IMPROVE trial (EVAR versus open repair for rAAA): there is a 30-day mortality rate of 51% in hypotensive patients with

SBP<70 mm Hg versus 34.1% in patients with SBP>70 mm Hg.[108] These findings suggest that SBP lower than 70 mm Hg could be harmful in patients with rAAA.[108]

Restrictive fluid resuscitation

Restrictive versus liberal approach to fluid resuscitation has been studied in conjunction with permissive hypotension strategy in different clinical situations. While in elective surgeries, lower complication rates, lower infection rates, and lower transfusion rates are observed in the restrictive fluid management group, compared to the liberal group,[109] meta-analyses in trauma and abdominal aortic surgery settings did not show benefit with a restrictive fluid strategy.[110,111] A small cohort study with rAAA showed that the rate of fluid infusion correlated with increased 30-day mortality independent of blood pressure.[112] Despite lack of strong evidence, the revised Advanced Trauma Life Support (ATLS) guidelines recommend restricting the initial resuscitation volume to 1 L of crystalloid, after which blood products should be given.[113]

Avoidance of hypothermia

Hypothermia has been known to impair platelet function and coagulation cascade. Even mild intraoperative hypothermia at a core temperature of 35° Celsius is associated with 16% increased blood loss and 22% increased risk of transfusion.[114,115] In addition, hypothermia is also associated with higher risks of perioperative cardiac events,[116] increased rates of wound infection,[117] and prolonged postoperative recovery.[118] Therefore, avoidance of intraoperative hypothermia with forced air warmer, fluid warmer, and adjustment of room temperature should be employed. Consideration for mild hypothermia for protection against spinal cord injury during TEVAR or EVAR has been studied in small cohorts but still requires further evaluation.[104]

Postoperative management

Resumption of anticoagulant The timing of the postoperative resumption of anticoagulants is a significant factor influencing postoperative bleeding.[18] As in preoperative decisions on when to stop these agents, the timing to restart anticoagulants depends on the risk assessment of bleeding versus thrombotic events. The resumption of these agents will need to be evaluated on an individual basis, subject to surgeon's or proceduralist's approval[18]. Oftentimes, heparin is required postoperatively for vascular graft patency.

Like LMWH, DOACs reach peak effect in a few hours, while warfarin takes 5–10 days to reach full effect. Therefore, LMWH and DOACs generally should not be started until 24–72 hours postprocedure, while warfarin can be reinitiated as soon as patients can tolerate oral medication, within 12–24 hrs after procedure.[18]

The BRIDGE trial has demonstrated safety in waiting 24–72 hours postprocedure before starting full anticoagulation.[119] Patients at high bleeding risk are recommended to wait 72 hours before restarting LMWH bridging. Safety in restarting rivaroxaban 6–8 hrs postoperatively,[120] apixaban 12–24 hrs postoperatively,[121] and lower dose dabigatran 1–4 hrs postoperatively[122] after knee or hip replacement surgeries have been demonstrated in orthopedic trials to prevent deep vein thrombosis or pulmonary embolism. Other than these trial protocols, there is overall a lack of study of when and at what doses the DOACs should be resumed postprocedure for atrial fibrillation or venous thromboembolism indications[18].

Reducing phlebotomy blood loss One common and preventable contributing factor to anemia is unnecessary phlebotomy during hospital stay.[123] A study has used mathematical modeling to estimate that a critically ill patient with an initial hemoglobin level of 11 g/dL will reach a hemoglobin level of 7 g/dL within 9–14 days of subjected to a daily blood loss of about 43 mL to diagnostic phlebotomies.[124] Studies have demonstrated the effectiveness of conservative strategies for decreasing phlebotomy blood loss in intensive care unit patients, such as utilizing pediatric-sized blood collection tubes, returning dead space volumes from arterial line tubing, and use of arterial line blood conservation devices.[125–127]

CLINICS CARE POINTS

- Patients presenting for elective vascular surgery should be assessed for preoperative anemia and treated appropriately before surgery is scheduled.
- Techniques for reducing surgical bleeding such as acute normovolemic hemodilution, maintaining normothermia after aortic cross-clamp removal, use of anti-fibrinolytics should be used in vascular surgery cases.
- Viscoelastic tests, such as thromboelastography and rotational thromboelastometry, are key to diagnosis and appropriate treatment of coagulopathies associated with vascular surgery.

DISCLOSURES

Nadia B. Hensley MD is on the scientific advisory board for Octapharma, USA and receives author royalties for uptodate.com

REFERENCES

1. Sandip N, Emma S, Luke B, et al. The Interplay between preoperative anemia and postoperative blood transfusion on survival following fenestrated aortic aneurysm repair. Ann Vasc Surg 2021;70:491–500.
2. Behrendt CA, Debus ES, Schwaneberg T, et al. Predictors of bleeding or anemia requiring transfusion in complex endovascular aortic repair and its impact on outcomes in health insurance claims. J Vasc Surg 2020;71(2):382–9.
3. Obi AT, Park YJ, Bove P, et al. The association of perioperative transfusion with 30-day morbidity and mortality in patients undergoing major vascular surgery. J Vasc Surg 2015;61(4):1000–9.e1.
4. Goodnough LT, Shander A. Patient blood management. Anesthesiology 2012; 116(6):1367–76.
5. Shander A, Van Aken H, Colomina MJ, et al. Patient blood management in Europe. Br J Anaesth 2012;109(1):55–68.
6. Richards T, Baikady RR, Clevenger B, et al. Preoperative intravenous iron to treat anaemia before major abdominal surgery (PREVENTT): a randomised, double-blind, controlled trial. The Lancet 2020;396(10259):1353–61.
7. Weltert L, D'Alessandro S, Nardella S, et al. Preoperative very short-term, high-dose erythropoietin administration diminishes blood transfusion rate in off-pump coronary artery bypass: a randomized blind controlled study. J Thorac Cardiovasc Surg 2010;139(3):621–6 [discussion: 626-627].
8. Shah A, Palmer AJR, Klein AA. Strategies to minimize intraoperative blood loss during major surgery. Br J Surg 2020;107(2):e26–38.
9. Klein AA, Collier T, Yeates J, et al. The ACTA PORT-score for predicting perioperative risk of blood transfusion for adult cardiac surgery. Br J Anaesth 2017; 119(3):394–401.
10. Chassot PG, Marcucci C, Delabays A. Perioper Antiplatelet Ther 2010;82(12):6.

11. Lewis SR, Pritchard MW, Schofield-Robinson OJ, et al. Continuation versus discontinuation of antiplatelet therapy for bleeding and ischaemic events in adults undergoing non-cardiac surgery. Cochrane Database Syst Rev 2018; 2018(7):CD012584.

12. Columbo JA, Lambour AJ, Sundling RA, et al. A Meta-analysis of the impact of aspirin, clopidogrel, and dual antiplatelet therapy on bleeding complications in noncardiac surgery. Ann Surg 2018;267(1):1–10.

13. Luni FK, Riaz H, Khan AR, et al. Clinical outcomes associated with per-operative discontinuation of aspirin in patients with coronary artery disease: a systematic review and meta-analysis. Catheter Cardiovasc Interv 2017;89(7):1168–75.

14. Keeling D, Tait RC, Watson H. Haematology the BC of S for. Peri-operative management of anticoagulation and antiplatelet therapy. Br J Haematol 2016;175(4): 602–13.

15. Chee YE, Liu SE, Irwin MG. Management of bleeding in vascular surgery. Br J Anaesth 2016;117:ii85–94.

16. Ansell J, Hirsh J, Hylek E, et al. Pharmacology and management of the vitamin K antagonists: American College of Chest Physicians Evidence-Based Clinical Practice Guidelines (8th Edition). Chest 2008;133(6 Suppl):160S–98S.

17. Doherty JU, Gluckman TJ, Hucker WJ, et al. 2017 ACC expert consensus decision pathway for periprocedural management of anticoagulation in patients with nonvalvular atrial fibrillation. J Am Coll Cardiol 2017;69(7):871–98.

18. Barnes GD, Mouland E. Peri-procedural management of oral anticoagulants in the DOAC Era. Prog Cardiovasc Dis 2018;60(6):600–6.

19. Douketis JD, Spyropoulos AC, Spencer FA, et al. Perioperative management of antithrombotic therapy. Chest 2012;141(2):e326S–50S.

20. Van Veen JJ. Management of peri-operative anti-thrombotic therapy. doi:10.1111/anae.12900

21. Heidbuchel H, Verhamme P, Alings M, et al. Updated European Heart Rhythm Association Practical Guide on the use of non-vitamin K antagonist anticoagulants in patients with non-valvular atrial fibrillation. Europace 2015;17(10): 1467–507.

22. Douketis JD, Healey JS, Brueckmann M, et al. Perioperative bridging anticoagulation during dabigatran or warfarin interruption among patients who had an elective surgery or procedure. Substudy of the RE-LY trial. Thromb Haemost 2015;113(3):625–32.

23. Cuker A, Burnett A, Triller D, et al. Reversal of direct oral anticoagulants: guidance from the Anticoagulation Forum. Am J Hematol 2019;94(6):697–709.

24. Forgie MA, Wells PS, Laupacis A, et al. For the international study of perioperative transfusion (ISPOT) Investigators. preoperative autologous donation decreases allogeneic transfusion but increases exposure to all red blood cell transfusion: results of a meta-analysis. Arch Intern Med 1998;158(6):610–6.

25. Carson JL, Stanworth SJ, Dennis JA, et al. Transfusion thresholds for guiding red blood cell transfusion. Cochrane Database Syst Rev 2021;12:CD002042.

26. Carson JL, Stanworth SJ, Alexander JH, et al. Clinical trials evaluating red blood cell transfusion thresholds: An updated systematic review and with additional focus on patients with cardiovascular disease. Am Heart J 2018;200:96–101.

27. Hovaguimian F, Myles PS. Restrictive versus liberal transfusion strategy in the perioperative and acute care settings: a context-specific systematic review and meta-analysis of randomized controlled trials. Anesthesiology 2016; 125(1):46–61.

28. Docherty AB, O'Donnell R, Brunskill S, et al. Effect of restrictive versus liberal transfusion strategies on outcomes in patients with cardiovascular disease in a non-cardiac surgery setting: systematic review and meta-analysis. BMJ 2016;352:i1351.

29. Ripollés Melchor J, Casans Francés R, Espinosa Á, et al. Restrictive versus liberal transfusion strategy for red blood cell transfusion in critically ill patients and in patients with acute coronary syndrome: a systematic review, meta-analysis and trial sequential analysis. Minerva Anestesiol 2016;82(5):582–98.

30. Dakour-Aridi H, Giuliano K, Locham S, et al. Perioperative blood transfusion in anemic patients undergoing elective endovascular abdominal aneurysm repair. J Vasc Surg 2020;71(1):75–85.

31. Friedman BA. An analysis of surgical blood use in United States hospitals with application to the maximum surgical blood order schedule. Transfusion 1979; 19:268–78.

32. Frank SM, Rothschild JA, Masear CG, et al. Optimizing preoperative blood ordering with data acquired from an anesthesia information management system. Anesthesiology 2013;118(6):1286–97.

33. Xiang Y, Chen X, Zhao J, et al. Endovascular treatment versus open surgery for isolated iliac artery aneurysms: a systematic review and meta-analysis. Vasc Endovascular Surg 2019;53(5):401–7.

34. Liu J, Xia J, Yan G, et al. Thoracic endovascular aortic repair versus open chest surgical repair for patients with type B aortic dissection: a systematic review and meta-analysis. Ann Med 2019;51(7–8):360–70.

35. Choi K, Han Y, Ko GY, et al. Early and late outcomes of endovascular aortic aneurysm repair versus open surgical repair of an abdominal aortic aneurysm: a single-center study. Ann Vasc Surg 2018;51:187–91.

36. Kakkos SK, Papazoglou KO, Tsolakis IA, et al. Open versus endovascular repair of inflammatory abdominal aortic aneurysms: a comparative study and meta-analysis of the literature. Vasc Endovascular Surg 2015;49(5–6):110–8.

37. Shiraev TP, Qasabian R, Tardo D, et al. Open versus endovascular repair of arch and descending thoracic aneurysms: a retrospective comparison. Ann Vasc Surg 2016;31:30–8.

38. Meybohm P, Choorapoikayil S, Wessels A, et al. Washed cell salvage in surgical patients: a review and meta-analysis of prospective randomized trials under PRISMA. Medicine (Baltimore) 2016;95(31):e4490.

39. Waters JH. Cell salvage in trauma. Curr Opin Anaesthesiol 2021;34(4):503–6.

40. Highmore W. Practical remarks on an overlooked source of blood-supply for transfusion in post-partum hæmorrhage, suggested by a recent fatal case. Lancet 1874;103(2629):89–90.

41. Frank SM, Sikorski RA, Konig G, et al. Clinical utility of autologous salvaged blood: a review. J Gastrointest Surg 2020;24(2):464–72.

42. Scott AV, Nagababu E, Johnson DJ, et al. 2,3-diphosphoglycerate concentrations in autologous salvaged versus stored red blood cells and in surgical patients after transfusion. Anesth Analg 2016;122(3):616–23.

43. Frank SM, Abazyan B, Ono M, et al. Decreased erythrocyte deformability after transfusion and the effects of erythrocyte storage duration. Anesth Analg 2013;116(5):975–81.

44. Salaria ON, Barodka VM, Hogue CW, et al. Impaired red blood cell deformability after transfusion of stored allogeneic blood but not autologous salvaged blood in cardiac surgery patients. Anesth Analg 2014;118(6):1179–87.

45. Clagett GP, Valentine RJ, Jackson MR, et al. A randomized trial of intraoperative autotransfusion during aortic surgery. J Vasc Surg 1999;29(1):22–30 [discussion: 30-31].
46. Mercer KG, Spark JI, Berridge DC, et al. Randomized clinical trial of intraoperative autotransfusion in surgery for abdominal aortic aneurysm. Br J Surg 2004; 91(11):1443–8.
47. Spark JI, Chetter IC, Kester RC, et al. Allogeneic versus autologous blood during abdominal aortic aneurysm surgery. Eur J Vasc Endovasc Surg 1997;14(6): 482–6.
48. Thompson JF, Webster JH, Chant AD. Prospective randomised evaluation of a new cell saving device in elective aortic reconstruction. Eur J Vasc Surg 1990;4(5):507–12.
49. Kelley-Patteson C, Ammar AD, Kelley H. Should the cell saver autotransfusion device be used routinely in all infrarenal abdominal aortic bypass operations? J Vasc Surg 1993;18(2):261–5.
50. Frank SM. Who benefits from red blood cell salvage?–Utility and value of intraoperative autologous transfusion. Transfusion 2011;51(10):2058–60.
51. Shander A, Hofmann A, Ozawa S, et al. Activity-based costs of blood transfusions in surgical patients at four hospitals. Transfusion 2010;50(4):753–65.
52. Farrer A, Spark JI, Scott DJ. Autologous blood transfusion: the benefits to the patient undergoing abdominal aortic aneurysm repair. J Vasc Nurs 1997; 15(4):111–5.
53. Takagi H, Sekino S, Kato T, et al. Intraoperative autotransfusion in abdominal aortic aneurysm surgery: meta-analysis of randomized controlled trials. Arch Surg 2007;142(11):1098–101.
54. Waters JH, Dyga RM, Waters JFR, et al. The volume of returned red blood cells in a large blood salvage program: where does it all go? Transfusion 2011;51(10): 2126–32.
55. Rollins KE, Trim NL, Luddington RJ, et al. Coagulopathy associated with massive cell salvage transfusion following aortic surgery. Perfusion 2012; 27(1):30–3.
56. Rudra P, Basak S. Coagulopathy during intraoperative cell salvage in a patient with major obstetric haemorrhage. Br J Anaesth 2011;106(2):280–1.
57. Heyns M, Knight P, Steve AK, et al. A single preoperative dose of tranexamic acid reduces perioperative blood loss: a meta-analysis. Ann Surg 2021; 273(1):75–81.
58. Hui S, Xu D, Ren Z, et al. Can tranexamic acid conserve blood and save operative time in spinal surgeries? A meta-analysis. Spine J 2018;18(8):1325–37.
59. Koh A, Adiamah A, Gomez D, et al. P107 safety and efficacy of tranexamic acid to minimise perioperative bleeding in extrahepatic abdominal surgery: a systematic review and meta-analysis. BJS Open 2021;5(Suppl 1). zrab032.106.
60. Sun L, An H, Feng Y. Intravenous tranexamic acid decreases blood transfusion in off-pump coronary artery bypass surgery: a meta-analysis. Heart Surg Forum 2020;23(1):E039–49.
61. Adler Ma SC, Brindle W, Burton G, et al. Tranexamic acid is associated with less blood transfusion in off-pump coronary artery bypass graft surgery: a systematic review and meta-analysis. J Cardiothorac Vasc Anesth 2011;25(1):26–35.
62. Dai Z, Chu H, Wang S, et al. The effect of tranexamic acid to reduce blood loss and transfusion on off-pump coronary artery bypass surgery: A systematic review and cumulative meta-analysis. J Clin Anesth 2018;44:23–31.

63. Wong J, George RB, Hanley CM, et al. Tranexamic acid: current use in obstetrics, major orthopedic, and trauma surgery. Can J Anaesth 2021;68(6):894–917.

64. Lee PL, Yang KS, Tsai HW, et al. Tranexamic acid for gastrointestinal bleeding: a systematic review with meta-analysis of randomized clinical trials. Am J Emerg Med 2021;45:269–79.

65. Taam J, Yang QJ, Pang KS, et al. Current evidence and future directions of tranexamic acid use, efficacy, and dosing for major surgical procedures. J Cardiothorac Vasc Anesth 2020;34(3):782–90.

66. Zhang Y, Bai Y, Chen M, et al. The safety and efficiency of intravenous administration of tranexamic acid in coronary artery bypass grafting (CABG): a meta-analysis of 28 randomized controlled trials. BMC Anesthesiol 2019;19:104.

67. Makhija N, Sarupria A, Kumar Choudhary S, et al. Comparison of epsilon aminocaproic acid and tranexamic Acid in thoracic aortic surgery: clinical efficacy and safety. J Cardiothorac Vasc Anesth 2013;27(6):1201–7.

68. Monaco F, Nardelli P, Pasin L, et al. Tranexamic acid in open aortic aneurysm surgery: a randomised clinical trial. Br J Anaesth 2020;124(1):35–43.

69. Spahn DR, Bouillon B, Cerny V, et al. The European guideline on management of major bleeding and coagulopathy following trauma: fifth edition. Crit Care 2019; 23(1):98.

70. American Society of Anesthesiologists Task Force on Perioperative Blood Management. Practice guidelines for perioperative blood management: an updated report by the American Society of Anesthesiologists Task Force on Perioperative Blood Management*. Anesthesiology 2015;122(2):241–75.

71. Kozek-Langenecker SA, Afshari A, Albaladejo P, et al. Management of severe perioperative bleeding: guidelines from the European Society of Anaesthesiology. Eur J Anaesthesiol 2013;30(6):270–382.

72. Desborough MJ, Oakland K, Brierley C, et al. Desmopressin use for minimising perioperative blood transfusion. Cochrane Database Syst Rev 2017;7: CD001884.

73. Desborough MJR, Oakland KA, Landoni G, et al. Desmopressin for treatment of platelet dysfunction and reversal of antiplatelet agents: a systematic review and meta-analysis of randomized controlled trials. J Thromb Haemost 2017;15(2): 263–72.

74. Grottke O, Levy JH. Prothrombin complex concentrates in trauma and perioperative bleeding. Anesthesiology 2015;122(4):923–31.

75. Chai-Adisaksopha C, Hillis C, Siegal DM, et al. Prothrombin complex concentrates versus fresh frozen plasma for warfarin reversal. A systematic review and meta-analysis. Thromb Haemost 2016;116(5):879–90.

76. Faulkner H, Chakankar S, Mammi M, et al. Safety and efficacy of prothrombin complex concentrate (PCC) for anticoagulation reversal in patients undergoing urgent neurosurgical procedures: a systematic review and metaanalysis. Neurosurg Rev 2021;44(4):1921–31.

77. Johansen M, Wikkelsø A, Lunde J, et al. Prothrombin complex concentrate for reversal of vitamin K antagonist treatment in bleeding and non-bleeding patients. Cochrane Database Syst Rev 2015;7:CD010555.

78. Holland L, Warkentin TE, Refaai M, et al. Suboptimal effect of a three-factor prothrombin complex concentrate (Profilnine-SD) in correcting supratherapeutic international normalized ratio due to warfarin overdose. Transfusion 2009;49(6): 1171–7.

79. Leissinger CA, Blatt PM, Hoots WK, et al. Role of prothrombin complex concentrates in reversing warfarin anticoagulation: a review of the literature. Am J Hematol 2008;83(2):137–43.

80. Simpson E, Lin Y, Stanworth S, et al. Recombinant factor VIIa for the prevention and treatment of bleeding in patients without haemophilia. Cochrane Database Syst Rev 2012;3:CD005011.

81. Chang Z, Chu X, Liu Y, et al. Use of recombinant activated factor VII for the treatment of perioperative bleeding in noncardiac surgery patients without hemophilia: a systematic review and meta-analysis of randomized controlled trials. J Crit Care 2021;62:164–71.

82. Fenger-Eriksen C, Jensen TM, Kristensen BS, et al. Fibrinogen substitution improves whole blood clot firmness after dilution with hydroxyethyl starch in bleeding patients undergoing radical cystectomy: a randomized, placebo-controlled clinical trial. J Thromb Haemost 2009;7(5):795–802.

83. Karlsson M, Ternström L, Hyllner M, et al. Prophylactic fibrinogen infusion reduces bleeding after coronary artery bypass surgery. A prospective randomised pilot study. Thromb Haemost 2009;102(1):137–44.

84. Rahe-Meyer N, Solomon C, Winterhalter M, et al. Thromboelastometry-guided administration of fibrinogen concentrate for the treatment of excessive intraoperative bleeding in thoracoabdominal aortic aneurysm surgery. J Thorac Cardiovasc Surg 2009;138(3):694–702.

85. Kozek-Langenecker S, Sørensen B, Hess JR, et al. Clinical effectiveness of fresh frozen plasma compared with fibrinogen concentrate: a systematic review. Crit Care 2011;15(5):R239.

86. Wikkelsø A, Lunde J, Johansen M, et al. Fibrinogen concentrate in bleeding patients. Cochrane Database Syst Rev 2013;8:CD008864.

87. Morrison GA, Koch J, Royds M, et al. Fibrinogen concentrate vs. fresh frozen plasma for the management of coagulopathy during thoraco-abdominal aortic aneurysm surgery: a pilot randomised controlled trial. Anaesthesia 2019;74(2):180–9.

88. Maslow A, Chambers A, Cheves T, et al. Assessment of heparin anticoagulation measured using i-STAT and hemochron activated clotting time. J Cardiothorac Vasc Anesth 2018;32(4):1603–8.

89. Falter F, MacDonald S, Matthews C, et al. Evaluation of Point-of-Care ACT Coagulometers and Anti-Xa Activity During Cardiopulmonary Bypass. J Cardiothorac Vasc Anesth 2020;34(11):2921–7.

90. Lequier L, Massicotte MP. Monitoring of anticoagulation in extracorporeal membrane oxygenation: is anti-Xa the new activated clotting time? Pediatr Crit Care Med 2015;16(1):87–9.

91. Dieplinger B, Egger M, Luft C, et al. Comparison between activated clotting time and anti-activated factor X activity for the monitoring of unfractionated heparin therapy in patients with aortic aneurysm undergoing an endovascular procedure. J Vasc Surg 2018;68(2):400–7.

92. Curry NS, Davenport R, Pavord S, et al. The use of viscoelastic haemostatic assays in the management of major bleeding: a British Society for Haematology Guideline. Br J Haematol 2018;182(6):789–806.

93. Collins PW, Cannings-John R, Bruynseels D, et al. Viscoelastometric-guided early fibrinogen concentrate replacement during postpartum haemorrhage: OBS2, a double-blind randomized controlled trial. Br J Anaesth 2017;119(3):411–21.

94. McNamara H, Kenyon C, Smith R, et al. Four years' experience of a ROTEM® -guided algorithm for treatment of coagulopathy in obstetric haemorrhage. Anaesthesia 2019;74(8):984–91.

95. Whiting P, Al M, Westwood M, et al. Viscoelastic point-of-care testing to assist with the diagnosis, management and monitoring of haemostasis: a systematic review and cost-effectiveness analysis. Health Technol Assess 2015;19(58): 1–228, v–vi.

96. Wikkelsø A, Wetterslev J, Møller AM, et al. Thromboelastography (TEG) or thromboelastometry (ROTEM) to monitor haemostatic treatment versus usual care in adults or children with bleeding. Cochrane Database Syst Rev 2016;8: CD007871.

97. Kim Y, Patel SS, McElroy IE, et al. A systematic review of thromboelastography utilization in vascular and endovascular surgery. J Vasc Surg 2022;75(3): 1107–15.

98. Bolliger D, Lancé MD, Siegemund M. Point-of-care platelet function monitoring: implications for patients with platelet inhibitors in cardiac surgery. J Cardiothorac Vasc Anesth 2021;35(4):1049–59.

99. Corredor C, Wasowicz M, Karkouti K, et al. The role of point-of-care platelet function testing in predicting postoperative bleeding following cardiac surgery: a systematic review and meta-analysis. Anaesthesia 2015;70(6):715–31.

100. Moon K, Nanaszko M, Levitt MR, et al. Carotid endarterectomy on antiplatelet agents in the era of point-of-care testing. World Neurosurg 2016;93:215–20.

101. Choi WS, Samman N. Risks and benefits of deliberate hypotension in anaesthesia: a systematic review. Int J Oral Maxillofac Surg 2008;37(8):687–703.

102. Paul JE, Ling E, Lalonde C, et al. Deliberate hypotension in orthopedic surgery reduces blood loss and transfusion requirements: a meta-analysis of randomized controlled trials. Can J Anaesth 2007;54(10):799–810.

103. Tran A, Yates J, Lau A, et al. Permissive hypotension versus conventional resuscitation strategies in adult trauma patients with hemorrhagic shock: A systematic review and meta-analysis of randomized controlled trials. J Trauma Acute Care Surg 2018;84(5):802–8.

104. Dijkstra ML, Vainas T, Zeebregts CJ, et al. Editor's choice - spinal cord ischaemia in endovascular thoracic and thoraco-abdominal aortic repair: review of preventive strategies. Eur J Vasc Endovasc Surg 2018;55(6):829–41.

105. Moreno DH, Cacione DG, Baptista-Silva JC. Controlled hypotension versus normotensive resuscitation strategy for people with ruptured abdominal aortic aneurysm. Cochrane Database Syst Rev 2018;6:CD011664.

106. Crawford ES. Ruptured abdominal aortic aneurysm. J Vasc Surg 1991;13(2): 348–50.

107. Chaikof EL, Dalman RL, Eskandari MK, et al. The Society for Vascular Surgery practice guidelines on the care of patients with an abdominal aortic aneurysm. J Vasc Surg 2018;67(1):2–77.e2.

108. IMPROVE Trial Investigators, Powell JT, Hinchliffe RJ, et al. Observations from the IMPROVE trial concerning the clinical care of patients with ruptured abdominal aortic aneurysm. Br J Surg 2014;101(3):216–24 [discussion: 224].

109. Schol PBB, Terink IM, Lancé MD, et al. Liberal or restrictive fluid management during elective surgery: a systematic review and meta-analysis. J Clin Anesth 2016;35:26–39.

110. Wang CH, Hsieh WH, Chou HC, et al. Liberal versus restricted fluid resuscitation strategies in trauma patients: a systematic review and meta-analysis of

randomized controlled trials and observational studies*. Crit Care Med 2014; 42(4):954–61.

111. Toomtong P, Suksompong S. Intravenous fluids for abdominal aortic surgery. Cochrane Database Syst Rev 2010;1:CD000991.

112. Dick F, Erdoes G, Opfermann P, et al. Delayed volume resuscitation during initial management of ruptured abdominal aortic aneurysm. J Vasc Surg 2013;57(4): 943–50.

113. ATLS Subcommittee, American College of Surgeons' Committee on Trauma, International ATLS working group. Advanced trauma life support (ATLS®): the ninth edition. J Trauma Acute Care Surg 2013;74(5):1363–6.

114. Rajagopalan S, Mascha E, Na J, et al. The effects of mild perioperative hypothermia on blood loss and transfusion requirement. Anesthesiology 2008; 108(1):71–7.

115. Reynolds L, Beckmann J, Kurz A. Perioperative complications of hypothermia. Best Pract Res Clin Anaesthesiol 2008;22(4):645–57.

116. Frank SM, Fleisher LA, Breslow MJ, et al. Perioperative maintenance of normothermia reduces the incidence of morbid cardiac events. A randomized clinical trial. JAMA 1997;277(14):1127–34.

117. Kurz A, Sessler DI, Lenhardt R. Perioperative normothermia to reduce the incidence of surgical-wound infection and shorten hospitalization. Study of Wound Infection and Temperature Group. N Engl J Med 1996;334(19):1209–15.

118. Lenhardt R, Marker E, Goll V, et al. Mild intraoperative hypothermia prolongs postanesthetic recovery. Anesthesiology 1997;87(6):1318–23.

119. Douketis JD, Spyropoulos AC, Kaatz S, et al. Perioperative bridging anticoagulation in patients with atrial fibrillation. N Engl J Med 2015;373(9):823–33.

120. Eriksson BI, Borris LC, Friedman RJ, et al. Rivaroxaban versus enoxaparin for thromboprophylaxis after hip arthroplasty. N Engl J Med 2008;358(26):2765–75.

121. Lassen MR, Raskob GE, Gallus A, et al. Apixaban or enoxaparin for thromboprophylaxis after knee replacement. N Engl J Med 2009;361(6):594 604.

122. Eriksson BI, Dahl OE, Rosencher N, et al. Dabigatran etexilate versus enoxaparin for prevention of venous thromboembolism after total hip replacement: a randomised, double-blind, non-inferiority trial. Lancet 2007;370(9591):949–56.

123. Shander A, Javidroozi M. Blood conservation strategies and the management of perioperative anaemia. Curr Opin Anaesthesiol 2015;28(3):356–63.

124. Lyon AW, Chin AC, Slotsve GA, et al. Simulation of repetitive diagnostic blood loss and onset of iatrogenic anemia in critical care patients with a mathematical model. Comput Biol Med 2013;43(2):84–90.

125. Harber CR, Sosnowski KJ, Hegde RM. Highly conservative phlebotomy in adult intensive care–a prospective randomized controlled trial. Anaesth Intensive Care 2006;34(4):434–7.

126. Siegal DM, Manning N, Jackson Chornenki NL, et al. Devices to reduce the volume of blood taken for laboratory testing in ICU patients: a systematic review. J Intensive Care Med 2020;35(10):1074–9.

127. MacIsaac CM, Presneill JJ, Boyce CA, et al. The influence of a blood conserving device on anaemia in intensive care patients. Anaesth Intensive Care 2003; 31(6):653–7.

Surgical Decision-Making and Outcomes in Open Versus Endovascular Repair for Various Vascular Diseases

Alana Keegan, MD[a], Caitlin W. Hicks, MD, MS[b],*

KEYWORDS

- Abdominal aorta • Carotid artery disease • CERAB • EVAR • TCAR • TEVAR
- Thoracic aorta • Peripheral arterial disease

KEY POINTS

- There has been a significant shift toward the use of endovascular therapy for the management of vascular disease over the past 30 years; however, open surgery remains a critical part of the vascular surgeon's armamentarium.
- Brief overview of the surgical and endovascular approaches for management of carotid occlusive disease, thoracic aortic dissection and aneurysm, abdominal aortic aneurysm, and suprainguinal and infrainguinal peripheral arterial disease.
- Patient-centered perioperative considerations when considering open versus endovascular therapy for the aforementioned disease processes.

INTRODUCTION
Disease History and Epidemiology

Over the past century, people have been fascinated with the ability to visualize the vascular anatomy. However, it was not until the 1960s that Dr Charles Dotter was able to transition these diagnostic imaging techniques into therapeutic capabilities. The first percutaneous transluminal angioplasty of a femoral artery was performed in 1964,[1] followed by the first endovascular aortic repair (EVAR) by Dr Juan Parodi in Buenos Aires approximately 30 years later. Today, approximately 80% of abdominal aortic aneurysms (AAAs) are treated endovascularly.[2] As endovascular therapy continues to advance, an increasingly large proportion of the current vascular surgeon's practice is dedicated to endovascular treatment. However, it is important to acknowledge that open surgical techniques will continue to be necessary for many patients for

[a] General Surgery, Sinai Hospital of Baltimore, 2435 West Belvedere Avenue, Suite 42, Baltimore, MD 21215, USA; [b] Division of Vascular Surgery and Endovascular Therapy, Johns Hopkins School of Medicine, 600 North Wolfe Street, Halsted 668, Baltimore, MD 21287, USA
* Corresponding author.
E-mail address: chicks11@jhmi.edu

Anesthesiology Clin 40 (2022) 627–644
https://doi.org/10.1016/j.anclin.2022.08.008
1932-2275/22/© 2022 Elsevier Inc. All rights reserved.

anesthesiology.theclinics.com

a wide variety of reasons and to understand the decision-making that goes into selecting an endovascular versus open repair approach.

The Nature of the Problem

With so many treatment options and modalities available to treat patients with vascular disease processes, how is it that vascular surgeons should decide which approach to use? It is important to weigh the pros and cons of endovascular and open techniques when evaluating each patient and to consider the disease process and surgical management they require. Although endovascular intervention has become widely used due to lower rates of periprocedural complications compared with open surgery, there are many circumstances in which an open procedure may be more beneficial.

Overall Considerations

There are certain patient-centered characteristics that should be considered when deciding whether to perform an endovascular or open procedure, regardless of the disease process that is being treated. The patient's age, frailty, functional status, cardiopulmonary status, and any uncontrolled comorbidities, such as diabetes and hypertension, must be taken into account. Endovascular interventions are typically less physiologically stressful than open operations so may be preferred in patients with more comorbidities, worse frailty, or poor functional status. In contrast, open operations have better longevity than endovascular interventions in many instances, so younger, fitter patients may benefit from a more physiologically stressful operation up front in order to maximize long-term gains.

The availability of a suitable vascular access site is also a critical consideration for any patient being considered for endovascular intervention. The vessel being accessed must have an adequate access point without prohibitive calcification and must have adequate diameter for the planned sheath; this is particularly relevant to women, who tend to have smaller diameter vessels that may not be of adequate caliber to accommodate a large-bore sheath. Access adequacy should be evaluated before any operative decision-making by using appropriate preoperative imaging.

DISCUSSION
Carotid Disease

Disease process and diagnosis

According to the US Centers for Disease Control and Prevention, there are approximately 800, 000 cerebrovascular accidents per year making stroke a leading cause of death and disability in patients older than 65 years.[3,4] Of these cerebrovascular events, 20% can be attributed to large vessel atherosclerotic disease, primarily of the carotid arteries.[3–6] Carotid artery stenosis can be recognized due to symptomatic presentation, or may be asymptomatic and found incidentally on imaging, or as a result of a carotid bruit on physical examination. In patients presenting with neurologic symptoms including stroke, transient ischemic attack, or amaurosis fugax, evaluation for carotid artery stenosis is indicated. Carotid duplex ultrasound is the imaging study of choice for carotid disease and can provide critical information regarding patient anatomy and flow velocity that corresponds to degree of stenosis and plaque characteristics. Duplex ultrasound, however, is limited in its ability to fully characterize calcified plaques and is unable to provide any information regarding intracranial carotid pathology, in which case computed tomographic angiography (CTA) (ideally) or magnetic resonance angiography is helpful. Digital subtraction angiography is reserved for cases in which the aforementioned studies are inconclusive, as it is an invasive imaging modality that is associated with a small risk of stroke.[5]

A brief overview of surgical approaches

Carotid endarterectomy. Carotid endarterectomy (CEA) is a procedure that directly removes the atherosclerotic plaque causing stenosis from the vessel lumen through an arteriotomy. CEA is the gold standard for management of both symptomatic and asymptomatic carotid occlusive disease. A brief summary of the procedure is as follows:

- The carotid sheath is accessed by a longitudinal incision along the medial border of the sternocleidomastoid.
- The distal common carotid artery, its bifurcation, and the internal and external carotid arteries are isolated, and control of the vessels is obtained proximal and distal to the area of disease.
- The surgeon must then decide whether to shunt blood flow around the area of stenosis to maintain cerebral perfusion through the internal carotid artery (ICA). Some surgeons practice routine shunting, others practice selective shunting, and others practice no shunting; there have been no data to support one approach over another, but consistent practice of one approach is typically favored.
- There are multiple techniques for plaque extraction. The two most described in the literature are the conventional endarterectomy and eversion endarterectomy techniques. In the conventional endarterectomy technique, a longitudinal arteriotomy is made extending from the distal common carotid artery onto the ICA, through which the plaque is elevated and removed. The arteriotomy is then closed with a patch to prevent restenosis. In the eversion endarterectomy technique, the ICA is transected at its origin from the common carotid artery, and the vessel is everted to expel the plaque.[5]

The North American Symptomatic Carotid Endarterectomy Trial (NASCET) was a landmark trial published in 1991 in which medical management alone was compared with medical management plus CEA in patients with symptomatic moderate (30%–69%) and severe (70%–99%) carotid artery stenosis. Patients with severe stenosis were found to have a 17% risk reduction in the incidence of ipsilateral stroke over a 2-year period following CEA compared with medical management alone; and those with moderate stenosis had a 6.5% risk reduction over a 5-year period compared with medical management alone.[5,7] The European Carotid Surgery Trial (ECST) revealed similar results favoring CEA for symptomatic patients over medical management alone (13.5% risk reduction over 3 years among patients with severe stenosis).[8] The Asymptomatic Carotid Atherosclerosis Study (ACAS) was a randomized controlled trial published in 1995 that evaluated the benefit of medical management alone compared with medical management plus CEA in patients with asymptomatic carotid artery stenosis between 60% and 99%. Patients undergoing CEA had a 5.9% risk reduction for ipsilateral stroke compared with medical management alone over a 5-year period, supporting the use of CEA in patients with asymptomatic carotid stenosis greater than 60%.[9] There is substantial debate about the contemporary relevance of the ACAS results because the trial was performed before the widespread use of statin therapy, but current professional guidelines still support the use of carotid revascularization for asymptomatic disease.[10]

Carotid artery stenting. There have been many advancements over the past four decades regarding endovascular alternatives for carotid occlusive disease management. In contrast to the carotid endarterectomy, carotid artery stenting (CAS) has been developed as a minimally invasive (endovascular) alternative for treatment of both symptomatic and asymptomatic carotid stenosis.[4,11] Carotid artery stenting was originally described via a percutaneous transfemoral approach (ie, TF-CAS) and was designed as a less invasive approach to carotid revascularization than CEA. The TF-CAS procedure is briefly performed as follows:

- The femoral artery is accessed using a sheath and then wires and catheters are advanced up through the aorta and aortic arch to select the common carotid artery on the affected side.
- Once carotid access is obtained, an embolic protection device is passed distal to the ICA lesion to protect the patient from any microemboli that may be produced during the procedure. Alternatives to the distal ICA filter include a distal ICA occlusive balloon or flow reversal using balloon occlusion of the common carotid artery inflow and the external carotid artery.
- Depending on the lesion characteristics, a balloon angioplasty is performed to allow for stent placement across the lesion. The stent is deployed across the lesion through the same sheath and may require postdeployment balloon angioplasty if the stenosis remains greater than 30%.

Early studies of TF-CAS in patients at high risk for CEA found that the intervention was limited by the high risk of plaque embolization to the brain. With the advent of embolic protection devices, as described earlier, the Stenting and Angioplasty with Protection in Patients at High Risk for Endarterectomy (SAPPHIRE) trial showed that TF-CAS was not inferior to CEA in the management of patients at high risk for CEA.[12] Subsequently, the Carotid Revascularization Endarterectomy versus Stenting Trial (CREST) found that a primary outcome of composite ipsilateral stroke, myocardial infarction, and death did not differ between patients with both symptomatic and asymptomatic carotid artery stenosis who underwent TF-CAS when compared with CEA; however, the risk of perioperative stroke was found to be higher in the TF-CAS group, whereas the risk of myocardial infarction was found to be lower.[11] The results from CREST also suggested that older patients (>70 years of age) had a significantly higher risk of stroke with TF-CAS compared with their younger counterparts. Currently, TF-CAS is only for carotid revascularization in patients who are considered high-risk for CEA,[13] which includes patients with the following:

- Class III or IV congestive heart failure
- Left ventricular ejection fraction less than 30%
- Recent myocardial infarction or unstable angina
- Contralateral carotid artery occlusion
- Recurrent stenosis following endarterectomy
- Previous neck surgery or radiation therapy to the head and neck
- Other conditions that were used to determine patients at high risk for CEA in carotid artery stenting trials such as the SAPPHIRE trial[12]

Transcarotid artery revascularization. Given the elevated risk of stroke with TF-CAS compared with CEA, transcarotid artery revascularization (TCAR) was developed as an alternative minimally invasive hybrid procedure in which flow in the carotid artery is reversed before stenting in order to protect against distal embolization of debris. Unlike TF-CAS, TCAR avoids manipulation of wires and catheters in the aortic arch, thereby theoretically reducing the risk of perioperative stroke. However, patients undergoing TCAR have to meet several other anatomic criteria (eg, appropriate length of common carotid artery to bifurcation, no common carotid artery disease, noncircumferential lesion calcification) in order to be eligible for the procedure. A brief summary of the steps of TCAR is as follows:

- A small incision is made at the base of the neck through which the common carotid artery is exposed.
- The exposed common carotid artery as well as the femoral vein are canalized and connected via an external filter–containing circuit to facilitate cerebral flow reversal.
- The common carotid artery is clamped proximal to the sheath, and flow reversal is initiated.
- A wire is used to cross the lesion in the ICA, and then a stent is placed across it.

The safety and efficacy of TCAR has been evaluated in the Safety and Efficacy Study for Reverse Flow Used during Carotid Artery Stenting Procedure (ROADSTER) 1 and 2 trials,[14,15] which suggest that TCAR has low rates of stroke and myocardial infarction. Based on data from the Vascular Quality Initiative, TCAR has been shown to be associated with a similar risk of perioperative and 1-year stroke/death and lower risk of myocardial infarction compared with CEA and a lower risk of perioperative stroke/death compared with TF-CAS. Although these data are promising, there are currently no randomized controlled trials (RCTs) comparing outcomes of TCAR with CEA or TFCAS, and long-term outcomes data are lacking.

- Key clinical points
  - CEA is considered the gold standard for carotid revascularization but also has the highest physiologic stress and myocardial infarctions risk compared with other approaches.
  - High-risk characteristics for CEA include both comorbidity and anatomic considerations.
  - The presence of favorable access site anatomy is critical to success of both TF-CAS and TCAR.
  - Severe arch atheroma precludes use of TF-CAS due to high stroke risk, whereas atherosclerotic disease of the common carotid artery precludes use of TCAR.

Thoracic Aorta

Disease process and diagnosis
Disease of the thoracic aorta includes both aneurysmal disease as well as aortic dissection. Unlike AAAs, which are usually caused by atherosclerotic disease, thoracic aortic aneurysms are more likely to be associated with intimal dissection secondary to shearing stress from uncontrolled hypertension, inflammation, trauma, and, in some circumstances, connective tissue disease. Patients with thoracic aortic disease may be asymptomatic and diagnosed incidentally, or they may present with distal ischemia or embolic symptoms, compressive symptoms, or even rupture.[16] The imaging modality of choice for both thoracic dissection and aneurysm is CTA, which is diagnostic and provides critical information regarding the patient's aortic anatomy for operative planning.[17] For patients presenting with thoracic or thoracoabdominal aortic aneurysms, operative repair is generally recommended when the aneurysm diameter is greater than 5.5 cm.[18,19] For patients with acute type B (descending) aortic dissections, operative repair is indicated for dissections complicated by such things as rupture or symptoms of malperfusion.[20] For acute uncomplicated type B aortic dissections, early management should focus on aggressive heart rate and blood pressure control with beta blockade or calcium channel blockade before consideration for operative intervention.

A brief overview of surgical approaches
Open repair. Open repair is technically the gold standard for repair of the thoracic aorta,[21] although there is an increasing push toward the use of endovascular repair,

given the high rates of early postoperative morbidity and mortality with open approaches. Open repair remains the first-line approach to thoracoabdominal aortic aneurysm repair, as complex endovascular devices are not currently commercially available. There are also data suggesting that the results with open repair are more durable, and patients have decreased rates of long-term mortality and return to the operating room for reinterventions that would be common after endovascular repair.[22] A brief overview of the procedural steps for an open thoracic/thoracoabdominal aortic aneurysm repair is as follows:

- Single lung ventilation is initiated, and the thoracic cavity is entered via a left posterolateral thoracotomy incision.
- The aorta is exposed by dividing the inferior pulmonary ligament and retracting the lung anteriorly.
- After control of the aorta proximal and distal to the extent of repair is obtained, the surgeon must decide whether to use the "clamp-and-sew" technique, in which the aorta is clamped while the anastomosis is created without visceral blood flow distally, or whether they will put the patient on partial left heart or full cardiopulmonary bypass.[17]
- The proximal anastomosis is created first, followed by the distal anastomosis and any necessary renovisceral anastomoses.

Despite higher rates of 30-day postoperative mortality with open, compared to endovascular thoracic aortic repair, retrospective analyses cite overall perioperative mortality in patients undergoing open repair to be as low as 3% in high volume centers. If patients survive the perioperative period, the 1- and 5-year survival rate can be greater than 70%.[23] This high survival likely reflects a treatment bias in the patients being selected for open repair, as this approach is very high risk and physiologically stressful, with associated complication rates ranging between 30% and 50%.[23]

Thoracic Endovascular Aortic Repair. In the mid-2000s, the Gore TAG trial compared TEVAR to open repair of thoracic aortic aneurysms and found that patients undergoing TEVAR had lower rates of perioperative cardiopulmonary complications and 30-day post operative mortality (2.1% with TEVAR compared to 11.7% in the open repair group). However, both groups experienced similar rates of perioperative stroke and spinal cord ischemia.[24,25] Multiple subsequent studies have confirmed the perioperative benefits with TEVAR, although longer term studies show consistently better freedom from reintervention with open repair.[26] A brief summary of the steps involved in TEVAR are follows:

- Percutaneous femoral artery access is obtained.
- Wire cannulation of the ascending aorta is achieved with a stiff wire.
- For cases involving a dissection, access via the true lumen is ensured using intravascular ultrasound before the stent graft is introduced via large bore sheath.
- For chronic aortic dissections and degenerative aneurysms, the stent graft is deployed with the intent to cover the entire descending thoracic aorta from an area of healthy tissue to an area of healthy tissue.
- For acute type B dissections, the goal is to ensure stent graft coverage of the most proximal intimal defect of the dissection.[17,25] The remaining aorta can be supported with bare metal dissection stents to stabilize the remainder of the dissection flap without excessive aortic coverage that may raise the risk of spinal cord injury.

To date, there are no RCTs that have been published that compare outcomes following TEVAR and open thoracic aortic repair. However, nonrandomized controlled studies have shown that in patients with favorable anatomy to support endovascular repair, TEVAR is noninferior and in some circumstances superior to open repair.[27] Favorable anatomy includes a noncalcified access site of adequate diameter to accommodate the large sheath required to deploy the stent graft, as well as a nontortuous aorta, and a 2-cm landing zone both proximal and distal to the proposed stent location. This landing zone allows the graft to form a good seal to prevent endoleak and stent migration.[20]

- Key clinical points
  - Open thoracic aortic repair remains the gold standard for management of chronic thoracoabdominal aortic disease due to the current lack of commercially available branched endovascular devices.
  - Open thoracic aortic repair is associated with higher risks of cardiopulmonary events and mortality in the perioperative period but has a lower risk of reintervention compared with TEVAR long-term.
  - Successful TEVAR requires a proximal and distal landing zone for the stent graft that is a minimum of 2 cm in length.
  - The presence of favorable access site anatomy is critical to the success of TEVAR.

Abdominal Aorta

Disease process and diagnosis
An AAA is described as a 50% increase in the diameter of the abdominal aorta when compared with its baseline measurement. It is caused, most often, by degeneration of the tunica media secondary to atherosclerosis.[28] Approximately 80% of AAAs occur distal to the takeoff of the renal arteries, and men are more frequently affected than women.[28] AAA rupture accounts for approximately 15,000 deaths annually in the United States.[2,28] Many patients found to have AAAs are asymptomatic and diagnosed secondary to incidental imaging findings. Current guidelines support AAA screening via duplex ultrasound for all men and women aged 65 to 75 years with a history of tobacco use, men 55 years or older with a family history of AAA, and women 65 years or older who have smoked or have a family history of AAA.[29] Abdominal duplex ultrasound can be used to serially monitor a patient with AAA who is undergoing nonoperative surveillance; however, it often will overestimate the diameter.[28] Criteria for consideration of AAA repair include diameter greater than 5.5 cm in men or greater than 5.0 cm in women, saccular aneurysm, and symptomatic aneurysms. In larger aneurysms nearing size criteria for repair, CTA is the imaging modality of choice for most surgeons, as it provides valuable insight into the extent of the aneurysm with relation to the iliac and renal vasculature, as well as other anatomic features that are important when considering repair.

A brief overview of surgical approaches
Open abdominal aortic aneurysm repair. Although open repair of AAAs is less commonly performed since the advent of the EVAR, there remains a role for its practice in vascular surgery today. The procedure can be briefly described as follows:

- The aorta is exposed by one of two methods: transabdominal, in which the patient is laying supine, or extended left retroperitoneal, in which the patient is in the right lateral decubitus position.
- If using a transabdominal approach, a left medial visceral rotation or division of the lesser omentum and gastrohepatic ligament is required to adequately expose the aorta.

- The patient is systemically anticoagulated and control of the aorta proximal and distal to the aneurysm is obtained.
- The aneurysm is incised longitudinally, and the proximal and distal anastomoses are completed in an end-to-end fashion.
- The aneurysm sac is closed over the graft at the completion of repair to prevent occurrence of an aorta-duodenal fistula.[23]

Multiple RCTs have been published comparing EVAR and standard open repair of AAA. The United Kingdom (UK) EVAR 1 trial found that EVAR was associated with significantly lower rates of perioperative mortality compared with open repair (1.8% compared with 4.3%), but that long-term overall and aneurysm-related mortality did not differ significantly between the two groups.[30] Similar results were published from the Open versus Endovascular Repair (OVER) trial, which found that, despite early mortality benefit with EVAR, 2-year mortality did not differ between groups.[31] All of these studies have focused on infrarenal AAA. Patients with juxtarenal or pararenal AAA are more complicated and require fenestrated endograft technology for repair. In patients with these more complex aneurysms, open repair may be preferred over an endovascular approach based on surgeon experience and access to complex endovascular repair options. One major limitation of EVAR (with or without fenestration) is the need for late reinterventions to address endoleaks, which occurs in up to 20% of patients.[30]

Endovascular aortic repair. Over the past three decades, EVAR has become the mainstay of surgical management for AAAs; it is estimated that 70% to 80% of aneurysms are now repaired endovascularly.[2,28] EVAR involves the following operative steps:

- Access to the bilateral common femoral vessels is obtained percutaneously.
- A series of sheaths and wires are used to gain access to the abdominal aorta, and the main body of the graft is inserted to just the level of the renal vessels (for infrarenal repair) or with alignment of the fenestrations with the renovisceral segment (for complex repairs).
- The main body of the stent graft is deployed from proximal to distal.
- The contralateral limb of the stent graft is then cannulated, and an iliac limb extension is placed, followed by deployment (and possible extension) of the remaining ipsilateral iliac limb. The bilateral iliac artery limbs are landed to obtain seal in the distal aspect of the common iliac arteries, taking care to preserve flow to the hypogastric arteries.
- A completion angiogram is performed to assess for leaks and adequate flow through the graft before the bilateral femoral arteriotomies are closed.[2]

In addition to ensuring bilateral femoral/iliac artery anatomy is favorable for access without significant atherosclerotic occlusive disease or calcification, aortoiliac anatomy must also be evaluated with CTA in all patients planned for EVAR. Aortic stent grafts are equipped with a set of Instructions for Use (IFU) created by the manufacturer. These instructions are slightly different for each device and describe the anatomic variations of the aorta for which they are proved to function. These anatomic criteria generally include aortic neck length, angulation, and diameter and iliac diameter characteristics (**Table 1**). Aortic neck length and angle are the most important criteria used to determine anatomic EVAR eligibility. These devices are occasionally used off-IFU in the management of ruptured AAA; however, outcomes have been shown to be inferior to those patients who received on-IFU care.[32]

The Dutch Randomized Endovascular Aneurysm Management (DREAM) trial was another RCT completed in Europe that compared EVAR and open aortic repair for management of AAA. The investigators found that EVAR was preferred due to lower perioperative morbidity and systemic complications.[33] The UK EVAR 2 trial was conducted as a follow-up to the EVAR 1 trial to determine if there is benefit for patients who were deemed too high risk to undergo open AAA repair to undergo EVAR. The results showed a decrease in the rates of aneurysm-related mortality with EVAR when compared with observation; however, there was no significant decrease in all-cause mortality.

- Key clinical points
  - EVAR is associated with better perioperative outcomes compared with open AAA repair, but long-term morality is similar.
  - The need for late reintervention is higher for EVAR compared with open repair. As such, patients require routine long-term imaging surveillance after EVAR that is not required after open repair. Aortic neck length and angle are the most important criteria used to determine anatomic EVAR eligibility.
  - The presence of a favorable access site is critical to the success of EVAR.
  - Open AAA repair should be considered in patients whose aortic anatomy that does not fit the IFU criteria set forth by stent graft manufacturers.
  - Patients at high risk for open AAA repair based on comorbidities should be considered for endovascular management.

Suprainguinal Peripheral Arterial Disease

Disease process and diagnosis
Peripheral arterial occlusive disease (PAOD) can be anatomically separated into suprainguinal and infrainguinal categories, in which suprainguinal disease primarily refers to occlusive disease of the infrarenal aorta and iliac arteries and infrainguinal disease refers to occlusive disease from the common femoral arteries distally. The most common cause of PAOD in the United States is atherosclerosis, so the risk factors for disease development and basis of medical management are directly related to this process. Tobacco use is the single most important risk factor contributing to disease development,[34,35] along with hyperlipidemia. Patients with aortoiliac occlusive disease can present with a range of symptoms ranging from no symptoms (asymptomatic, most common) to claudication to chronic limb-threatening ischemia.[35] The severity of these symptoms depends on the distribution and severity of the PAOD, as well as the activity

Table 1
Endovascular stent graft instructions for use (IFU) in repair of abdominal aortic aneurysms as determined by the manufacturer.

Device	Neck Length (mm)	Neck Diameter (mm)	Infrarenal Angle (°)	Suprarenal Angle (°)
Cook Zenith	15	18–32	60	45
Endologix AFX	15	18–32	60	N/A
Endologix Ovation	10	16–30	60	N/A
Endologix Ovation[a]	7	16–30	45	N/A
Gore Excluder	15	19–29	60	N/A
Medtronic Endurant	10[a]	19–32	60	N/A

[a] Endologix Ovation has 2 separate criteria for neck length based on degree of infrarenal angulation.
Data from Zarkowsky DS et al. 2021.[32]

level of the patient. Although aortoiliac occlusive disease can often be diagnosed following a thorough history and physical examination, obtaining an ankle-brachial index is the best initial test to confirm the presence of PAOD. This involves calculating the ratio between the patient's highest brachial artery systolic pressure and their posterior tibial artery systolic pressure and a value of less than 0.9 is considered abnormal. The first-line management of asymptomatic PAOD and claudication is medical optimization (ie, antiplatelet therapy, statin therapy, smoking cessation, and supervised exercise therapy).[36] Lower extremity revascularization via either an open or endovascular approach is reserved for patients who have persistent lifestyle-limiting symptoms despite maximal medical therapy and for patients with chronic limb-threatening ischemia (ie, rest pain or tissue loss). Of those patients who require an intervention, preoperative imaging before intervention is common, particularly in patients suspected to have suprainguinal disease. Although conventional angiography is still considered the gold standard for diagnosis of PAOD, CTA is quickly becoming the most widely used modality for preoperative assessment and operative planning.[34]

A brief overview of surgical approaches

Anatomic and extra-anatomic revascularization. Although the use of endovascular techniques in the management of suprainguinal PAOD have increased drastically in recent years, open anatomic bypass remains the gold standard for treatment. Anatomic revascularization refers to the use of endarterectomy or bypass to restore in-line arterial flow of the normal anatomy (eg, aortobifemoral bypass). Extra-anatomic bypass refers to revascularization of distal arteries from a proximal source that differs from normal anatomic flow (eg, axillofemoral bypass). Extra-anatomic procedures are usually reserved for patients who are contraindicated for or would not otherwise tolerate an extensive open vascular procedure. Because it remains the gold standard for management of suprainguinal PAOD, the authors focus on aortobifemoral bypass for the purposes of this paper. A brief description of the procedure is as follows:

- After the patient is prepped and draped, the femoral arteries are exposed via cutdown, and proximal and distal control is obtained. Care must be taken to obtain control of both the superficial femoral artery and profunda femoris.
- Aortic exposure is then obtained via a midline laparotomy incision.
- Retroperitoneal tunnels are then constructed for the bypass graft limbs using blunt dissection, taking care to tunnel the limbs posterior to the ureters to prevent a late ilio-ureteral fistula.
- The patient is systemically anticoagulated and the aorta cross-clamped.
- The aortic anastomosis is completed before the grafts are tunneled through the previously made tracts toward the groin where the femoral anastomosis is performed.
- Once both anastomoses have been completed, distal revascularization of the lower extremities is ensured and the incisions closed.

An aortobifemoral bypass surgery has relatively low perioperative mortality risk, and studies have shown patency rates ranging between 80% and 95% at 5 years and 75% and 80% at 10 years.[34,37] However, the operation is time-consuming, and an aortic cross-clamp is required, so patients must have the appropriate physiologic reserve. For patients who may not tolerate a large open operation, an endovascular approach may be more appropriate as long as the anatomy is amenable to it. The Trans-Atlantic Inter-Society Consensus for the management of PAD (TASC II) has made recommendations regarding the management of aortoiliac lesions and femoropopliteal lesions. The aortoiliac lesions have been split into four types based on location and length of the segment, type A, B, C, and D (Appendix A). Per these guidelines, endovascular intervention is recommended for type A and B lesions, whereas open repair is recommended for the more complex type C and D lesions.[34]

Iliac artery stenting. As noted previously, over the last several decades, endovascular therapy has become commonplace in the management of both acute and chronic PAOD, and open surgery is often reserved for patients without anatomy that is amenable to percutaneous angioplasty and stenting. An iliac stenting procedure can be described as follows:

- Femoral arterial access is obtained using a micropuncture needle, and a sheath is introduced into the vessel and advanced to the level of the lesion.
- Once the lesion is identified, it is traversed, and a balloon-expandable stent is placed across it extending from healthy artery to healthy artery.
- The arterial access site is then controlled using a closure device or appropriate manual pressure.[34]

Rates of iliac artery stent patency have been shown to be upward of 95% initially and approximately 75% at 5 years.[38] Unfortunately, despite excellent long-term patency results with isolated iliac disease, results are much less favorable when the aortic bifurcation is included in the diseased segment. Previously, surgeons had used two separate bare stents in the bilateral common iliac arteries that would meet at the bifurcation, referred to as "kissing stents." This technique unfortunately proved to have low rates of long-term graft patency.[38] Following the conclusion of the COB-EST Trial, which showed that covered endovascular stent grafts were superior to bare metal stents,[39] covered endovascular reconstruction of the aortic bifurcation (CERAB) was introduced as an alternative endovascular procedure.

Studies have found primary patency rates following CERAB to be approximately 86% to 87.5% at 1 year[40,41] and greater than 83% at 5 years.[42] In a study directly comparing CERAB with aortobifemoral bypass, both procedures were found to have 100% technical success without significant difference in length of surgery, patency of the graft at 12 months, or 30-day mortality. However, patients who underwent CERAB had shorter intensive care unit length of stay and fewer postoperative complications than those who underwent aortobifemoral bypass.[43] It should be noted that the use of commercially available iliac stent grafts for CERAB is currently off-label.

- Key clinical points
  - The decision to perform an open anatomic, open extra-anatomic, or endovascular revascularization largely depends on the patients' risk factors for surgery as well as their anatomy and pattern of disease.
  - The TASC II classification and guidelines recommend endovascular repair for type A and B aortoiliac lesions and open repair for type C and D aortoiliac lesions (see Appendix A).
  - The presence of adequate bilateral femoral artery access sites is crucial to performing iliac artery stent placement or CERAB.
  - CERAB and aortobifemoral bypass have similar rates of graft patency and mortality in the short and mid-term, although CERAB is associated with fewer postoperative complications.

Infrainguinal Peripheral Arterial Disease

Disease process and diagnosis

Infrainguinal PAOD encompasses both femoropopliteal and tibioperoneal occlusive disease. Similar to suprainguinal PAOD, the most common cause of the disease process is atherosclerosis. However, there has been a notable increase in tibioperoneal disease over the past two decades, likely due to the increasing prevalence of risk factors such as diabetes. Patients with infrainguinal PAOD often present with lower extremity claudication or chronic limb-threatening ischemia (CLTI). CLTI can take the form of rest pain, ulceration, or gangrene. These patients should undergo a thorough history and physical examination, and ankle-brachial indices (ABIs) should be obtained. An ABI less than 0.4 is thought to coincide with CLI, although many patients with CLTI in the setting of diabetes will have noncompressible vessels leading to falsely elevated ABI values. In these patients, toe pressure may be more accurate, with less than 60 mm Hg corresponding to ischemia. Other diagnostic imaging that may useful is arterial duplex imaging or CTA. [44,45] As noted earlier, TASC II has also created classification criteria and guidelines for femoropopliteal disease based on location and length of the segment affected (Appendix B). Per these guidelines, endovascular intervention is recommended for type A, B, and C lesions, whereas open repair is recommended for the more complex type D lesions. [34]

A brief overview of surgical approaches
Lower extremity bypass grafting. For many years, open surgical therapy has been the gold-standard treatment of infrainguinal PAOD and, despite the widespread use and increasing effectiveness of endovascular techniques, is still commonly performed. Open lower extremity bypass grafting is the technique of choice for patients with extensive disease as defined by the TASC II criteria. A good bypass requires adequate inflow and outflow. Most often the inflow vessel of choice is the common femoral artery, but the surgeon may also use the external iliac artery, superficial femoral artery, or above-knee popliteal artery depending on the pattern of disease. The outflow vessel should be the least diseased, most proximal vessel with adequate inline flow to the foot. The conduit of choice is autologous vein, ideally great saphenous vein followed by small saphenous vein or an upper extremity vein. If a patient does not have available autologous vein, synthetic conduits (ie, polytetrafluoroethylene or Dacron) may be used, ideally with an adjunct procedure such as a distal vein patch for any target below the knee. Once the appropriate conduit is determined, the procedure may proceed as follows:

- The great saphenous vein is harvested to an adequate length (if applicable).
- Incisions are made over the inflow and outflow vessels of choice, and the arteries are isolated. A tunneling device is used to bluntly create a tunnel for the bypass either subcutaneously or in an anatomic configuration. Counter incisions are made as needed along the course of the tunnel.
- The patient is systemically anticoagulated and the proximal anastomosis performed.
- The conduit is oriented appropriately and passed through the tunnel to the distal target, where the distal anastomosis is completed.
- Distal reperfusion is ensured before the end of the case.

When saphenous vein grafts are used, open bypass grafts have a 70% to 75% patency at 5 years depending on the distal target, with an approximate 80% limb salvage rate.[44] The Bypass versus Angioplasty in Severe Ischemia of the Leg (BASIL) trial was a multicenter RCT conducted to evaluate the efficacy of treating with angioplasty versus bypass grafting first for patients with CLTI secondary to infrainguinal disease. The BASIL trial found that, for as long as 2 years following intervention, there was no significant difference in amputation-free survival between the two groups.[46] In follow-up to this trial, a by-treatment-received analysis was conducted and found that the rate of early technical failure of angioplasty was much higher than for bypass. In addition, they found that after

2 years following intervention, patients who underwent lower extremity bypass using an autologous vein conduit had improved amputation-free and overall survival compared with patients undergoing endovascular revascularization.[47] Based on these data, younger patients with greater than 2 years of life expectancy and available autogenous vein are recommended for bypass.[36] However, one of the major criticisms of the BASIL trial is that endovascular interventions were limited to plain balloon angioplasty, which is known to have inferior patency outcomes compared with other newer technologies. There are currently two similar RCTs ongoing to compare open lower extremity bypass with endovascular revascularization for lower extremity disease.

Percutaneous vascular intervention. Endovascular interventions, otherwise known as percutaneous vascular interventions (PVIs), are increasingly commonplace in the United States and can be applied to patients with both lifestyle-limiting claudication and CLTI. PVI is minimally invasive, can be performed on an outpatient basis, and involves immediate symptomatic improvement with minimal recovery time. Interventions include plain or drug-coated balloon angioplasty, plain or drug-coated stenting, atherectomy, or a combination of all three. A brief overview of the steps for PVI is briefly described:

- After an access site is identified, a micropuncture needle is used to gain access to the femoral artery, usually on the contralateral side to the lesion.
- Wires and sheaths are used to access the infrarenal aorta and select the contralateral iliac artery in an "up-and-over" technique.
- The lesion is traversed, and an intervention (balloon angioplasty, atherectomy, stent placement) is performed.
- The access site vessel is closed, and manual pressure is held to obtain hemostasis.

Primary stenting, when compared with angioplasty alone, has been found to have greater rates of patency at 1 and 2 years postprocedure.[44] Drug-coated technology (either balloon or stenting) is associated with better patency than non–drug-coated interventions,[48,49] but there is some controversy around a possible increase in mortality and major amputation with drug-coated technologies.[50,51] There is currently no evidence to support the routine use of atherectomy in patients with PAOD, as patency outcomes are similar to that of angioplasty with significantly higher complication rates and cost burden.[52,53]

- Key clinical points
  - The TASC II classification and guidelines recommend endovascular repair for type A to C and open repair for type D femoropopliteal lesions (see Appendix B).
  - Results from the BASIL trial suggest that patients with CLTI who have greater than 2 years life expectancy and available autologous vein may have better outcomes with lower extremity bypass compared to an endovascular balloon angioplasty. There are a number of newer endovascular technologies that have not been evaluated compared with open lower extremity bypass, although RCTs are currently under way.
  - Percutaneous vascular interventions are minimally invasive with short recovery times, although long-term patency is better with open bypass.

SUMMARY

The practice of vascular surgery in the 21st century is always changing and ever expanding. The advancement of endovascular capabilities has made minimally invasive repair of even the largest of arteries possible with durable outcomes and fewer complications compared with traditional open surgery. It is of the utmost importance that clinicians recognize the pros and cons of both open and endovascular management of vascular disease in the context of important patient-centered factors and that they are able to apply them to their practice in order to provide optimal outcomes. In general, endovascular interventions are less physiologically stressful and have shorter recovery times with fewer perioperative complications compared with open surgery, but long-term outcomes tend to be relatively similar across approaches. For most disease processes, patient risk status and disease anatomy are the primary factors in determining whether an open or endovascular approach to surgery is warranted.

CLINICS CARE POINTS

- The decision regarding open versus endovascular intervention in vascular surgery depends on many factors, including patient comorbidities, disease location and anatomy, vascular access, and the overarching goal of treatment.
- For carotid revascularization, carotid endarterectomy is the gold standard, but transfemoral or transcarotid artery stenting are endovascular alternatives currently indicated for use in high-risk patients with appropriate anatomy.
- For thoracic and abdominal aortic aneurysm repair, endovascular therapy has better short-term outcomes but more long-term reinterventions.
- When treating suprainguinal or infrainguinal peripheral artery disease, the decision to proceed with open surgery or endovascular therapy depends largely on the severity of disease being treated, in addition to underlying patient risk factors.
- In general, endovascular interventions have shorter recovery times and fewer perioperative complications but are associated with reduced longevity compared with open surgery.

DISCLOSURE

C.W. Hicks is a speaker for Cook Medical Inc., and W.L. Gore & Associates, Inc, and receives grant support from the NIH/NIDDK (K23DK124515), Society for Vascular Surgery, and American College of Surgeons.

REFERENCES

1. Payne MM. Charles Theodore Dotter. The father of intervention. Tex Heart Inst J 2001;28(1):28–38.
2. Cambria RP, Prushik SG. Endovascular Treatment of Abdominal Aortic Aneurysms. In: Cameron JL, Cameron AM, editors. Current surgical therapy. 13th edition. Philadelphia: Elsevier; 2020. p. 905–11.
3. Centers for Disease Control and Prevention. In: National Center for Chronic Disease Prevention and Health Promotion, Division for Heart Disease and Stroke Prevention. 2021. Available at: https://www.cdc.gov/stroke/facts.htm. Accessed February 5, 2022.
4. Garrido DE, Ramirez DE, O'Mara CS. Balloon Angioplasty and Stents in Carotid Artery Occlusive Disease. In: Cameron JL, Cameron AM, editors. Current surgical therapy. 13th edition. Philadelphia: Elsevier; 2020. p. 939–46.
5. Holscher CM, Abularrage CJ. Carotid Endarterectomy. In: Cameron JL, Cameron AM, editors. Current surgical therapy. 13th edition. Philadelphia: Elsevier; 2020. p. 928–39.

6. Duncan A, Scallan O. Carotid artery disease: Do women present differently than men?. In: Hicks CW, Harris LM, editors. Vascular Disease in Women, an overview of the literature and treatment recommendations. London: Elsevier; 2022. p. 81-7.
7. North American Symptomatic Carotid Endarterectomy Trial Collaborators. Beneficial Effect of Carotid Endarterectomy in Symptomatic Patients with High-Grade Carotid Artery Stenosis. N Eng J Med 1991;325:445-53.
8. Warlow CP. Symptomatic patients: the European Carotid Surgery Trial (ECST). J Mal Vasc 1993;18(3):198-201.
9. Endarterectomy for asymptomatic carotid artery stenosis. Executive Committee for the Asymptomatic Carotid Atherosclerosis Study. JAMA 1995;273(18):1421-8.
10. Ricotta JJ, Aburahma A, Ascher E, et al. Updated Society for Vascular Surgery guidelines for management of extracranial carotid disease. J Vasc Surg 2011; 54:1-31.
11. Brott TG, Hobson RW, Howard G, et al. Stenting versus Endarterectomy for Treatment of Carotid Artery Stenosis. N Engl J Med 2010;363:11-23.
12. Yadav JS, Wholey MH, Knutz RE, et al. Protected Carotid-Artery Stenting versus Endarterectomy in High Risk Patients. N Engl J Med 2004;351:1493-501.
13. Phurrough S, Salive M, Hogarth R, et al. Coverage Decision Memorandum for Carotid Artery Stenting: CAG-00085R. In: Medicare Coverage Database. Available at: NCA - Carotid Artery Stenting (CAG-00085R) - Decision Memo (cms.gov). Accessed March 1, 2022.
14. Kwolek CJ, Jaff MR, Leal JI, et al. Results of the ROADSTER multicenter trial of transcarotid stenting with dynamic flow reversal. J Vasc Surg 2015;62(5): 1227-34.
15. Kashyap VS, Schneider PA, Foteh M, et al. Early Outcomes in the ROADSTER 2 Study of Transcarotid Artery Revascularization in Patients with Significant Carotid Artery Disease. Stroke 2020;51:2620-9.
16. Kiguchi MM, Salazar D. Thoracic aortic dissection repair in women. In: Hicks CW, Harris LM, editors. Vascular Disease in Women, an overview of the literature and treatment recommendations. London: Elsevier; 2022. p. 21-30.
17. Assi R, Steinberg T, Vallabhajosyula P. Management of Descending Thoracic and Thoracoabdominal Aortic Aneurysms. In: Cameron JL, Cameron AM, editors. Current surgical therapy. 13th edition. Philadelphia: Elsevier; 2020. p. 917-21.
18. Hiratzka LF, Creager MA, Isselbacher EM, et al. Surgery for Aortic Dilatation in Patients With Bicuspid Aortic Valves: A Statement of Clarification From the American College of Cardiology/American Heart Association Task Force on Clinical Practice Guidelines. Circulation 2016;133(7):680-6.
19. Erbel R, Aboyans V, Boileau C, et al. ESC Guidelines on the diagnosis and treatment of aortic diseases: Document covering acute and chronic aortic diseases of the thoracic and abdominal aorta of the adult. The Task Force for the Diagnosis and Treatment of Aortic Diseases of the European Society of Cardiology (ESC) [published correction appears in Eur Heart J. 2015 Nov 1;36(41):2779]. Eur Heart J 2014;35(41):2873-926.
20. Nation DA, Wang GJ. TEVAR: Endovascular Repair of the Thoracic Aorta. Semin Intervent Radiol 2015;32(3):265-71.
21. Hong JC, Coselli JS. Open repair remains the gold standard. JTCVS Tech 2021; 10:16-23.
22. Chiu P, Goldstone AB, Schaffer JM, et al. Endovascular Versus Open Repair of Intact Descending Thoracic Aortic Aneurysms. J Am Coll Cardiol 2019;73: 643-51.

23. Goodney PP, Travis L, Lucas FL, et al. Survival After Open Versus Endovascular Thoracic Aortic Aneurysm Repair in an Observational Study of the Medicare Population. Circulation 2011;124:2661–9.

24. Cho JS, Haider SE, Makaroun MS. Endovascular therapy of thoracic aneurysms: Gore TAG trial results. Semin Vasc Surg 2006;19(1):18–24.

25. Beaulieu RJ, Black JH. Management of Acute Aortic Dissection. In: Cameron JL, Cameron AM, editors. Current surgical therapy. 13th edition. Philadelphia: Elsevier; 2020. p. 922–8.

26. McCarthy A, Gray J, Sastry P, et al. Systematic review of endovascular stent grafting versus open surgical repair for the elective treatment of arch/descending thoracic aortic aneurysms. BMJ Open 2021;11(3):e043323.

27. Patterson BO, Thompson MM. The Value of TEVAR Trials. 2014. In: Endovascular today. Available at: The Value of TEVAR Trials - Endovascular Today (evtoday.com). Accessed March 1, 2022.

28. Perler B. Open Repair of Abdominal Aortic Aneurysms. In: Cameron JL, Cameron AM, editors. Current surgical therapy. 13th edition. Philadelphia: Elsevier; 2020. p. 901–5.

29. US Preventive Services Task Force. Screening for Abdominal Aortic Aneurysm: US Preventive Services Task Force Recommendation Statement. JAMA 2019; 322(22):2211–8.

30. The United Kingdom EVAR Trial Investigators. Endovascular versus Open Repair of Abdominal aortic Aneurysm. N Engl J Med 2010;362:1863–71.

31. Lederle FA, Kyriakides TC, Stroupe KT, et al. Open versus Endovascular Repair of Abdominal Aortic Aneurysm. N Engl J Med 2019;380:2126–35.

32. Zarkowsky DS, Sorber R, Ramirez JL, et al. Aortic Neck IFU Violations During EVAR for Ruptured Infrarenal Aortic Aneurysms are Associated with Increased In-Hospital Mortality. Ann Vasc Surg 2021;75:12–21.

33. Prinssen M, Verhoeven ELG, Buth J, et al. A Randomized Trial Comparing Conventional and Endovascular Repair of Abdominal Aortic Aneurysms. N Engl J Med 2004;351:1607–18.

34. Blas JV, Taylor SM. Aortoiliac Occlusive Disease. In: Cameron JL, Cameron AM, editors. Current surgical therapy. 13th edition. Philadelphia: Elsevier; 2020. p. 968–76.

35. Heaton J, Khan YS. Aortoiliac occlusive disease. [Updated 2021 Aug 23]. In: StatPearls [Internet]. Treasure Island (FL): StatPearls Publishing; 2022. Available at: https://www.ncbi.nlm.nih.gov/books/NBK559086/.

36. Gerhard-Herman MD, Gornik HL, Barrett C, et al. 2016 AHA/ACC Guideline on the Management of Patients With Lower Extremity Peripheral Artery Disease: A Report of the American College of Cardiology/American Heart Association Task Force on Clinical Practice Guidelines [published correction appears in J Am Coll Cardiol. 2017 Mar 21;69(11):1521]. J Am Coll Cardiol 2017;69(11):e71–126.

37. Velazquez-Ramirez G, Rosenberg ML. Suprainguinal peripheral artery disease: Open management. In: Hicks CW, Harris LM, editors. Vascular Disease in Women, an overview of the literature and treatment recommendations. London: Elsevier; 2022. p. 185–202.

38. Goverde PCJM, Grimme FAB, Verbruggen P JEM, et al. Covered Endovascular Reconstruction of Aortic Bifurcation (CERAB) technique: A new approach in treating extensive aortoiliac occlusive disease. J Cardiovasc Surg (Torino) 2013;54: 383–7.

39. Mwipatayi BP, Sharma S, Daneshmand A, et al. Durability of the balloon-expandable covered versus bare-metal stents in the Covered versus Balloon

Expandable Stent Trial (COBEST) for the treatment of aortoiliac occlusive disease. J Vasc Surg 2016;64:83–94.

40. Borghese O., Ferrer C., Coscarella C., et. al. Two-year single centre results with covered endovascular reconstruction of aortic bifurcation (CERAB) in the treatment of extensive aorto-iliac occlusive disease. *Vascular.* 30 (3), 2022, 500-508.

41. Taeymans K, Jebbink EG, Holewijn S, et al. Three year outcome of the covered endovascular reconstruction of the aortic bifurcation technique for aortoiliac occlusive disease. J Vasc Surg 2018;67:1438–47.

42. de Cort BA, Salemans PB, Fritschy WM, et al. Long-Term Outcome for Covered Endovascular Reconstruction of Aortic Bifurcation for Aortoiliac Disease: A Single-Center Experience. J Endovasc Ther 2021;28(6):906–13.

43. Gouveia e Melo R, Fernandes e Fernandes R, Garrido P, et al. Comparison Between Aortobifemoral Bypass and Covered Endovascular Reconstruction of Aortic Bifurcation for Aortoiliac Obstructive Disease: Short-term and Midterm Results. J Vasc Surg 2018;68(5S):E137.

44. AbuRahma AF, AbuRahma ZT. Femoropopliteal Occlusive Disease. In: Cameron JL, Cameron AM, editors. Current surgical therapy. 13th edition. Philadelphia: Elsevier; 2020. p. 976–83.

45. Beaulieu RJ, Reifsnyder T. Management of Tibioperoneal Arterial Occlusive Disease. In: Cameron JL, Cameron AM, editors. Current surgical therapy. 13th edition. Philadelphia: Elsevier; 2020. p. 983–8.

46. BASIL Trial Participants. Bypass versus angioplasty in severe ischemia of the leg (BASIL): multicentre, randomized controlled trial. Lancet 2005;366(9501): 1925–34.

47. Bradbury AW, Adam DJ, Bell J, et al. Bypass versus Angioplasty in Severe Ischemia of the Leg (BASIL) trial: Analysis of amputation and overall survival by treatment received. J Vasc Surg 2010;51(5):18–31.

48. Teichgräber U, Lehmann T, Aschenbach R, et al. Drug-coated Balloon Angioplasty of Femoropopliteal Lesions Maintained Superior Efficacy over Conventional Balloon: 2-year Results of the Randomized EffPac Trial. Radiology 2020; 295(2):478–87.

49. Schroeder H, Werner M, Meyer DR, et al. Low-Dose Paclitaxel-Coated Versus Uncoated Percutaneous Transluminal Balloon Angioplasty for Femoropopliteal Peripheral Artery Disease: One-Year Results of the ILLUMENATE European Randomized Clinical Trial (Randomized Trial of a Novel Paclitaxel-Coated Percutaneous Angioplasty Balloon). Circulation 2017;135(23):2227–36.

50. Katsanos K, Spiliopoulos S, Kitrou P, et al. Risk of Death Following Application of Paclitaxel-Coated Balloons and Stents in the Femoropopliteal Artery of the Leg: A Systematic Review and Meta-Analysis of Randomized Controlled Trials. J Am Heart Assoc 2018;7(24):e011245.

51. Katsanos K, Spiliopoulos S, Teichgräber U, et al. Editor's Choice - Risk of Major Amputation Following Application of Paclitaxel Coated Balloons in the Lower Limb Arteries: A Systematic Review and Meta-Analysis of Randomised Controlled Trials. Eur J Vasc Endovasc Surg 2022;63(1):60–71.

52. Zia S, Juneja A, Shams S, et al. Contemporary outcomes of infrapopliteal atherectomy with angioplasty versus balloon angioplasty alone for critical limb ischemia. J Vasc Surg 2020;71(6):2056–64.

53. Hicks CW, Holscher CM, Wang P, et al. Use of Atherectomy During Index Peripheral Vascular Interventions. JACC Cardiovasc Interv 2021;14(6):678–88.

APPENDIX A: THE TRANS-ATLANTIC INTER-SOCIETY CONSENSUS FOR THE MANAGEMENT OF PAD (TASC II) CLASSIFICATION FOR AORTOILIAC OCCLUSIVE DISEASE

Type A
- Unilateral (UL) or bilateral (BL) stenosis of the common iliac artery (CIA)
- UL or BL single short segment stenosis of external iliac artery (EIA) ($\leq$3 cm)

Type B
- Short segment stenosis of the infrarenal aorta ($\leq$3 cm)
- UL CIA occlusion
- Single or multiple stenoses totaling 3 to 10 cm involving the EIA without extension into the common femoral artery (CFA)
- Unilateral EIA occlusion

Type C
- BL CIA occlusion
- BL EIA stenoses totaling 3 to 10 cm long without extension into CFA
- UL EIA stenosis extending into CFA
- UL EIA occlusion involving origin of internal iliac artery (IIA) and/or CFA
- Heavily calcified UL EIA occlusion

Type D
- Infrarenal aortoiliac occlusion
- Diffuse disease involving the aorta and BL iliac arteries
- Multiple stenoses involving the UL CIA, EIA, and/or CFA
- UL occlusions of both CIA and EIA
- BL occlusions of EIA

APPENDIX B: THE TRANS-ATLANTIC INTER-SOCIETY CONSENSUS FOR THE MANAGEMENT OF PAD (TASC II) CLASSIFICATION FOR FEMOROPOPLITEAL OCCLUSIVE DISEASE

Type A
- Single stenosis $\leq$10 cm in length
- Single occlusion $\leq$5 cm in length

Type B
- Multiple stenoses or occlusions, each $\leq$5 cm in length
- Single stenosis or occlusion $\leq$15 cm in length and not involving the infrageniculate popliteal artery
- Single or multiple stenoses in the absence of continuous tibial vessel flow
- Single popliteal stenosis

Type C
- Multiple stenoses or occlusions totaling greater than 15 cm with or without heavy calcification
- Recurrent stenoses or occlusions that need treatment after 2 endovascular interventions

Type D
- Chronic total occlusions of the common femoral artery (CFA) or superficial femoral artery (SFA)
- Chronic total occlusion of the popliteal artery and proximal trifurcation

Monitoring During Vascular Surgery

Joshua Roach, MD[a],*, Stephanie Cha, MD[b]

KEYWORDS

- Vascular • surgery • Intraoperative monitors • Cerebrospinal fluid drainage
- Monitoring

KEY POINTS

- Complex vascular surgeries can result in severe clinical complications, including acute cardiac injury, stroke, spinal cord injury, and death.
- Although all vascular surgeries should include monitoring of pulse oximetry, capnography, blood pressure, temperature, and 5-lead electrocardiography, additional monitoring modalities commonly used include cerebrospinal fluid drainage, somatosensory and motor-evoked potentials, transesophageal echocardiography, and cerebral oximetry.
- Use of specialized monitoring may reduce the risk of complications following vascular surgery, such as using cerebrospinal fluid drainage to prevent spinal cord injury in patients undergoing thoracic aortic repair.

INTRODUCTION

The American Society of Anesthesiologists (ASA) has set forth clear guidelines for the basic monitoring of all general anesthetics that include continually evaluating the patient's oxygenation, ventilation, circulation, and temperature.[1] When using an anesthesia machine, inspired gas analysis using an oxygen analyzer with a low oxygen concentration limit alarm should occur. Pulse oximetry, electrocardiography, arterial blood pressure monitoring at least every 5 min, and a quantitative method to assess the adequacy of ventilation, typically in the form of capnography, should be used. Circulatory function should be continually evaluated by detection of pulse or pulse plethysmography or oximetry. As clinically significant changes in body temperature are likely, temperature monitoring is advised.[2] Complex vascular surgery such as aortic repairs and carotid endarterectomies (CEAs)/stenting may require additional or more invasive monitoring as changes in hemodynamics may occur frequently and

[a] Department of Anesthesiology & Critical Care Medicine, Johns Hopkins University School of Medicine, 2440 North Berkshire Road, Charlottesville, VA 22901, USA; [b] Department of Anesthesiology & Critical Care Medicine, Johns Hopkins University School of Medicine, 1800 Orleans Street, Suite 6216, Baltimore, MD 21287, USA
* Corresponding author.
E-mail address: jroach8@jhmi.edu

Anesthesiology Clin 40 (2022) 645–655
https://doi.org/10.1016/j.anclin.2022.08.009   anesthesiology.theclinics.com
1932-2275/22/© 2022 Elsevier Inc. All rights reserved.

rapidly. In addition, specialized monitoring may reduce the risk for certain procedure-specific complications such as spinal cord ischemia (SCI) or insufficient somatic or cerebral oxygenation during cases assisted by left-heart bypass. The response to these monitoring modalities requires a multi-disciplinary approach, of which the anesthesiologist must take a lead role. Here we aim to discuss some of the monitors used in these procedures including lumbar drains, spinal somatosensory evoked potentials (SSEPs), transesophageal echocardiography (TEE), and cerebral oximetry.

Lumbar Drains for Open and Endovascular Aortic Repair

Brief overview

In the 1960s, it was shown in dog models that draining cerebrospinal fluid decreased SCI during aortic cross-clamp by increasing SC perfusion pressure.[3,4] Dasmahapatra and colleagues[5] discovered that the degree of SC ischemia was directly related to cerebrospinal fluid (CSF) pressure (p = .0092), and negatively related to the percent change in CSF pressure (p = 0.028) by measuring SSEPs during interval cross-clamping of a canine aorta. McCullough and colleagues[6] showed successful CSF drainage in 24 human patients undergoing nondissecting thoracoabdominal aortic aneurysm (TAAA) repairs, and showed a decrease in SCI after aortic cross-clamp. A subsequent prospective randomized clinical trial by Coselli and colleagues[7] showed an 80% relative risk reduction of postoperative neurologic deficits following TAAA repair performed with lumbar CSF drainage, although they were unable to show a difference in mortality. Finally, Safi and colleagues[8] performed a retrospective analysis that included 1,004 TAAA repairs between 1991 and 2003 and showed that long-term survival was improved with CSF drainage and persisted after adjustment for age, extent of aneurysm, and preoperative renal function. These results have been reproduced not only in open TAAAs, but in thoracic endovascular aortic repair (TEVAR) as well.[9]

Indications and risk factors

The 2010 American College of Cardiology Foundation (ACCF)/American Heart Association (AHA)/American Society of Anesthesiology (ASA) guidelines recommend CSF drainage as an spinal cord (SC) protective strategy for open and endovascular thoracic aortic repair for patients at increased risk for SCI injury.[10] Similarly, the 2015 European Association for Cardiothoracic Surgeons recommend considering CSF drainage for TEVAR procedures, but only with Level IIaC evidence (expert opinion).[11] Increased surgical risk factors for SC ischemia following TEVAR include the following: (1) total aortic coverage >20 cm, (2) concomitant abdominal aortic or prior aortic aneurysm repair, (3) coverage of two or more vascular territories, (4) left subclavian artery coverage, (5) procedure urgency, (6) coverage of hypogastric artery, (7) use of three or more stents, (8) longer procedure duration, and (9) excessive blood loss. Increased patient risk factors include age, perioperative hypotension (mean arterial pressure (MAP) <70), renal insufficiency, chronic obstructive pulmonary disease, hypertension, and degenerative aneurysms.[12]

Limitations and complications

Risks of lumbar CSF drain placement include headache, development of spinal or epidural hematoma, infection, retained catheter, persistent CSF leak, and intracerebral hemorrhage (ICH). Numerous small studies outline complications that vary widely across studies because of the experience level of the proceduralist, timing of drain placement, and whether the placement was done blindly or under fluoroscopic guidance. Estrera and colleagues[13] performed a retrospective observational study of 1,105 patients who underwent CSF drainage for thoracic aorta repairs at a single institution and found that catheter-related complications occurred in 1.5% of patients. The most common complication was CSF leak with a spinal headache (0.54%), ICH (.45%), and isolated headache (.2%). Other complications included fractured catheter and meningitis. A smaller single-center retrospective study of 81 patients by Hanna and colleagues[14] showed a catheter-related minor complication rate of 11.1% which included spinal headache, puncture site bleeding, and clinically insignificant subdural hematoma. These patients often require systemic anticoagulation, and one should refer to the American Society of Regional Anesthesia (ASRA) and Pain Medicine guidelines before attempting to place a lumbar drain for any patient requiring anticoagulation to reduce the risk for ICH, hematoma, and subsequent SC ischemia.

Lumbar drain placement and management
Ideally, lumbar drains are placed in awake patients to allow for patient feedback, such perceived laterality and development of paresthesia, to guide placement and prevent neuraxial injury. Lumbar drains are often placed in the upright position with lumbar flexion, but can also be placed in the lateral decubitus position if the patient is unable to sit upright, and this may even minimize the hydrostatic CSF column and therefore CSF loss. However, midline spinal structures may be more difficult to identify in this position. Once placed and secured, the CSF drain transducer should be zeroed at the level of the external auditory meatus as a surrogate for the Circle of Willis, regardless of patient positioning. It is suggested that CSF pressure should be maintained below 15 mm Hg, but may be lowered to 10 mm Hg if there is a loss of SSEPs or MEPs.[13] CSF drains freely against a pressure column to maintain these goals, but should typically never exceed 15 mL/h to minimize the risk for ICH. Postoperatively the drain should be left in for up to 3 days while draining to a CSF pressure of less than 10 mm Hg if there are no neurologic complications. Ideally, the patient should be able to participate in a neurological examination every hour in the immediate postoperative period, the frequency of which may be relaxed if the examination remains normal. In the case of an abnormal neurologic examination, the surgical team should be immediately notified and the patient sent for computed tomography (CT) or MRI to assess for spinal hematoma or ICH, depending on clinical presentation.[15]

Neuromonitoring for Carotid Artery and Aortic Surgery

"Awake" monitoring
Ischemic stroke is one of the most feared complications from carotid surgery, with an incidence of 2.3% in CEA and 4.1% in carotid artery stenting (CAS).[16] Therefore, it is critical to monitor cerebral perfusion intraoperatively. The most reliable way to detect clinically significant ischemia is by evaluation of gross neurologic examination and level of consciousness under "awake" surgical techniques, performed under deep or superficial cervical plexus nerve blocks.[17] "Awake" monitoring is associated with an increased sensitivity and specificity for ischemia detection over electroencephalography (EEG) and stump pressure transduction.[18] Disadvantages include risk of patient anxiety, airway obstruction, conversion to general anesthesia because of inadequate regional anesthesia, and inadvertent nerve or vascular injury during regional block placement.[17] Recent clinical trials have not shown a benefit in mortality, length of hospital stay, death, or quality of life when compared with general anesthesia,[19] and "awake" monitoring has largely fallen out of favor, replaced monitoring techniques that can be performed under general anesthesia.

Somatosensory evoked potentials
SSEPs evaluate the integrity of ascending sensory neural pathways (dorsal column-medial lemniscus), and motor-evoked potentials (MEPs) evaluate the integrity of

descending motor neural pathways. This can be useful when monitoring for SCI in aortic surgery as well as thromboembolic stroke and hypoperfusion during carotid clamping during CEA procedures. SSEPs are more commonly used as it allows the anesthesiologist to use neuromuscular blockade, something that is avoided when using MEPs. Essentially, a stimulus is applied to a peripheral nerve such as the posterior tibial or common peroneal nerve, and an electric stimulus is repeatedly administered. An electrode placed on the scalp will then detect those stimuli and after hundreds of repetitions, will report an average of their latency and amplitues.[1] A decrease in amplitude and/or an increase in latency may indicate an interruption in that neural pathway and should prompt a discussion between the surgeon, anesthesiologist, and neuromonitoring technologist. However, many common medications and perioperative circumstances may also cause abnormal neural signaling, and this must be taken into consideration.

Indications
Detecting thromboembolic events and inadequate collateral circulation during carotid cross-clamp may prompt immediate intervention, such as raising the mean arterial blood pressure or inserting a shunt to minimize perioperative stroke risk. A meta-analysis by Reddy and colleagues[20] of patients undergoing CEA identified SSEP "change" (most often, decrease in amplitude by >50% and increase in latency by >10%) as a predictor for 30-day perioperative stroke risk. Similarly, a meta-analysis by Nwachuku and colleagues[21] examined 4,557 patients undergoing CEA with SSEP monitoring and found that the odds of observing an SSEP change among those with neurologic deficits were 14 times higher than those without neurologic deficits.

The utility of using MEPs and SSEPs in aortic surgery (particularly TEVARs) is less convincing due to the results of clinical trials showing high rates of both false positive and false negative results. This could be due to common perioperative factors such as large volume blood loss and resuscitation, hypotension, and the use of large-bore lower extremity perfusion cannulas. Weigang and colleagues[22] showed a change in SSEPs/MEPs refractory to treatment with no post-neurologic deficit (false positive), and one patient with delayed paresis with unchanged intraoperative neuromonitoring (IONM; false negative). A subsequent study by Schurink and colleagues[23] of 10 patients undergoing TEVAR with MEPs reported >50% reduction in MEPs in 20% of patients. The procedure was then carried out in stages to minimize SCI by allowing collaterals to develop in between surgeries. One patient (10%) developed lower limb paralysis although there were no significant MEP changes intraoperatively. Subsequent studies have shown more encouraging results-Banga and colleagues[24] reported a 6% rate of SCI with a 63% intraoperative change in SSEPs/MEPs due to intraoperative intervention (increase blood pressure or CSF drainage).

Complications and limitations
Intraoperative complications due to neuromonitoring are rare. IONM may increase intracranial pressure (ICP) and induce seizures according to the American Clinical Neurophysiology Society (ACNS),[25] so relative contraindications include patients with cerebral vascular clips, pacemakers, history of epilepsy, and history of increased intracranial pressure.[25,26] In addition, MEPs cause muscle contraction in the distribution of the area being tested, so bite blocks should be used when monitoring the facial nerve.

Selection of anesthetic is important when IONM is used as many common anesthetic agents interfere with IONM and mimic nerve ischemia. MEPs are generated and propagated via the pyramidal tract so neuromuscular blockade cannot be used when this modality is used. Inhaled halogenated agents cause a dose-dependent decrease in amplitude and increase in latency, so intravenous anesthesia should be considered. IONM interference may also be precipitated by hypotension, mechanical compression of neural tissue, hypocapnia, and hypothermia. IONM also requires expert technologists, which carries additional expense.

Electroencephalography. EEG monitoring has been used for decades in identifying cerebral ischemia during carotid surgery.[17] EEG provides real-time feedback that allows the surgeon to determine if a shunt is necessary to prevent cerebral ischemia. In the operative setting, an EEG specialist continually monitors brainwave activity from electrodes placed preoperatively and notifies the surgeon and anesthesiologist if abnormalities occur. Indications of ischemia include brain wave slowing, attenuation, or loss of signal transduction.[27] A retrospective analysis by Woodworth and colleagues[28] of 1411 patients, showed selective shunting guided by EEG combined with SSEP monitoring decreased the rate of stroke from 4% to 1% when compared with routine shunting. They further surmised that a surgical volume of 200 cases was needed to decrease the risk of stroke by twofold, with an odds ratio of 0.38; 95% confidence interval of 0.20–0.74; $P < 0.01$. The advantages thus include real-time evaluation of cortical blood flow integrity and subsequent reduction in cerebral ischemia. Disadvantages of EEG monitoring include the cost and availability of an EEG technician to be available throughout the surgery, and the sensitivity of EEG to hypothermia, anesthetic agents, and interference from previous strokes. Virtually all inhaled halogenated anesthetics mimic ischemia by decreasing brainwave amplitude and frequency to some degree, and intravenous sedatives such as benzodiazapines, barbituates, and propofol cause a dose-dependent reduction of EEG, albeit to a lesser extent than halogenated inhalants.[29] It should also be noted that EEG monitors primarily monitor activity in the cerebral cortex, not deeper structures such as the brainstem.[17] Therefore, when using EEG as a monitoring modality, it is important to maintain a stable core temperature, limit the use of halogenated agents, and communicate with the EEG technician any changes made to the anesthetic regimen.

Transesophageal Echocardiography in Vascular Surgery

Brief overview

Side and colleagues[30] first used an esophageal ultrasound probe in an awake patient to visualize aortic blood flow, and subsequently surmised that "beat to beat changes in the flow pattern and peak velocity and acceleration can be of considerable value to the surgeon by giving immediate warning of deteriorating cardiac efficiency." Frazin and colleagues[31] used Motion- or "M"-mode to evaluate cardiac structures such as the left atrium and aorta and then validated their findings by comparison to transthoracic echocardiography (TTE). Matsuzaki and colleagues used an endoscopy-like TEE probe on 35 patients, most of which had coronary artery disease to record the motion of the left ventricle and compare them to healthy adult controls. They found that compared with ventriculography, TEE was more sensitive than TTE in detecting wall motion abnormalities.[32,33] Subsequently, introduction of a phased-array transducer at the tip of the probe allowed greater manipulation and superior cardiac imaging, marking the start of TEE imaging for the diagnosis of structural heart disease.[33]

Indications

TEE is increasingly used to help guide surgeons and anesthesiologists in their management of complex vascular patients, particularly aortic dissections and TAAAs. The 2010 ACCF/AHA guidelines stated that "urgent and definitive imaging of the aorta using transesophageal echocardiogram... is recommended to identify or exclude thoracic aortic dissection in patients at high risk for the disease by initial screening" with level B evidence. Furthermore, "TEE may be used when the nature of the planned surgery or the patient's known or suspected cardiovascular pathology might result in severe hemodynamic or pulmonary compromise."[10] The decision to use TEE should therefore be guided not only by the nature of the surgery, but also by the patient's medical background and perioperative circumstances as judged by the treating physician.[34] A basic TEE examination will not only provide baseline cardiac function, but is also helpful in (1) assisting surgeons in cannulation, (2) identifying the true and false lumen during a dissection repair, (3) monitoring for wall motion abnormalities and left ventricular function during the extreme increase in afterload caused by aortic cross-clamping, (4) differentiating cardiomyopathy from hypovolemia in the setting of hypoperfusion from massive bleeding (which includes right ventricular function), and (5) monitoring for pericardial effusions, pleural effusions, and hemothorax.

Complications and limitations
TEE is generally safe and is a minimally invasive procedure in trained hands. Minor complications include sore throat, dental damage, and trauma to lips and gums, whereas more severe complications include inadvertent tracheal placement with subsequent extubation and/or respiratory distress, esophageal variceal rupture, bleeding, and esophageal or gastric perforation. It has been reported that the rate of TEE-related morbidity rages from 0.2 to 1.2%.[35] According to the American Society of Echocardiography (ASE), contraindications include esophageal stricture, diverticulum, tumor, and recent esophageal or gastric surgery.[36] Therefore, a careful history and physical must be undertaken before probe placement that includes ruling out prior esophageal surgeries, esophageal dysmotility, esophageal strictures, and poor dentition.

Cerebral Oximetry

Brief overview
It is well established that neurologic injury such as stroke and neurocognitive dysfunction is a common complication of vascular surgery due to cerebral ischemia and hypoxia, and that conventional hemodynamic monitoring may not adequately assess cerebral perfusion.[18] Near-infrared spectroscopy (NIRS) uses infrared light on the relative transparency of the scalp and skull, and the differential absorption capacity of oxy- and deoxy-hemoglobin to quantify regional oxygen saturation of hemoglobin continuously in real-time.[37] In practice, electrode sensors are placed over the frontotemporal regions of the brain allowing for estimation of the oxy-hemoglobin saturation associated with the white matter of the watershed areas between the anterior cerebral artery and the middle cerebral artery.

Indications
NIRS application was first described by Jöbsis[38], and has been studied extensively over the past four decades with mixed results in different surgical populations. It has been previously reported that cerebral ischemia occurs when regional brain oxygen saturation (rSO2) falls below 20% of baseline,[39] which is measured before preoxygenation of patients during induction of anesthesia. Therefore, it is suggested that intervention occur when rSO2 drops below 20% of baseline when baseline rSO2 is > 50%, or when rSO2 drops below 15% of baseline in patients with baseline rSO2 < 50%.[40] In 2002, a randomized controlled study of 200 patients by Murkin and colleagues[41] showed that cerebral oximetry monitoring decreased intensive care unit length of stay, mortality, major organ damage, and stroke rate in patients undergoing coronary artery bypass surgery. Since then, many studies have failed to reproduce those results, and in 2017 a meta-analysis that included 15 studies showed that data favored against using cerebral oximetry in cardiac surgery due to its lack of

clinical significance, cost, and limitations.[40] CEA surgery, however, involves the unique phenomenon of occluding one side of the brain's oxygen supply during cross-clamp of the carotid artery. Cerebral oximetry can be considered during this period to determine if a shunt around the occlusion may be needed to maintain adequate brain oxygenation due to a dysfunctional Circle of Willis. A small study by Fassiadis and colleagues[42] showed that cerebral oximetry correlated well with the mean flow velocity obtained by measuring stump pressures, and because stump pressures were unable to be reliably monitored in over 30% of patients, cerebral oximetry may be a superior method of monitoring. These results were reproduced in a trial by Ali and colleagues[43] who also showed that cerebral oximetry was more accurate in predicting need for shunt compared with stump pressures. To date, there are no clinical trials that show a clear correlation between cerebral oximetry and stump pressures, or other forms of neuromonitoring, specifically EEG and SSEP monitoring.[44]

Complications and limitations
Although there are no true complications of using NIRS, there are several limitations. The rSO2 measurement is independent of weight, height, and gender, but because the position of the probe measures rSO2 of the underlying anatomy, measurements can be inaccurate if congenital, structural, or traumatic skull defects are present.[45] It should also be noted that NIRS only measures approximately 1 cm of brain tissue, so exact placement along the watershed regions is prone to human error. Another great limitation of cerebral oximetry is that it likely reflects primarily cerebral venous blood, not arterial blood. Therefore although it may reflect regional changes in oxygen consumption or delivery, it does not directly or specifically sample arterial oxygenation. Furthermore, due to the minute area of brain tissue being monitored, strokes of the posterior circulation or brainstem will go undetected.[40] As these spectrometers are unable to differentiate between the various forms of hemoglobin (carboxyhemoglobin, fetal hemoglobin, methemoglobin etc.), atypical hemoglobin forms and molecules with similar absorption peaks (bilirubin and biliverdin) may confound readings.[39]

DISCUSSION

The complications of vascular surgery carry significant morbidity. Carotid and open/endovascular aortic surgeries may be complicated by devastating SCI, stroke, and myocardial infarction due to common perioperative events including cardiovascular collapse, hemorrhage, increased afterload from aortic cross-clamp, and disruption of SC blood flow due to graft placement. In the case of carotid surgery, the tightly controlled autoregulatory mechanisms for blood flow and oxygenation are often impaired following carotid cross-clamp, which may result in long-term injuries including cognitive impairment, psychological distress, postoperative delirium, and debilitating strokes.[39] Although standard ASA monitors and arterial waveform analysis may not be adequately sophisticated to prevent neurologic injury, the use of subspecialized monitoring modalities discussed in this review is still controversial. Although there are clear indications for lumbar drains and electrophysiologic monitoring during open and endovascular aortic repair, recommended indications for the use of TEE are less defined and leave room for interpretation. Cerebral oximetry provides a noninvasive estimate of cerebral oxygenation, but remains an evolving technology, and should be used adjunctively with conventional forms of monitoring. In the future, we recommend additional, high-quality investigations to guide the management of these monitoring techniques across vascular surgery populations. The well-informed anesthesiologist should be familiar with all monitoring modalities, and understand the indications as well as limitations associated with each.

CLINICS CARE POINTS

- Consider cerebrospinal fluid drainage in any patient undergoing open or thoracic aortic repair with increased risk for spinal cord ischemia.

- Discuss goals of cerebrospinal fluid drainage with the surgical team. Often cerebrospinal fluid pressure should be maintained below 15 mm Hg and less than 15 mL/h.

- During carotid endarterectomy, discuss any significant change in somatosensory evoked potentials with the surgical team, and whether temporary carotid shunting is indicated.

- When using intraoperative neuromonitoring, remember that motor-evoked potentials are impaired by neuromuscular blocking agents. In addition, many commonly used anesthetics (ie, propofol and halogenated agents) as well as common intraoperative events (ie, hypotension, hypothermia) can cause a dose-dependent impairment in amplitude and latency of evoked potentials.

- When monitoring cerebral oximetry, consider interventions to augment cerebral blood flow when regional brain oxygen saturation falls below 20% baseline.

DISCLOSURE

The authors have no relevant disclosures.

REFERENCES

1. Papworth D. Intraoperative monitoring during vascular surgery. Anesthesiol Clin North America 2004;22(2):223–50, vi.
2. American Society of Anesthesiologists. Standards for basic anesthetic monitoring. https://www.asahq.org/standards-and-guidelines/standards-for-basic-anesthetic-monitoring. [Accessed April 2022].
3. BLAISDELL FW, COOLEY DA. The mechanism of paraplegia after temporary thoracic aortic occlusion and its relationship to spinal fluid pressure. Surgery 1962;51:351–5. PMID: 13869747.
4. Miyamoto K, Ueno A, Wada T, et al. A new and simple method of preventing spinal cord damage following temporary occlusion of the thoracic aorta by draining the cerebrospinal fluid. J Cardiovasc Surg 1960;1:188–97.
5. Dasmahapatra HK, Coles JG, Wilson GJ, et al. Relationship between cerebrospinal fluid dynamics and reversible spinal cord ischemia during experimental thoracic aortic occlusion. J Thorac Cardiovasc Surg 1988;95(5):920–3. Available at: http://www.ncbi.nlm.nih.gov/pubmed/3361940.
6. McCullough JL, Hollier LH, Nugent M. Paraplegia after thoracic aortic occlusion: influence of cerebrospinal fluid drainage. Experimental and early clinical results. J Vasc Surg 1988;7(1):153–60. Available at: http://www.ncbi.nlm.nih.gov/pubmed/3336121.
7. Coselli JS, LeMaire SA, de Figueiredo LP, et al. Paraplegia after thoracoabdominal aortic aneurysm repair: is dissection a risk factor? Ann Thorac Surg 1997;63(1):28–35 [discussion: 35-6].
8. Safi HJ, Hess KR, Randel M, et al. Cerebrospinal fluid drainage and distal aortic perfusion: reducing neurologic complications in repair of thoracoabdominal aortic aneurysm types I and II. J Vasc Surg 1996;23(2):223–8 [discussion: 229].
9. Hnath JC, Mehta M, Taggert JB, et al. Strategies to improve spinal cord ischemia in endovascular thoracic aortic repair: outcomes of a prospective cerebrospinal fluid drainage protocol. J Vasc Surg 2008;48(4):836–40.

10. Hiratzka LF, Bakris GL, Beckman JA, et al. 2010 ACCF/AHA/AATS/ACR/ASA/SCA/SCAI/SIR/STS/SVM Guidelines for the diagnosis and management of patients with thoracic aortic disease. A Report of the American College of Cardiology Foundation/American Heart Association Task Force on Practice Guidelines, A. J Am Coll Cardiol 2010;55(14):e27–129.

11. Etz CD, Weigang E, Hartert M, et al. Contemporary spinal cord protection during thoracic and thoracoabdominal aortic surgery and endovascular aortic repair: a position paper of the vascular domain of the European Association for Cardio-Thoracic Surgery. Eur J Cardiothorac Surg 2015;47(6):943–57.

12. Awad H, Ramadan ME, El Sayed HF, et al. Spinal cord injury after thoracic endovascular aortic aneurysm repair. Can J Anaesth 2017;64(12):1218–35.

13. Estrera AL, Sheinbaum R, Miller CC, et al. Cerebrospinal fluid drainage during thoracic aortic repair: safety and current management. Ann Thorac Surg 2009; 88(1):9–15 [discussion: 15].

14. Hanna JM, Andersen ND, Aziz H, et al. Results with selective preoperative lumbar drain placement for thoracic endovascular aortic repair. Ann Thorac Surg 2013; 95(6):1968–74 [discussion: 1974-5].

15. Estrera AL, Miller CC, Huynh TTT, et al. Preoperative and operative predictors of delayed neurologic deficit following repair of thoracoabdominal aortic aneurysm. J Thorac Cardiovasc Surg 2003;126(5):1288–94.

16. Brott TG, Hobson RW, Howard G, et al. Stenting versus endarterectomy for treatment of carotid-artery stenosis. N Engl J Med 2010;363(1):11–23.

17. Li J, Shalabi A, Ji F, et al. Monitoring cerebral ischemia during carotid endarterectomy and stenting. J Biomed Res 2017;31(1). https://doi.org/10.7555/JBR.31. 20150171.

18. Hans SS, Jareunpoon O. Prospective evaluation of electroencephalography, carotid artery stump pressure, and neurologic changes during 314 consecutive carotid endarterectomies performed in awake patients. J Vasc Surg 2007;45(3): 511–5.

19. General anaesthesia versus local anaesthesia for carotid surgery (GALA): a multicentre, randomised controlled trial. Lancet 2008;372(9656):2132–42.

20. Reddy RP, Brahme IS, Karnati T, et al. Diagnostic value of somatosensory evoked potential changes during carotid endarterectomy for 30-day perioperative stroke. Clin Neurophysiol 2018;129(9):1819–31.

21. Nwachuku EL, Balzer JR, Yabes JG, et al. Diagnostic value of somatosensory evoked potential changes during carotid endarterectomy: a systematic review and meta-analysis. JAMA Neurol 2015;72(1):73–80.

22. Weigang E, Hartert M, Siegenthaler MP, et al. Perioperative management to improve neurologic outcome in thoracic or thoracoabdominal aortic stent-grafting. Ann Thorac Surg 2006;82(5):1679–87.

23. Schurink GWH, De Haan MW, Peppelenbosch AG, et al. Spinal cord function monitoring during endovascular treatment of thoracoabdominal aneurysms: implications for staged procedures. J Cardiovasc Surg (Torino) 2013;54(1 Suppl 1):117–24. Available at: http://www.ncbi.nlm.nih.gov/pubmed/23443596.

24. Banga PV, Oderich GS, Reis de Souza L, et al. Neuromonitoring, cerebrospinal fluid drainage, and selective use of iliofemoral conduits to minimize risk of spinal cord injury during complex endovascular aortic repair. J Endovasc Ther 2016; 23(1):139–49.

25. Legatt AD, Emerson RG, Epstein CM, et al. ACNS Guideline: Transcranial Electrical Stimulation Motor Evoked Potential Monitoring. J Clin Neurophysiol 2016; 33(1):42–50.

26. Ghatol D, Widrich J. Intraoperative Neurophysiological Monitoring. 2022. http://www.ncbi.nlm.nih.gov/pubmed/33085350. [Accessed April 2022].

27. Arnold M, Sturzenegger M, Schäffler L, et al. Continuous intraoperative monitoring of middle cerebral artery blood flow velocities and electroencephalography during carotid endarterectomy. A comparison of the two methods to detect cerebral ischemia. Stroke 1997;28(7):1345–50. https://doi.org/10.1161/01.str.28.7.1345.

28. Woodworth GF, McGirt MJ, Than KD, et al. Selective versus routine intraoperative shunting during carotid endarterectomy: a multivariate outcome analysis. Neurosurgery 2007;61(6):1170–6 [discussion: 1176-7].

29. Sloan TB. Anesthetic effects on electrophysiologic recordings. J Clin Neurophysiol 1998;15(3):217–26.

30. Side CD, Gosling RG. Non-surgical assessment of cardiac function. Nature 1971;232(5309):335–6.

31. Frazin L, Talano JV, Stephanides L, et al. Esophageal echocardiography. Circulation 1976;54(1):102–8.

32. Matsuzaki M, Matsuda Y, Ikee Y, et al. Esophageal echocardiographic left ventricular anterolateral wall motion in normal subjects and patients with coronary artery disease. Circulation 1981;63(5):1085–92.

33. Orihashi K. The history of transesophageal echocardiography: the role of inspiration, innovation, and applications. J Anesth 2020;34(1):86–94.

34. Fayad A, Shillcutt SK. Perioperative transesophageal echocardiography for noncardiac surgery. Can J Anaesth 2018;65(4):381–98.

35. Purza R, Ghosh S, Walker C, et al. Transesophageal echocardiography complications in adult cardiac surgery: a retrospective cohort study. Ann Thorac Surg 2017;103(3):795–802.

36. Shanewise JS, Cheung AT, Aronson S, et al. ASE/SCA guidelines for performing a comprehensive intraoperative multiplane transesophageal echocardiography examination: recommendations of the American Society of Echocardiography Council for Intraoperative Echocardiography and the Society of Cardiovasc. Anesth Analg 1999;89(4):870–84.

37. Scheeren TWL, Schober P, Schwarte LA. Monitoring tissue oxygenation by near infrared spectroscopy (NIRS): background and current applications. J Clin Monit Comput 2012;26(4):279–87.

38. Jöbsis FF. Noninvasive, infrared monitoring of cerebral and myocardial oxygen sufficiency and circulatory parameters. Science 1977;198(4323):1264–7.

39. Edmonds HL, Ganzel BL, Austin EH. Cerebral oximetry for cardiac and vascular surgery. Semin Cardiothorac Vasc Anesth 2004;8(2):147–66.

40. Raza SS, Ullah F, Chandni, et al. Cerebral Oximetry Use For Cardiac Surgery. J Ayub Med Coll Abbottabad. 29(2):335-339. http://www.ncbi.nlm.nih.gov/pubmed/28718260. [Accessed April 2022].

41. Murkin JM, Adams SJ, Novick RJ, et al. Monitoring brain oxygen saturation during coronary bypass surgery: a randomized, prospective study. Anesth Analg 2007;104(1):51–8.

42. Fassiadis N, Zayed H, Rashid H, et al. Invos Cerebral Oximeter compared with the transcranial Doppler for monitoring adequacy of cerebral perfusion in patients undergoing carotid endarterectomy. Int Angiol 2006;25(4):401–6. Available at: http://www.ncbi.nlm.nih.gov/pubmed/17164748.

43. Ali AM, Green D, Zayed H, et al. Cerebral monitoring in patients undergoing carotid endarterectomy using a triple assessment technique. Interact Cardiovasc Thorac Surg 2011;12(3):454–7.

44. Friedell ML, Clark JM, Graham DA, et al. Cerebral oximetry does not correlate with electroencephalography and somatosensory evoked potentials in determining the need for shunting during carotid endarterectomy. J Vasc Surg 2008; 48(3):601–6.
45. Tan ST. Cerebral oximetry in cardiac surgery. Hong Kong Med J = Xianggang Yi Xue Za Zhi 2008;14(3):220–5. Available at: http://www.ncbi.nlm.nih.gov/pubmed/18525092.

Abdominal Aortic Aneurysms (Etiology, Epidemiology, and Natural History)

Michael P. Calgi, BS[a], John S. McNeil, MD[b],*

KEYWORDS

- Abdominal aortic aneurysm • Vascular surgery • Vascular anesthesiology
- Tobacco use

KEY POINTS

- The incidence of the abdominal aortic aneurysm has decreased worldwide due to reductions in tobacco use.
- Male sex and advanced age, among others, are risk factors for the development of an abdominal aortic aneurysm, and most screening guidelines were designed accordingly.
- Unfortunately, outcomes for those outside this demographic are worse, with women at greater risk for mortality from aortic rupture and African Americans at greater risk for re-rupture.
- Endovascular repair is now more common than open repair; although both are considered high-risk, outcomes are significantly better when performed electively rather than after rupture, highlighting the importance of effective screening.
- Recent advances include the use of artificial intelligence to more accurately measure the diameter using computed tomography and a further understanding of genetics in abdominal aortic aneurysm predisposition; a pharmacologic treatment to slow growth however is still missing.

INTRODUCTION/HISTORY/DEFINITIONS/BACKGROUND

The abdominal aorta is the portion of the descending aorta between the diaphragm and the common iliac artery bifurcation. A retroperitoneal structure, it courses through the diaphragm at the aortic hiatus, typically at the level of T12, and gradually tapers in diameter until dividing into the iliac arteries at L4. Important embryonic differences

[a] University of Virginia School of Medicine, 200 Jeanette Lancaster Way, Charlottesville, VA 22903, USA; [b] Department of Anesthesiology, University of Virginia School of Medicine, PO Box 800710, Charlottesville, VA 22908-0710, USA
* Corresponding author.
E-mail address: jsm6j@virginia.edu

Anesthesiology Clin 40 (2022) 657–669
https://doi.org/10.1016/j.anclin.2022.08.010
1932-2275/22/© 2022 Elsevier Inc. All rights reserved.
anesthesiology.theclinics.com

Abbreviations	
AAA	Abdominal aortic aneursym

exist between the portion of the descending aorta that is thoracic and the portion that is abdominal, with the former possessing neural-crest derived smooth muscle cells with additional elastic lamellae (**Table 1**) to better withstand greater pulse pressure.[1]

An abdominal aortic aneurysm (AAA) is the most common site of an arterial aneurysm. It is defined as dilation greater than 50% of the expected aortic diameter; clinically, this is often simplified to > 3 cm. Classification is by relation to the mesenteric and renal arteries. Approximately 85% are located below the renal arteries (infrarenal); infrequently they involve the mesenteric arteries (suprarenal), the renal arteries (pararenal), or are just distal to the renal arteries (juxtarenal). Most AAAs are fusiform, meaning they involve the whole circumference of the artery; saccular aneurysms, which bulge on just one side, have a higher risk of rupture. The first documented evidence of dilation of this vessel dates back to second century AD, when Antyllus diagnosed (and surgically treated) the first AAA.[2]

Nature of the Problem

Aneurysmal development is likely multifactorial but centers around a systemic inflammatory response linked to several clear risk factors. Histologically, AAA tissue shows a variety of perturbations including inflammation, oxidative stress, and extracellular matrix degradation.[3] These changes have been found to occur with tobacco use, especially in the tunica media. An animal study using implanted tobacco osmotic minipumps found that tobacco damaged the elastic lamella of major arteries, and that effect was more pronounced in the abdominal aorta than the thoracic.[4] Alternatively, some researchers believe the immune system may play a role in AAA development, with antibodies created after a bacterial or viral infection later attacking aortic proteins that mimic the microorganism.[1,5] Irrespective of mechanism, cell counts in aneurysmal tissue have shown decreased vascular smooth cells but an increased number of stem cells; the latter suggests that the tissue may be attempting to heal itself and may provide an avenue for future therapy.[1]

Epidemiology

In the twentieth century, AAA was a disease on the rise, with steadily climbing rates of incidence and mortality.[6,7] However, by the twenty-first century these trends reversed around the world.[8–10] A 25-year prevalence study in the UK with screening abdominal ultrasound performed in more than 80,000 65-year-old men showed a decrease in prevalence from 5.0% in 1991% to 1.3% in 2015.[9] This finding is consistent with other modern studies which show a prevalence between 1.3% and 3.0% in similar patient

Table 1	
Three layers of an artery	
Tunica Adventitia	Outermost, connective tissue layer that is predominantly collagen and fibroblasts, provides structure and prevents excess expansion when blood pressure increases
Tunica media	Middle, contractile tissue layer that provides elasticity, primarily smooth muscle cells, and elastic lamellae
Tunica intima	Innermost and thinnest, the endothelial layer that is in direct contact with blood

populations that are considered to be high risk.[8,9,11] Although the decrease in prevalence may be due to several factors, it is most often attributed to reduced tobacco use, which is the most significant modifiable risk factor for AAA development.[8] Mean annual incidence of AAA development is currently estimated to be around 0.4% in western populations.[12] In men, the incidence of acute events secondary to AAA such as hemodynamic instability, severe abdominal pain, or limb ischemia is positively correlated with both age and tobacco use. Two-thirds of these acute events occur in patients over the age of 75 and more than 96% occur in patients with a smoking history.[13]

A lack of direct screening data outside of the older male demographic makes the determination of general population prevalence challenging. Currently, the United States Preventative Services Task Force (USPSTF) recommends a one-time screening abdominal ultrasound for men age 65 to 75 with a smoking history. Recommendations for male non-smokers are selective, with screening decisions deferred to clinical judgment while testing for women is either recommended against or without the recommendation in cases of a positive smoking history.[14] These guidelines stem from older studies that argued for the cost-effectiveness and mortality benefits of testing when disease prevalence was higher than currently reported.[15] Notably, most AAAs detected from screening are small and at low risk for rupture (rAAA), which may further inform decision-making regarding testing recommendations in the future.[16] Thus, efforts to determine general population prevalence have relied on algorithms and regression analyses to generate predictions based on the prevalence of known concomitant risk factors and their strength of association with AAA. One such study, applying data obtained on more than 3 million patients evaluated for the disease, estimated there are 1.1 million Americans with AAA, or a 1.4% prevalence in all Americans age 50 to 84.[9] Individuals that fall under the existing USPSTF guidelines as being recommended for screening would only account for approximately 30% of the estimated national prevalence. Identification of more subtle risk factors for development, expansion, and rupture of AAA could reveal insights into the presentation of the estimated remaining 70% of Americans.

Risk Factors

Sex and age
It is well-established that male sex and increasing age are strong independent risk factors for the development of AAA.[10–12,17] Individuals over the age of 75 have a 3 to 8 times greater risk of having an AAA than those between 65 and 74.[11,12] These aneurysms are rare in individuals less than 50; thus, the prevailing approach remains that there is not a significant mortality benefit to screening individuals before age 65. One-third of all acute AAA events occur after age 85, with that proportion expected to increase in the future due to aging populations.[13] Interestingly, the increasing prevalence with age does not seem to be correlated with increasing aneurysm size.[10] Male sex is associated with a 2.7 to 3.8 times greater risk of AAA than the female sex over age 65.[11,12] Indeed, incidence of hospitalizations related to acute AAA is significantly higher for men than women, even when controlling for other comorbidities.[18] This trend does not hold, however, with morbidity and mortality. Of total hospitalizations for AAA, multiple studies confirm women account for roughly 30%,[18,19] yet almost 54% of females presenting to a hospital with rAAA die compared with 42% of males. When adjusting for covariates, females have a 14% to 44% greater risk of in-hospital mortality compared with males when repair of an rAAA is performed.[18] More research needs to be performed into why such a difference exists. Leading hypotheses currently include differences in screening practices, anatomic variances, and the use of historically male aortic size thresholds for informing management.[18–20]

Tobacco use

Smoking status is the most important modifiable risk factor for the development of AAA and a significant risk factor for acute AAA events.[10–13,19] In recent studies, approximately 80% of all patients diagnosed with AAA were ever-smokers.[10,12,13] When age-matched nonsmokers were compared with those that smoked at least one pack per day, the latter group had a greater than 13 times increased risk of AAA.[12] A positive dose-dependent relationship exists between pack years and AAA, and an inverse association occurs with years since smoking cessation.[10] For example, patients who quit smoking for greater than 10 years will have less than half the risk of patients that quit only 2 years ago. A systematic review of prospective studies showed that relative risk of AAA formation returns to non-smoker levels after 25 years of smoking cessation.[21] Although there is a lack of equivalent studies in humans, murine models exposed to e-cigarette vapors have shown aortic wall changes consistent with AAA formation similar to changes seen with conventional cigarettes.[22,23] Smoking status has also been linked to increased growth rates of small AAA, leading to quicker disease progression.[24,25]

Race and family history

A positive family history, and to a lesser extent certain races, have been strongly associated with the development of AAA.[10,11,26,27] African Americans, Hispanics, and Asians have shown lower prevalence of AAA when compared with non-Hispanic whites and Native Americans, after controlling for other risk factors.[10] Non-Hispanic whites, specifically, have a greater risk of hospitalization and mortality from acute AAA events.[26] In a recent study, no differences in mortality have been found between different races in the perioperative window following elective AAA repair, overall and when controlling for surgery type.[28] However, African Americans have higher rates of delayed re-rupture following surgery and subsequent return for reintervention.[28,29]

A significantly greater prevalence of AAA has been reported in first-degree relatives of affected patients compared with the general population, regardless of environmental exposure history, familial risk with AAA is likely quite high. Prevalence is almost 10-fold higher in brothers and almost 4-fold higher in sisters of individuals with AAA when compared with a 65-year-old control.[27] This trend has been reproduced in twin studies.[30] The genetic entity contributing to familial forms of AAA is thought to likely be different than those genes that increase risk in the sporadic form of the disease, as the vast majority of patients with AAA do not report a family history.[30] Genetics research has yet to uncover high-risk genes specifically for AAA, although genome-wide association studies (GWAS) and family-based linkage analyses have identified over 30 single-nucleotide polymorphisms (SNPs) associated with the disease.[31,32] Interestingly, some SNPs significantly associated with AAA have also been implicated in coronary artery disease, although more research is needed to determine if these findings are contributory to pathogenesis or present due to concurrent heart disease. The highly penetrant, rare, monogenetic disorders such as Marfan syndrome, Ehlers-Danlos syndrome, and others seem to be more closely linked to thoracic aortic aneurysms than AAA.[31]

Other factors

Many patients with AAA have other vascular comorbidities. More than 25% have CAD, 15% have a history of peripheral artery disease (PAD), and close to two-thirds have dyslipidemia.[10,11,13] However, a consistent dose–response relationship has not been established between atherosclerotic disease burden and AAA diameter,[33] making it unclear whether concurrence is due to causation or merely similar risk factors.

Evidence pointing toward both diseases sharing a different pathogenesis include lower atherosclerotic burden in patients with familial AAA rather than sporadic AAA,[34] and diabetes mellitus (DM) having a negative association with AAA but a positive association with cardiovascular disease.[35] However, further studies have proposed the protective effects of DM lie within treatment regimens, with patients using metformin having slower growing aneurysms and less acute events.[36] Hypertension is less associated with AAA development but is a significant predictor of acute AAA events after age 85, becoming more important than smoking status.[18]

Diets high in antioxidants, such as fruits, vegetables, and nuts, have been associated with decreased incidence of AAA development and rupture.[10,37] These findings are more pronounced in women than men. Similarly, increased physical activity seems to reduce the risk of AAA development in multiple studies, although specific dose–response relationships are unclear.[10,38] No medications have yet been shown to reduce the risk of rupture or AAA growth in randomized clinical trials for AAA patients,[39,40] and several drugs studied prospectively have actually been found to increase rate of aneurysmal growth (doxycycline, angiotensin-converting enzyme (ACE)-inhibitors).[41,42] Statins, potentially via an anti-inflammatory effect, seem to be beneficial but have only been studied retrospectively.[43] As aforementioned, metformin, while currently only explored in observational studies in diabetic patients, seems to show an ability to limit growth and rupture.[44] Clinical trials to evaluate the efficacy of metformin use in the non-diabetic population are currently underway, with results expected in the next few years.[45–48]

Natural history

The natural history and progression of AAAs follow a classic course, with a subclinical stage, then progression with potential for clinical detection, and an eventual resolution resulting in either repair or death secondary to rupture with acute severe hemorrhage. The subclinical phase is marked by cellular and subcellular changes that weaken the aortic wall and predispose it toward aneurysm formation. AAAs are most commonly detected incidentally or via screening efforts, as unruptured AAAs are generally asymptomatic during development.[13,14,38] Once AAAs rupture or reach a state indicating a high risk of rupture, patients must undergo surgical repair to prevent mortality.

Progression and detection

Weakening of the abdominal aortic wall via aneurysm pathogenesis leads to progressive enlargement, which is positively correlated with rupture risk. This phenomenon is also supported biomechanically, as widening vessel diameter increases peak wall stress and places greater tension on an already weakened aorta.[49] Aneurysm size has historically been one of the main predictors of further growth and rupture risk.[50] Likelihood of rupture is low in patients with aneurysms less than 5 cm in diameter, with a cumulative 1-year risk of less than 1%. Yearly rupture risk increases to 5.3% for AAA greater than 5.5 cm and 6.3% for those greater than 7.0 cm.[51] Similarly, larger aneurysm size is associated with an increased growth rate; each 0.5 cm increase over baseline AAA diameter results in a 0.59 mm per year increase in size.[50] At the time of diagnosis when classic screening of elderly males is used, more than 90% of patients with AAA present with a diameter of less than 5.5 cm, indicating low rupture risk.[8,14]

Other intrinsic characteristics of an AAA may influence early rupture and accelerated progression. Those individuals with small AAAs and a positive family history have faster growth and subsequently higher rupture risk, likely secondary to differences in pathogenesis.[52] Finite element analysis and modeling of wall stress have revealed that factors such as aneurysm shape and wall strength can significantly influence rupture and may be more sensitive measures than diameter.[53,54] Computational modeling of wall stress has revealed that women experience a higher proportion of aneurysms with elevated peak wall stress.[55] Interestingly, the female sex remains an independent predictor of rupture after controlling for wall stress, suggesting other mechanisms beyond relative aorta size differences contribute to varying outcomes between sexes.

Non-rAAAs present asymptomatically for the vast majority of patients; the presence of symptoms is uncommon and is associated with a greater risk of rupture and then a two-fold increase in perioperative mortality compared with asymptomatic AAA repair.[56] When symptoms do occur, abdominal, back, or flank pain are most often reported. This pain commonly mimics cholecystitis, appendicitis, or pancreatitis, and thus a high index of suspicion is necessary.[57] Co-occurrence of spinal degeneration in the at-risk demographic may also mask back pain from AAA. Case reports have noted expanding aneurysms can cause symptoms of mass effect, such as focal neurologic deficits from nerve root compression; the femoral nerve is most commonly affected.[58] In addition, AAAs may create a blood flow environment conducive to thrombus formation that may occasionally lead to acute thrombosis and bilateral lower limb ischemia.[59,60] In rare circumstances, mycotic aneurysms may form from hematogenous seeding and show exceedingly high rupture rates of approximately 75% at the time of repair.[61] In less than 1% of AAAs, a fistula may form between the aorta and inferior vena cava leading to symptoms of syncope, high output heart failure, and renal insufficiency.

Owing to the frequent asymptomatic presentation of AAAs, most of these aneurysms are diagnosed non-acutely by physical examination, routine screening, or as incidental findings on abdominal imaging.[57] Abdominal palpation and auscultation are limited by aneurysm size and the patient's body habitus. Palpation of a pulsatile abdominal mass is a moderately sensitive marker for AAA diagnosis, with the sensitivity of 68% and specificity of 75%.[62] Auscultation of an abdominal bruit is more specific (95%) but is infrequently heard, with a sensitivity of only 11%.[63] The use of abdominal ultrasound as a screening tool, as recommended by USPSTF guidelines, has a sensitivity of 95% and specificity approaching 100%.[61] The Society for Vascular Surgery recommends further regular ultrasound screening at 3-year, 12-month, or 6-month intervals, depending on aneurysm size, to monitor for growth.[57] However, effective ultrasound measuring is operator dependent, and computed tomography remains the gold standard for quantifying aneurysm size and instability[64] (**Fig. 1**). Diameters measured on computed tomography are typically approximately 5 mm greater than those measured with ultrasound; the former allows aortic diameter measurement

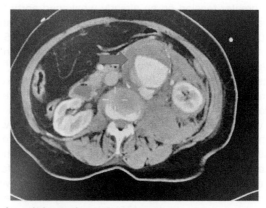

Fig. 1. CT image of an abdominal aortic aneurysm.

in any plane, whereas the latter is limited to anterior-posterior and transverse planes.[65] Three-dimensional computed tomography reconstructions are now created to aid in surgical planning for repair (**Fig. 2**).

Abdominal imaging may also reveal incidental AAAs, with one survey of 80,000 images showing a 1.4% aneurysm detection rate in an elderly population receiving ultrasound, computed tomography (CT), and MRI for other purposes.[66] However, in one study, only 16% of patients with incidental AAAs on imaging went on to receive appropriate monitoring. Incidental detection and subsequent appropriate observation or referral is therefore an area for potential improvement in mitigating rAAA. A robust imaging biomarker protocol for predicting AAA growth or rupture in humans does not currently exist [67] although artificial intelligence is being studied as a novel method for determining diameter on CT imaging.[68]

Resolution: Rupture and Repair

Clinical outcomes

Rupture is the most significant complication of AAAs, with a mortality rate often quoted at greater than 70%.[69] Approximately 37% of patients with rAAAs die in the community before presenting to the hospital, although this statistical is likely underreported due to inherent difficulties of confirming rAAA without an autopsy. Approximately 40% of rAAA patients reach the hospital but experience mortality before initiation of surgery. The yearly incidence of fatal rAAA in the general population of the United States is estimated to be 15 per 1 million.[70] The classic presentation of rAAA consists of acute onset back and/or abdominal pain accompanied by symptoms of shock. Notably, however, pain may only be present in half of these patients.[71] Other initial symptoms of rAAA are significantly less prevalent and include

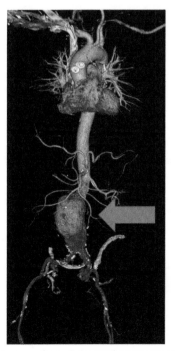

Fig. 2. 3D reconstructed CT image of an abdominal aortic aneurysm.

presentations such as transient lower limb paralysis, paresthesias in the femoral nerve distribution, and pelvic ecchymoses.[72,73] Rupture most commonly causes extravasation of blood into the retroperitoneal space, with bleeding extending up to the pararenal spaces and then the intraperitoneal space with massive hemorrhage.[61,74] In cases of anterior aneurysm rupture, extravasation into the much larger intraperitoneal space is more likely.

Surgical techniques

Rupture can either be treated emergently or, ideally, prevented via elective surgical intervention. Current guidelines for intervention by the Society for Vascular Surgery[57] state that symptomatic aneurysms warrant immediate CT evaluation of rupture status with subsequent emergent repair if ruptured. If the AAA is symptomatic but unruptured, surgery can be briefly delayed to permit optimization of coexisting medical conditions in an intensive care unit setting. Recommendations for elective asymptomatic repair are less defined, with surgical indications including enlarged aneurysm size (greater than 5.5 cm) and accelerated growth rate (greater than 1 cm per year).[75,76] Current research, especially in computational modeling, is working to uncover more reliable metrics of rupture risk to triage elective AAA repair.[77]

Surgical interventions are either classified as open (**Fig. 3**) or endovascular aneurysm repair (EVAR). EVAR has been steadily displacing open repair as the primary form of unruptured and rAAA repair, with some form of endovascular intervention now comprising more than 80% of the total elective caseload in the United States in 2013.[57,78] Although EVAR has previously been associated with lower perioperative mortality, recent studies have found insignificant differences in perioperative and long-term mortality rates.[79,80] However, patients undergoing EVAR have a slightly higher

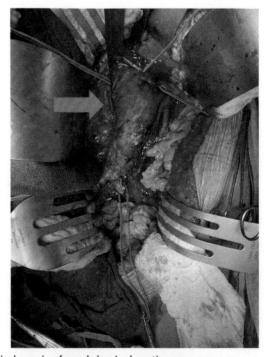

Fig. 3. Open surgical repair of an abdominal aortic aneurysm.

risk of requiring secondary procedures following initial intervention among studies since 2010 (12.9% vs 7.5%).[81] Major postoperative complications from both procedures may include ischemic colitis (23% of EVAR vs 42% of open cases), abdominal compartment syndrome (approximately 7%), and multisystem organ failure (approximately 3% of all cases).[57]

DISCLOSURE

No funding is involved with this manuscript. The content is solely the responsibility of the authors.

CONFLICTS OF INTEREST

M.P Calgi: None. J.S McNeil: None.

CLINICAL TRIAL NUMBER/REGISTRY URL

Not applicable.

CONTRIBUTIONS

M.P Calgi: This author created and edited the article. J.S McNeil: This author created and edited the article.

ACKNOWLEDGMENTS

The authors would like to thank Dr. Darrin Clouse for his assistance with manuscript preparation and for providing figures.

REFERENCES

1. Kuivaniemi H, Ryer EJ, Elmore JR, et al. Understanding the pathogenesis of abdominal aortic aneurysms. Expert Rev Cardiovasc Ther 2015;13(9):975–87.
2. Livesay JJ, Messner GN, Vaughn WK. Milestones in the treatment of aortic aneurysm: Denton A. Cooley, MD, and the Texas Heart Institute. Tex Heart Inst J 2005; 32(2):130–4.
3. Boddy AM, Lenk GM, Lillvis JH, et al. Basic research studies to understand aneurysm disease. Drug News Perspect 2008;21(3):142–8.
4. Azarbal AF, Repella T, Carlson E, et al. A Novel Model of Tobacco Smoke-Mediated Aortic Injury. Vasc Endovascular Surg 2022;56(3):244–52. https://doi.org/10.1177/15385744211063054. Epub 2021 Dec 27. PMID: 34961389.
5. Hinterseher I, Gäbel G, Corvinus F, et al. Presence of Borrelia burgdorferi sensu lato antibodies in the serum of patients with abdominal aortic aneurysms. Eur J Clin Microbiol Infect Dis 2012;31(5):781–9.
6. Filipovic M, Goldacre MJ, Roberts SE, et al. Trends in mortality and hospital admissions for abdominal aortic aneurysm in England and Wales, 1979-1999. Br J Surg 2005;92(8):968–75.
7. Gillum RF. epidemiology of aortic aneurysm in the United States. J Clin Epidemiol 1995;48(11):1289–98.
8. Svensjö S, Björck M, Gürtelschmid M, et al. Low prevalence of abdominal aortic aneurysm among 65-year-old Swedish men indicates a change in the epidemiology of the disease. Circulation 2011;124:1118–23.

9. Oliver-Williams C, Sweeting MJ, Turton G, et al. Lessons learned about prevalence and growth rates of abdominal aortic aneurysms from a 25-year ultrasound population screening programme. Br J Surg 2018;105(1):68–74.

10. Kent KC, Zwolak RM, Egorova NN, et al. Analysis of risk factors for abdominal aortic aneurysm in a cohort of more than 3 million individuals. J Vasc Surg 2010;52(3):539–48.

11. Summers KL, Kerut EK, Sheahan CM, et al. Evaluating the prevalence of abdominal aortic aneurysms in the United States through a national screening database. J Vasc Surg 2021;73(1):61–8.

12. Forsdahl SH, Singh K, Solberg S, et al. Risk factors for abdominal aortic aneurysms: A 7-year prospective study: The Tromsø study, 1994-2001. Circulation 2009;119(16):2202–8.

13. Howard DPJ, Banerjee A, Fairhead JF, et al. Population-based study of incidence of acute abdominal aortic aneurysms with projected impact of screening strategy. J Am Heart Assocaiton 2015;4(8):e001926.

14. Final Recommendation Statement: Abdominal Aortic Aneurysm: Screening. Uspreventiveservicestaskforce.org. Published December 10, 2019. Accessed December 22, 2021. Available at: https://www.uspreventiveservicestaskforce. org/uspstf/recommendation/abdominal-aortic-aneurysm-screening#citation35

15. Thompson SG, Ashton HA, Gao L, et al. Screening men for abdominal aortic aneurysm: 10 year mortality and cost effectiveness results from the randomized Multicentre Aneurysm Screening Study. BMJ 2009;338:b2307.

16. Mohansson M, Hansson A, Brodersen J. Estimating overdiagnosis in screening for abdominal aortic aneurysm: Could a change in smoking habits and lowered aortic diameter tip the balance of screening towards harm? BMJ 2015;350:h825.

17. Ashton HA, Buxton MJ, Day NE, et al. The Multicentre Aneurysm Screening Study (MASS) into the effect of abdominal aortic aneurysm screening on mortality in men: A randomised controlled trial. Lancet 2002;260(9345):1531–9.

18. Stuntz M, Audibert C, Su Z. Persisting disparities between sexes in outcomes of ruptured abdominal aortic aneurysm hospitalizations. Nat Scientific Rep 2017;7: 17994.

19. Kühnl A, Erik A, Trenner M, et al. Incidence, treatment and mortality in patients with abdominal aortic aneurysms: An analysis of hospital discharge data from 2005-2014. Deutsches Ärzteblatt Int 2017;114(22–23):391–8.

20. Sciria CT, Osorio B, Wang J, et al. Sex-based disparities in outcomes with abdominal aortic aneurysms. Am J Cardiol 2021;155:135–48.

21. Aune D, Schlesinger S, Norat T, et al. Tobacco smoking and the risk of abdominal aortic aneurysm: A systematic review and meta-analysis of prospective studies. Scientific Rep 2018;8(1):14786.

22. Mulorz J, Mulorz P, Wagenhaeuser MU, et al. E-cigarette vapor accelerates abdominal aortic aneurysm in mice [446]. Arterioscler Thromb Vasc Biol 2019; 39:A446. Available at: https://www.ahajournals.org/doi/abs/10.1161/atvb.39. suppl_1.446.

23. Clayton S, DeVallance E, Branyan K, et al. Vaping to vascular damage: The role of e-cigarettes on vascular function. FASEB J 2018;31(51):lb651.

24. MacSweeney ST, Ellis M, Worrell PC, et al. Smoking and growth rate of small abdominal aortic aneurysms. Lancet 1994;344(8923):651–2.

25. Blanchard JF, Armenian HK, Friesen PP. Risk factors for abdominal aortic aneurysm: Results of a case-control study. Am J Epidemiol 2000;151(6):575–83.

26. Li SR, Rietz KM, Gabriel L. The epidemiology of race- and sex-specific hospitalizations for abdominal aortic aneurysms [10519]. Circulation 2021;144(1). Available at: https://www.ahajournals.org/doi/abs/10.1161/circ.144.suppl_1.10519.
27. Linné A, Lindström D, Hultgren R. High prevalence of abdominal aortic aneurysms in brothers and sisters of patients despite a low prevalence in the population. J Vasc Surg 2012;56(2):305–10.
28. Deery SE, O'Donnell TFX, Shean KE, et al. Racial disparities in outcomes after intact abdominal aortic aneurysm repair. J Vasc Surg 2018;67(4):1059–67.
29. Marcaccio C, de Guerre L, Patel P, et al. Racial and ethnic differences in long-term outcomes after elective endovascular repair of abdominal aortic aneurysm. J Vasc Surg 2021;74(3):160–1. https://doi.org/10.1016/j.jvs.2021.06.244.
30. Joergensen TMM, Christensen K, Lindholt JS, et al. Editor's choice - high heritability of liability to abdominal aortic aneurysms: A population based twin study. Eur J Vasc Endovascular Surg 2016;52(1):41–6.
31. Pinard A, Jones GT, Milewicz DM. Genetics of thoracic and abdominal aortic diseases. Circ Res 2019;124(4):588–606.
32. Singh TP, Field MA, Bown MJ, et al. Systematic review of genome-wide association studies of abdominal aortic aneurysm. Atherosclerosis 2021;327:39–48. https://doi.org/10.1016/j.atherosclerosis.2021.05.001.
33. Takagi H, Umemoto T. Coronary. Coronary artery disease and abdominal aortic aneurysm growth. Vasc Med 2016;21(3):199–208.
34. van de Luijtgaarden KM, Gonçalves FB, Hoeks SE, et al. Lower atherosclerotic burden in familial abdominal aortic aneurysm. J Vasc Surg 2014;59(3):589–93.
35. Aune D, Schlesinger S, Norat T, et al. Diabetes mellitus and the risk of abdominal aortic aneurysm: A systematic review and meta-analysis of prospective studies. J Diabetes Its Complications 2018;32(12):1169–74.
36. Yuan Z, Heng Z, Lu Y, et al. The protective effect of metformin on abdominal aortic aneurysm: A systematic review and meta-analysis. Front Endocrinol 2021;12:721213.
37. Kaluza J, Stackelberg O, Harris HR, et al. Anti-inflammatory diet and risk of abdominal aortic aneurysm in two Swedish cohorts. Heart 2019;105(24):1876–83.
38. Aune D, Sen A, Kobeissi E, et al. Physical activity and the risk of abdominal aortic aneurysm: A systemic review and meta-analysis of prospective studies. Nat Scientific Rep 2020;10(1):22287.
39. Kokje VBC, Hamming JF, Lindeman JHN. Editor's choice – pharmaceutical management of small abdominal aortic aneurysms: A systematic review of the clinical experience. Eur J Vasc Endovascular Surg 2015;50(6):702–13.
40. Golledge J, Moxon JV, Singh TP, et al. Lack of an effective drug therapy for abdominal aortic aneurysm. J Intern Med 2020;288(1):6–22.
41. Meijer CA, Stijnen T, Wasser MN, et al. Doxycycline for stabilization of abdominal aortic aneurysms: a randomized trial. Ann Intern Med 2013;159(12):815–23.
42. Sweeting MJ, Thompson SG, Brown LC, et al. Use of angiotensin converting enzyme inhibitors is associated with increased growth rate of abdominal aortic aneurysms. J Vasc Surg 2010;52(1):1–4.
43. Karrowni W, Dughman S, Hajj GP, et al. Statin therapy reduces growth of abdominal aortic aneurysms. J Investig Med 2011;59(8):1239–43.
44. Thanigaimani S, Singh TP, Unosson J, et al. Editor's choice – Association between metformin prescription and abdominal aortic aneurysm growth and clinical events: A systematic review and meta-analysis. Eur J Vasc Endovascular Surg 2021;62(5):747–56.

45. Metformin Therapy in Non-diabetic AAA Patients (MetAAA). Clinicaltrials.gov. Published April 25, 2018. Updated October 24, 2019. Available at: https://clinicaltrials.gov/ct2/show/NCT03507413. Accessed January 27, 2022.
46. Limiting AAA With Metformin (LIMIT) Trial (LIMIT). Clinicaltrials.gov Published Au'gust 5, 2020. Updated September 8, 2021. Available at: https://clinicaltrials.gov/ct2/show/NCT04500756. Accessed January 27, 2022.
47. Metformin for Abdominal Aortic Aneurysm Growth Inhibition (MAAAGI). Clinicaltrials.gov. Published January 13, 2020. Updated September 30, 2021. Available at: https://clinicaltrials.gov/ct2/show/NCT04224051. Accessed January 27, 2022.
48. Moxon JV, Parr A, Emeto TI, et al. Diagnosis and monitoring of abdominal aortic aneurysm: Current status and future prospects. Curr Probl Cardiol 2011;35(10):512–48.
49. Speelman L, Hellenthal FA, Pulinx B, et al. The influence of wall stress on AAA growth and biomarkers. Eur J Vasc Endovascular Surg 2010;39(4):410–6.
50. Thompson SG, Bown MJ, Sweeting MJ, et al. Surveillance intervals for small abdominal aortic aneurysms: A meta-analysis. JAMA 2013;309(8):806–13.
51. Parkinson F, Ferguson S, Lewis P, et al. Rupture rates of untreated large abdominal aortic aneurysms in patients unfit for elective repair. J Vasc Surg 2015;61(6):1606–12.
52. Akai A, Watanabe Y, Hoshina K, et al. Family history of aortic aneurysm is an independent risk factor for more rapid growth of small abdominal aortic aneurysms in Japan. J Vasc Surg 2015;61(2):287–90.
53. Hall AJ, Busse EF, McCarville DJ, et al. Aortic wall tension as a predictive factor for abdominal aortic aneurysm rupture: Improving the selection of patients for abdominal aortic aneurysm repair. Ann Vasc Surg 2000;14(2):152–7.
54. Doye BJ, Bappoo N, Syed MBJ, et al. Biomechanical assessment predicts aneurysm related events in patients with abdominal aortic aneurysm. Eur J Vasc Endovascular Surg 2020;60(3):365–73.
55. Fillinger MF, Marra SP, Raghavan ML, et al. Prediction of rupture risk in abdominal aortic aneurysm during observation: Wall stress versus diameter. J Vasc Surg 2003;37(4):724–32.
56. Soden PA, Zettervall SL, Ultee KHJ, et al. Outcomes for symptomatic abdominal aortic aneurysms in the American College of Surgeons National Surgical Quality Improvement Program (NSQIP). J Vasc Surg 2016;64(2):297–305.
57. Chaikoff EL, Dalman RL, Eskandari MK, et al. The Society for Vascular Surgery practice guidelines on the care of patients with an abdominal aortic aneurysm. J Vasc Surg 2018;67(1):2–77.
58. Wilberger JE Jr. Lumbosacral radiculopathy secondary to abdominal aortic aneurysms: Report of three cases. J Neurosurg 1983;58(6):965–7.
59. El-Kayali A, Al-Salman MMS. Unusual presentation of acute bilateral lower limb ischemia (thrombosis of abnormal aortic aneurysm). Ann Saudi Med 2001;21(5–6).
60. Li H, Chan YC, Cui D, et al. Acute thrombosis of an infrarenal abdominal aortic aneurysm presenting as bilateral critical lower limb ischemia. Vasc Endovascular Surg 2020;55(2):186–8.
61. Kumar Y, Hooda K, Li S, et al. Abdominal aortic aneurysm: Pictorial review of common appearances and complications. Ann Translation Med 2017;5(12):256.
62. Fink HA, Lederle FA, Roth CS, et al. The accuracy of physical examination to detect abdominal aortic aneurysm. Arch Intern Med 2000;160(6):833–6.
63. Lederle FA, Walker JM, Reinke DB. Selective screening for abdominal aortic aneurysms with physical examination and ultrasound. Arch Intern Med 1988;148(8):

1753–6. Available at: https://jamanetwork.com/journals/jamainternalmedicine/article-abstract/610308.

64. Wadgaonkar AD, Black JH 3rd, Weihe EK, et al. Abdominal aortic aneurysms revisted: MDCT with multiplanar reconstructions for identifying indicators of instability in the pre- and postoperative patient. Radiographics 2015;35(1):254–68.

65. Fadel BM, Mohty D, Kazzi BE, et al. Ultrasound Imaging of the Abdominal Aorta: A Comprehensive Review. J Am Soc Echocardiogr 2021;34(11):1119–36.

66. van Walraven C, Wong J, Morant K, et al. Incidence, follow-up, and outcomes of incidental abdominal aortic aneurysms. J Vasc Surg 2010;52(2):282–9.

67. Jalalzadeh H, Indrakusuma R, Planken RN, et al. Inflammation as a predictor of abdominal aortic aneurysm growth and rupture: A systematic review of imaging biomarkers. Eur J Vasc Endovascular Surg 2016;52(3):333–42.

68. Lareyre F, Chaudhuri A, Flory V, et al. Automatic measurement of maximal diameter of abdominal aortic aneurysm on computed tomography angiography using artificial intelligence [published online ahead of print, 2021 Dec 22]. Ann Vasc Surg 2021;S0890-5096(21):00963–8.

69. Reimerink JJ, van der Laan MJ, Koelemay MJ, et al. Systematic review and meta-analysis of population-based mortality from ruptured abdominal aortic aneurysm. Br J Surg 2013;100(11):1405–13.

70. Abdulameer H, Taii HA, Al-Kindi SG, et al. Epidemiology of fatal ruptured aortic aneurysms in the United States (1999-2016). J Vasc Surg 2019;69(2):278–384.

71. Akkersdijk GJM, van Bockel JH. Ruptured abdominal aortic aneurysm: Initial misdiagnosis and the effect on treatment. Eur J Surg 1998;164(1):29–34.

72. Banerjee A. Atypical manifestations of ruptured abdominal aortic aneurysms. Postgrad Med J 1993;69(807):6–11.

73. Metcalfe D, Sugand K, Thrumurthy SG, et al. Diagnosis of ruptured abdominal aortic aneurysm: A multicentre cohort study. Eur J Emerg Med 2016;23(5):386–90.

74. Vu K, Kaitoukov Y, Morin-Roy F, et al. Rupture signs on computed tomography, treatment, and outcome of abdominal aortic aneurysms. Insights into Imaging 2014;5(3):281–93.

75. Cao P, De Rango P, Verzini F, et al. Comparison of surveillance versus aortic endografting for small aneurysm repair (CAESAR): Results from a randomised trial. Eur J Vasc Endovascular Surg 2011;41(1):13–25.

76. Lederle FA, Johnson GR, Wilson SE, et al. Rupture rate of large abdominal aortic aneurysms in patients refusing or unfit for elective repair. JAMA 2002;287(22):2968–72.

77. Kontopodis N, Pantidis D, Dedes A, et al. The – not so – solid 5.5 cm threshold for abdominal aortic aneurysm repair: Facts, misinterpretations, and future directions. Front Surg 2016;3:1–6.

78. Suckow BD, Goodney PP, Columbo JA, et al. National trends in open surgical, endovascular, and branched-fenestrated endovascular aortic aneurysm repair in Medicare patients. J Vasc Surg 2017;67(6):1690–7.

79. Lederle FA, Kyriakides TC, Stroupe KT, et al. Open versus endovascular repair of abdominal aortic aneurysm. New Year J Med 2019;380:2126–35.

80. Lieberg J, Kadatski KG, Kals M, et al. Five-year survival after elective open and endovascular aortic aneurysm repair. Scand J Surg 2021;0(0):1–7.

81. Li B, Khan S, Salata K, et al. A systematic review and meta-analysis of the long-term outcomes of endovascular versus open repair of abdominal aortic aneurysm. J Vasc Surg 2019;70(3):954–69.

Thoracic and Thoracoabdominal Aneurysms
Etiology, Epidemiology, and Natural History

Ryan T. Downey, MD[a],*, Rebecca A. Aron, MD[b]

KEYWORDS

- Thoracic aneurysm • Thoracoabdominal aneurysms • Aneurysmal disease

KEY POINTS

- Thoracic aneurysms and thoracoabdominal aneurysms are common and often clinically silent until complications occur. The majority are diagnosed incidentally.
- Dissection and rupture are the most common complications of thoracic aortic aneurysms (TAAs) and thoracoabdominal aortic aneurysms (TAAAs) and are associated with high mortality.
- TAAs and TAAAs in younger patients without significant cardiovascular risk factors often have a genetic basis some of which include Marfan, Ehlers–Danlos, Loeys–Dietz, and bicuspid aortic valve.
- Most TAAs grow slowly over time. Factors that may accelerate growth include chronic dissection, larger aneurysm size, bicuspid aortic valve disease, and Marfan syndrome.
- Symptomatic aneurysms should be treated regardless of size.

INTRODUCTION: THORACIC AND THORACOABDOMINAL ANEURYSMS

Thoracic aortic aneurysms (TAAs) and thoracoabdominal aortic aneurysms (TAAAs) are often clinically silent but potentially fatal. For many patients, the first presentation of a TAA is death because of the high mortality rate of related complications including aortic dissection and rupture. Despite advancements in treatment, aneurysms of the thoracic aorta account for a significant number of deaths in the United States. According to the Centers for Disease Control and Prevention, aortic aneurysms (thoracic and abdominal) were the 16th leading cause of death among individuals 60 years and older between 1999 and 2019.[1] The presence of a TAA/TAAA may have implications for anesthetic

[a] Department of Radiology, The University of Nebraska Medical Center, 981045 Nebraska Medical Center, Omaha, NE 68198-1045, USA; [b] Department of Anesthesiology, The University of Nebraska Medical Center, 4202 Emile Street, Omaha, NE 68198-1045, USA
* Corresponding author.
E-mail address: ryan.downey@unmc.edu

Anesthesiology Clin 40 (2022) 671–683
https://doi.org/10.1016/j.anclin.2022.08.011
1932-2275/22/© 2022 Elsevier Inc. All rights reserved.
anesthesiology.theclinics.com

Abbreviations	
SMA	superior mesenteric artery
IMA	inferior mesenteric artery
TGF	transforming growth factor
AV	aortic valve
ACE	angiotensin-converting enzyme
ARBs	angiotensin receptor blockers

management. Therefore, anesthesiologists must be knowledgeable about the physiologic considerations and potential complications of thoracic aneurysmal disease.

BACKGROUND: AORTIC ANATOMY

The normal aortic wall is composed of three layers: the tunica intima, the tunica media, and the tunica adventitia. The intima is the thin, innermost layer composed of endothelial cells, subendothelial connective tissue, and an internal elastic lamina. The media is the largest component of the aortic wall and is composed of packed layers of smooth muscle cells and an extracellular matrix of structural proteins, notably elastin and collagen. The adventitia is composed predominantly of connective tissue with a few small vessels (vasa vasorum) which are the blood supply to the cells of the aortic wall.[2,3] The media is responsible for most of the mechanical properties of the aorta, though the adventitia provides some support.[3]

Anatomically, the thoracic aorta is divided into four parts[4,5]:

1. The *aortic root* extends from the annulus (or ventriculo-aortic junction) to the sinotubular junction and includes the aortic valve leaflets and attachments along with the sinuses of Valsalva that give rise to the coronary arteries.
2. The *ascending aorta* begins at the sinotubular junction and extends to the aortic arch at the origin of brachiocephalic artery.
3. The *aortic arch* is the short segment which begins at the origin of the brachiocephalic artery and ends at the left subclavian artery, giving rise to the brachiocephalic artery, left common carotid, and left subclavian artery.
4. The *descending aorta* begins at the left subclavian artery origin and extends to the level of the diaphragm.

Fig. 1 summarizes the relevant anatomy.

The aorta gradually tapers from the root to the diaphragmatic hiatus. The aortic size varies by age, gender, and body size, but in general, the diameter of the ascending aortic diameter for adults should not exceed 4 cm, and the diameter of the descending aorta should not exceed 3 cm.[6] **Table 1** summarizes the mean aortic diameters by location and sex.[7]

A common pathology of the aorta is the development of an aneurysm.[2] A true aneurysm is dilation of all three layers of the vessel wall more than 50% of the expected normal diameter. Ectasia is dilation of less than 50% of the normal arterial diameter. TAAs can involve one or more segments of the thoracic aorta, whereas TAAAs involve the descending aorta and a portion of the abdominal aorta.[8] Approximately, 60% of TAAs involve the aortic root or ascending aorta, 10% involve the arch, 10% involve the thoracoabdominal aorta, and 40% involve the descending aorta.[9] Fusiform and saccular are the two major aneurysm morphologies. The morphology type may have implications for treatment. With the more common fusiform aneurysms, all sides of the aortic wall dilate relatively symmetrically. With saccular aneurysms, aortic dilation is eccentric with focal ballooning of only a portion of the aortic wall.[10]

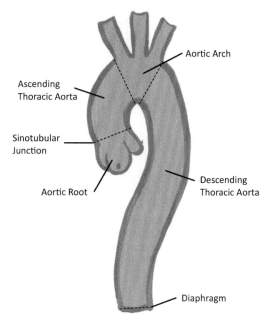

Fig. 1. Thoracic aortic aneurysm.

Although there is no widely applied classification system for TAAs, the *Crawford Classification* system is a commonly used classification system for TAAAs.[11] **Fig. 2** shows an example of a TAAA.

- *Type I* aneurysms extend from the origin of the left subclavian artery to the suprarenal abdominal aorta.
- *Type II* aneurysms extend from the left subclavian artery to the aortic bifurcation.
- *Type III* aneurysms involve the distal half of the descending aorta to the aortic bifurcation.
- *Type IV* aneurysms involve the entire abdominal aorta from the diaphragm to the aortic bifurcation.

ETIOLOGY AND RISK FACTORS
Degenerative

Most of the TAAs are degenerative in nature (and also referred to idiopathic or sporadic) and develop in patients with risk factors for atherosclerosis (eg, smoking and hypertension).[4] The pathogenesis is not fully understood; however, protein

Table 1		
Mean aortic diameters by sex		
Mean Aortic Diameter	**Male (cm)**	**Female (cm)**
Ascending aorta	3.4	3.1
Aortic arch	3.0	2.7
Descending aorta	2.5	2.3

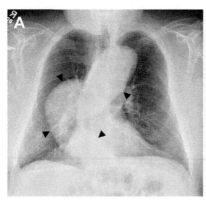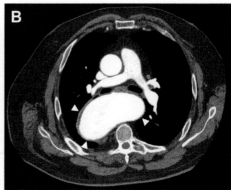

Fig. 2. Chest radiograph (*A*) and axial computed tomography angiography image (*B*) in a 66-year-old man with a large TAAA detected incidentally on a screening ultrasound of the abdominal aorta. The descending thoracic aorta is dilated (*arrowheads*), measuring up to 6.8 cm. The aneurysm extends from the left subclavian artery to the aortic bifurcation (not shown) consistent with a Crawford type II TAAA.

degradation and mechanical forces are thought to cause cystic medial degeneration of the aortic wall which leads to smooth muscle cell dropout and elastic fiber loss. This process results in a weakened aortic wall and loss of elasticity, which then leads to dilation. Cystic medial degeneration occurs normally with aging, but hypertension and other atherosclerosis risk factors accelerate this process.[4,9] A large prospective 20-year cohort study that followed 8000 Japanese men in Hawaii found that risk factors predictive of atherosclerosis were also associated with aortic aneurysms. The incidence of aortic aneurysms increased steadily with age after 60 years in this study. The investigators also found that aneurysms were associated with hypertension, smoking, and hypercholesterolemia.[12]

Familial/Genetic

TAAs that occur in younger patients without significant cardiovascular risk factors often have a genetic basis. Genetically mediated aortic aneurysms may be part of a syndrome. For example, patients with syndromic disorders of connective tissue, including Marfan, Ehlers–Danlos, and Loeys–Dietz, are prone to develop TAAs and comprise approximately 10% to 15% of all heritable TAAs.[13] On the other hand, some patients may develop TAAs linked to a genetic mutation that only affects the cardiovascular system without abnormalities in other organ systems. These include bicuspid aortic valve (BAV) with TAA and familial TAA.[13,14]

Marfan Syndrome

Marfan syndrome is a rare autosomal dominant disorder of the connective tissues caused by mutations in the fibrillin-1 gene that can lead to abnormalities in multiple organs including the thoracic aorta. Skeletal changes (eg, long slender digits, anterior chest deformity, scoliosis), ocular findings (lens dislocation), and cardiovascular manifestations (aortic root, proximal ascending aorta and pulmonary artery aneurysms, myxomatous mitral valve disease) may be evident. The cardiovascular system is the primary cause of morbidity and mortality in Marfan syndrome. The age of onset of aortic dilation varies in Marfan patients, but most patients have aortic dilation before the age of 18 with progressive dilation over time. Dilation most commonly occurs at the sinuses of Valsalva but can affect any part of the aorta. The rate of progression of aortic dilation is highly variable among patients. If the dilation involves the aortic annulus, secondary aortic regurgitation may occur. A significant risk of dissection or rupture occurs when the aortic diameter reaches 5 cm in adults.[4,15]

Loeys–Dietz Syndrome

Loeys–Dietz syndrome (LDS) is another autosomal dominant connective tissue disorder with multisystem involvement with characteristic features of hypertelorism, bifid/broad uvula or cleft palate and aortic aneurysms, and/or generalized arterial tortuosity. Mutations in the genes for the TGF-beta receptors lead to overproduction of collagen, loss of elastin, and disarrayed elastic fibers, which result in the typical phenotypic abnormalities. Diagnosis is confirmed through analysis of the gene mutations of TGF-beta genes. Importantly, patients with Loeys–Dietz may have widespread arterial involvement and are at high risk for aneurysms, including aortic aneurysms, which are prone to dissect or rupture at smaller aortic diameters and at younger ages compared with other connective tissue disorders.[16]

The more aggressive natural history of this syndrome was described by Williams and colleagues in a retrospective review of medical records of all LDS patients from The Johns Hopkins Medical Institutions in Baltimore, Maryland and Ghent University Hospital in Ghent, Belgium. Before surgical intervention, six patients (9%) died of aneurysm rupture or dissection despite several of these patients having aortic diameters less than 4.5 cm and being as young as 6 months old. Aortic aneurysm surgery was performed on 21 LDS patients (30%) and the mean age at operation for the cohort was 16 years (range 0.8–40 years). This cohort included 14 children and 2 adults; 80% of the surgeries were for aortic root aneurysms. The remaining surgeries were for arch pseudoaneurysms, type A dissections, and type A/B dissection. Preoperative and postoperative vascular imaging also revealed that close to two-thirds had aneurysm disease in many locations including the thoracic aorta, abdominal aorta, pulmonary artery, coronary arteries, vertebral arteries, carotid arteries, subclavian arteries, splenic arteries, celiac artery, superior mesenteric artery and inferior mesenteric artery.. Multiple surgical interventions were required in 33% of patients.[16] Unlike Marfan syndrome, which has a relatively favorable prognosis with a median survival of 70 years, Loeys–Dietz has a more aggressive vascular course with a median survival of only 37 years.[14]

Ehlers–Danlos Syndrome, Vascular Form

Ehlers–Danlos syndrome (EDS) is a group of rare genetic disorders of the connective tissue which has 13 subtypes. Although some subtypes are associated with only mild symptoms, the vascular EDS (EDS type IV) can have life-threatening complications such as aortic dissection or rupture. Vascular EDS is autosomal dominant and characterized by arterial, intestinal, and/or uterine fragility. Major diagnostic criteria for the disorder are (1) arterial aneurysms, dissection, or rupture, (2) intestinal rupture, (3) uterine rupture during pregnancy, and (4) family history of vascular EDS.[17] In one large study that reviewed the medical and surgical complications in 220 index patients with vascular EDS and 199 of their affected relatives, arterial complications were the most frequent first complication (46%). In addition, of the 131 deaths, most (79%) were due to arterial rupture with the majority (76%) involving thoracic or abdominal arteries. Even though most patients survived the first and second major complications, vascular EDS type IV was associated with early death. The median survival for the entire cohort was only 48 years with the age of death ranging from 6 to 73 years.[18]

Bicuspid Aortic Valve

BAV is the most common congenital cardiac defect in adults, affecting 0.5% to 2% of people, and is responsible for more deaths and complications than all other congenital cardiac defects combined. BAV is highly heritable with a prevalence of 9% among first-degree relatives of patients with BAV. The genetics of BAV are not fully understood, but mutations in multiple genes have been implicated. Aortic valvular disease, specifically, aortic regurgitation and aortic stenosis, is the most common complication of BAV. However, patients with BAV are also prone to develop TAAs, which occur in up to 50%.[19,20] Aortic dilation begins in childhood and progressively increases over time. Although altered hemodynamics is thought to contribute to aortic dilation, dilation of the aortic root or ascending aorta is prevalent even in the absence of aortic valvular disease.[21,22] Patients with a bicuspid valve who underwent isolated aortic valve replacements continue to be at risk for aortic complications, suggesting an aortopathy depends on more than just the hemodynamic alterations related to the bicuspid valve.[19,20]

Other Genetic Syndromes

Other genetic syndromes are associated with thoracic aortic aneurysmal disease. These include familial thoracic aneurysms and dissections, autosomal dominant polycystic kidney disease, Turner syndrome (associated also with coarctation of the aorta, BAV), neurofibromatosis, Noonan syndrome, tuberous sclerosis, homocystinuria, and neurofibromatosis.[23]

Mycotic Aneurysms

Infection is a rare but important cause of TAA/TAAA. Infected or mycotic aortic aneurysms can develop through several mechanisms: (1) hematogenous spread of infectious microemboli to the vasa vasorum, often in the setting of bacterial endocarditis, (2) infection of a preexisting intimal defect or atherosclerotic plaque by circulating pathogens, (3) contiguous involvement of the aorta by an adjacent source of infection, or (4) direct inoculation of the aortic wall, such as by penetrating trauma or iatrogenic injury.[24] Infection will destroy and weaken the aortic wall potentially leading to pseudoaneurysm formation. If untreated, infected aortic aneurysms often rapidly enlarge and rupture.[25]

Infected TAAs are most often due to bacterial infection, commonly *Staphylococcus* and *Streptococcus* species in Western countries, though rare reports of aortic aneurysms secondary to fungal infection have been described.[25] In one of the largest retrospective reviews of 32 patients with infected TAAs treated at a large hospital in Taiwan, *Salmonella* (57%) was the most common microorganism followed by *Staphylococcus aureus* (14%) and *Mycobacterium tuberculosis* (11%). The mortality rate of infected TAAs is high. In this series, the mortality rate was 57% with medical treatment alone and 28% in patients who underwent surgery.[26]

Chronic Aortic Dissection

TAA/TAAA may also develop as a result of a chronic thoracic aortic dissection. Most Stanford type A dissections (discussed in a later section) are treated surgically. However, medical management with antihypertensive therapy and surveillance imaging is the treatment of choice for uncomplicated Stanford type B dissections. After a dissection occurs, the tunica media may atrophy and undergo pathological changes including fibrosis, smooth muscle cell loss, and fragmentation of the elastin fibers. The adventitia and subadventitia may also become inflamed and fibrotic over time, compromising blood flow through the vasa vasorum. These changes can lead to weakening of the aortic wall and progressive dilation. The rate of aortic enlargement in the setting of dissection is the greatest immediately after dissection but plateaus over time. Continued patency of the false lumen of the dissection is also associated with higher rates of aortic enlargement and decreased long-term survival.[27]

EPIDEMIOLOGY

The true incidence and prevalence of TAA/TAAAs are not certain because of the silent nature of the disease. Some aneurysms are incidentally detected by imaging such as echocardiography, chest radiograph, or chest computed tomography. Many are not discovered until urgent intervention is necessary. Still others are probably never recognized in patients who die suddenly of their complications. Consequently, the true incidence may be higher than reported in the literature. Nonetheless, studies have attempted to better define the epidemiology of thoracic aortic aneurysmal disease. A 2021 review and large meta-analysis of population-based studies assessed available worldwide studies and found the pooled incidence of TAA at 5.3 per 100,000 individuals per year and a prevalence of 0.16%.[28]

The incidence and prevalence of aortic aneurysms involving the thoracic and abdominal aorta are more poorly defined because the investigators have historically combined TAAs and TAAAs in epidemiological studies and few studies have looked at TAAAs alone. Nonetheless, TAAAs are probably less common than TAAs. Evidence for this comes from a large retrospective study looking at 45,000 individuals in a Midwestern community over 30 years. This study found TAAs in 72 residents with the majority of aneurysms (67) isolated to the thoracic aorta and the minority (5) involving the abdominal aorta.[29] Another large retrospective study analyzing 44,332 autopsy reports over a 28 year period in a city in Sweden found asymptomatic TAAs in 205 patients, approximately 5% of which were thoracoabdominal.[30]

NATURAL HISTORY
Aneurysm Expansion

Most TAAs grow slowly over time. In a large retrospective study of 1600 patients tracking TAAs over a 10-year period, the average growth rate was 0.1 cm/year. The rate of growth for descending aortic aneurysms was faster than for ascending aortic aneurysms, growing at 0.19 cm/year versus 0.07 cm/year. Aneurysm growth rate was also faster for larger aneurysms.[31] Most TAAAs grow at a similar rate as TAAs. In the largest case series to date following 907 patients with descending thoracic and TAAAs over a 5-year period, descending TAAs and TAAAs had a mean growth of 0.19 cm/year with increased growth rates observed with larger initial aortic sizes.[32] **Table 2** summarizes the mean growth rates for each type of aneurysm.

Table 2 Mean growth rates for aneurysm by location	
Type of Aneurysm	Mean Growth Rate
Ascending aortic aneurysm	0.07 cm/year
Descending aortic aneurysm	0.19 cm/year
Thoracoabdominal aortic aneurysm	0.19 cm/year

Box 1
Factors that accelerate aneurysm growth rate

Chronic dissection

Increased aneurysm size

Bicuspid aortic valve

Marfan syndrome

Box 1 lists other factors that may accelerate aneurysm growth rates. For example, in a study of 230 patients with TAAs treated at large medical center over an 11-year period, patients with chronic dissections had a significantly higher rate of growth, with smaller (4.0 cm) aneurysms growing at a rate of 0.28 cm/year and larger (8.0 cm) aneurysms growing at 0.56 cm/year[33] Faster growth rates of TAAs in the setting of BAV and Marfan syndrome have been observed in several studies as well.[34]

Clinical Manifestations

Although TAA/TAAAs are often clinically silent, a few patients may experience symptoms relating to the mass effect of the aneurysm on adjacent structures in the chest. Compression of the tracheobronchial tree may produce cough, dyspnea, and wheezing. Compression of the esophagus may result in dysphagia or odynophagia. Hoarseness may occur if the recurrent laryngeal nerve is compressed. If the aneurysm becomes large enough, back pain may ensue due to mass effect on the spine.[9] Aneurysms involving the aortic root may cause AI leading to dyspnea, syncope, angina, or heart failure.[4]

The most devastating complications of TAAs/TAAAs are dissection or rupture, which have high mortality rates. As an aortic aneurysm enlarges, the aortic wall weakens and becomes prone to dissection or rupture. Aortic dissection is the result of a tear of intima and usually involves the proximal thoracic aorta. Flowing blood enters the aortic wall and separates the media into two layers: an inner layer composed of the intima and a portion of the media and an outer layer composed of a portion of the media and the adjacent adventitia.[2] The dissection may progress antegrade or retrograde along the aortic wall and lead to reentry of blood into the true lumen. The tear may involve branch vessels of the aorta and lead to malperfusion syndromes, cardiac tamponade, or aortic insufficiency.[35] If the tear extends through the outer wall, blood quickly escapes the aorta and aortic wall rupture ensues, which is almost always fatal if not treated immediately.[2]

Because the anatomic extent of the aortic dissections has management ramifications, various classification systems have been developed. One of the more widely used and most simple classification systems is the *Stanford classification*[35]:

- *Type A* dissection involves the ascending aorta and may extend to the arch or descending aorta.
- *Type B* dissections involve the descending thoracic aorta distal to the left subclavian artery.

The *DeBakey classification* is based on the site of origin of the intimal tear and is divided into four types[35]:

- *Type I* involves the ascending aorta, arch, and descending thoracic aorta and with or without involvement of the abdominal aorta.

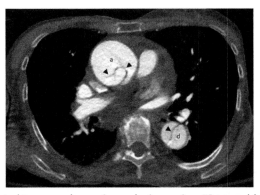

Fig. 3. Axial computed tomography angiography image in a 72-year-old woman with acute chest pain shows a Stanford type A dissection involving the ascending (a) and descending (d) thoracic aorta. The ascending thoracic aorta is dilated, and the dissection flap is visible as a small curvilinear filling defect (*arrowheads*).

- *Type II* involves only the ascending aorta.
- *Type IIIa* involves the descending thoracic aorta distal to the left subclavian and proximal to the celiac trunk.
- *Type IIIb* involves the thoracoabdominal aorta distal to the left subclavian artery.

The Societies of Vascular and Thoracic Surgeons recommend another classification system that is similar to the Stanford system but more specifically describes the distal extent of the dissection.[36]

The mortality rate of aortic dissections has historically remained high. Type A aortic dissections are more deadly than type B and are typically managed surgically. **Fig. 3** shows an example of a type A dissection. According to a study analyzing the data from the International Registry of Acute Aortic Dissection, the mortality of untreated type A dissections was 58%, whereas the mortality of type A dissections managed surgically was 26%. On the other hand, the mortality of type B dissections managed medically was 10.7%. The most common causes of death among patients who died of type A dissection were rupture and cardiac tamponade followed by visceral ischemia. For patients with type B dissections who died, aortic rupture was the most common cause of death followed by visceral ischemia.[37]

Management

Studies have consistently shown that the risks of thoracic aortic dissection and rupture increase with an increasing aneurysm size. Elefteriades found that by the time an aneurysm of the ascending thoracic aorta reaches 6 cm, the yearly rate of dissection, rupture, and/or death becomes 14.1% compared with a yearly rate of 6.5% at 5 cm and 5.3% at 4 cm.[31] A study specifically examining descending TAAs and TAAAs found a similar high yearly rate of dissection, rupture, and/or death at 19% for aneurysms 6 cm or greater. Interestingly, the same group found that dissections of the descending TAAs and TAAAs occurred at smaller diameters, whereas rupture more frequently occurred at larger diameters.[32]

Because of the catastrophic risks associated with TAAs, asymptomatic patients with aneurysms of the ascending aorta or arch measuring 5.5 cm or greater generally should be considered for surgical repair. No firm recommendations exist for the appropriate size for surgical repair of descending TAAs or TAAAs.[4] However, some investigators have suggested an aneurysm size threshold of 5.0 to 5.5 cm for intervention.[32] In patients with TAAs/TAAAs which are rapidly enlarging or symptomatic or who have an underlying connective disorder, intervention is indicated at smaller diameters.[4,38]

Medical Treatment Recommendations

For patients who may present with TAA/TAAA or for complications related to TAA/ TAAA such as aortic dissection, medical management is important. Aortic wall stress if determined by the velocity of ventricular contraction (dP/dt), the heart rate, and blood pressure. Maintaining adequate perfusion while addressing these three areas may be critical, in particular in patients with dissection to minimize the risk for propagation. Recommendations for patients with chronic thoracic aortic disease include BP goals less than 140/90 (without diabetes) or 130/80 (with diabetes or chronic kidney disease). Beta blockers or ACE inhibitors or ARBS are recommended. For patients with acute dissection, multisociety guidelines suggest a heart rate target less than 60 bpm and a systolic blood pressure between 100 and 120 mm Hg.[4] Initial treatment with beta blockers such as short-acting esmolol infusion or IV propanolol, metoprolol, or labetalol may be good options. In patients who cannot tolerate beta blockers, non-dihydropyridine calcium channel blockers such as verapamil or diltiazem are recommended as an acceptable alternative. Caution should be used with beta blockers in patients with significant aortic regurgitation. Vasodilators may also be needed to control blood pressure and short-acting agents such as nicardipine or nitroglycerine may be most appropriate. It is important to consider establishing beta blockade before vasodilator treatment to prevent reflex tachycardia or increased inotropy that may lead to increased aortic wall sheer stress.[4] Pain control may also be appropriate to decrease the sympathetic outflow.

SUMMARY

The etiology, epidemiology, and natural history of thoracic aneurysm and thoracoabdominal aneurysmal disease were described. The following summarizes key points regarding patients with TAA/TAAAs.

- TAA and TAAAs are common, are often clinically silent until complications occur, and are often diagnosed incidentally.
- Dissection and rupture are the most common complications of TAA/TAAAs and are associated with high mortality.
- Most of the TAA and TAAAs are degenerative and develop in patients with risk factors for atherosclerosis.
- TAAs and TAAAs in younger patients without significant cardiovascular risk factors often have a genetic basis some of which include Marfan, Ehlers–Danlos, Loeys–Dietz, and BAV.
- Most TAAs grow slowly over time. Factors that may accelerate growth include chronic dissection, larger aneurysm size, BAV and connective tissue disease.
- Size cutoffs beyond which complications and fatal events significantly increase guide when surgical or endovascular intervention should be considered.
- Symptomatic aneurysms should be treated regardless of size.
- For patients who present with TAA/TAAAs, maintaining adequate perfusion while avoiding increases in aortic wall stress, tachycardia, and hypertension is essential.

CLINICS CARE POINTS

- Most authors and guidelines suggest a size threshold of 5 to 5.5 cm for intervention for TAA/TAAA. In patients with aneurysms that have underlying connective tissue disease, aneurysms that are enlarging rapidly, or are symptomatic, intervention is indicated at a smaller size.

- Medical management of TAA/TAAAs include minimizing aortic wall stress by limiting the velocity of ventricular contraction (dP/dt), heart rate, and blood pressure while maintaining adequate perfusion.

- For patients with an acute dissection, heart rate target is less than 60 bpm and systolic blood pressures should be between 100 and 120 mm Hg.

DISCLOSURE

The authors have no commercial or financial conflict of interest and no funding source.

REFERENCES

1. Centers for Disease Control and Prevention. 20 Leading Causes of Death, United States, 1999 - 2019, All Races, Both Sexes. 2022. Available at: https://wisqars.cdc.gov/cgi-bin/broker.exe. Accessed April 6, 2022.

2. Bäck M, Gasser TC, Michel J-B, et al. Biomechanical factors in the biology of aortic wall and aortic valve diseases. Cardiovasc Res 2013;99(2):232–41.

3. Singh M, Ziganshin BA, Elefteriades JA. Aortic Aneurysm. In: Vasan RS, Sawyer DB, editors. Encyclopedia of cardiovascular research and medicine. Oxford: Elsevier; 2018. p. 123–42.

4. Hiratzka LF, Bakris GL, Beckman JA, et al. 2010 ACCF/AHA/AATS/ACR/ASA/SCA/SCAI/SIR/STS/SVM guidelines for the diagnosis and management of patients with Thoracic Aortic Disease: a report of the American College of Cardiology Foundation/American Heart Association Task Force on Practice Guidelines, American Association for Thoracic Surgery, American College of Radiology, American Stroke Association, Society of Cardiovascular Anesthesiologists, Society for Cardiovascular Angiography and Interventions, Society of Interventional Radiology, Society of Thoracic Surgeons, and Society for Vascular Medicine. Circulation 2010;121(13):e266–369.

5. Senser EM, Misra S, Henkin S. Thoracic aortic aneurysm: a clinical review. Cardiol Clin 2021;39(4):505–15.

6. Agarwal PP, Chughtai A, Matzinger FR, et al. Multidetector CT of thoracic aortic aneurysms. Radiographics 2009;29(2):537–52.

7. Rylski B, Desjardins B, Moser W, et al. Gender-related changes in aortic geometry throughout life. Eur J Cardiothorac Surg 2014;45(5):805–11.

8. Johnston KW, Rutherford RB, Tilson MD, et al. Suggested standards for reporting on arterial aneurysms. Subcommittee on Reporting Standards for Arterial Aneurysms, Ad Hoc Committee on Reporting Standards, Society for Vascular Surgery and North American Chapter, International Society for Cardiovascular Surgery. J Vasc Surg 1991;13(3):452–8.

9. Isselbacher EM. Thoracic and abdominal aortic aneurysms. Circulation 2005;111(6):816–28.

10. Nathan DP, Xu C, Pouch AM, et al. Increased wall stress of saccular versus fusiform aneurysms of the descending thoracic aorta. Ann Vasc Surg 2011;25(8):1129–37.

11. Crawford ES, Coselli JS. Thoracoabdominal aneurysm surgery. Semin Thorac Cardiovasc Surg 1991;3(4):300–22.
12. Reed D, Reed C, Stemmermann G, et al. Are aortic aneurysms caused by atherosclerosis? Circulation 1992;85(1):205–11.
13. Bhandari R, Kanthi Y. The genetics of aortic aneurysms. Am Coll Cardiol 2018;. https://www.acc.org/latest-in-cardiology/articles/2018/05/02/12/52/the-genetics-of-aortic-aneurysms.
14. Bhandari R, Aatre RD, Kanthi Y. Diagnostic approach and management of genetic aortopathies. Vasc Med 2020;25(1):63–77.
15. Tinkle BT, Saal HM. Health supervision for children with Marfan syndrome. Pediatrics 2013;132(4):e1059–72.
16. Williams JA, Loeys BL, Nwakanma LU, et al. Early surgical experience with Loeys-Dietz: a new syndrome of aggressive thoracic aortic aneurysm disease. Ann Thorac Surg 2007;83(2):S757–63 [discussion: S785-790].
17. Byers PH. Vascular ehlers-danlos syndrome. In: Adam MP, Ardinger HH, Pagon RA, et al, editors. GeneReviews(®). Seattle (WA): University of Washington, Seattle Copyright © 1993-2022, University of Washington, Seattle. GeneReviews is a registered trademark of the University of Washington, Seattle. All rights reserved.; 1993. p. 1–16.
18. Pepin M, Schwarze U, Superti-Furga A, et al. Clinical and genetic features of Ehlers-Danlos syndrome type IV, the vascular type. N Engl J Med 2000; 342(10):673–80.
19. Siu SC, Silversides CK. Bicuspid aortic valve disease. J Am Coll Cardiol 2010; 55(25):2789–800.
20. Verma S, Siu SC. Aortic dilatation in patients with bicuspid aortic valve. N Engl J Med 2014;370(20):1920–9.
21. Blais S, Meloche-Dumas L, Fournier A, et al. Long-term risk factors for dilatation of the proximal aorta in a large cohort of children with bicuspid aortic valve. Circ Cardiovasc Imaging 2020;13(3):e009675.
22. Grattan M, Prince A, Rumman RK, et al. Predictors of bicuspid aortic valve-associated aortopathy in childhood: a report from the MIBAVA consortium. Circ Cardiovasc Imaging 2020;13(3):e009717.
23. Cury M, Zeidan F, Lobato AC. Aortic disease in the young: genetic aneurysm syndromes, connective tissue disorders, and familial aortic aneurysms and dissections. Int J Vasc Med 2013;2013:267215.
24. Lopes RJ, Almeida J, Dias PJ, et al. Infectious thoracic aortitis: a literature review. Clin Cardiol 2009;32(9):488–90.
25. Lee WK, Mossop PJ, Little AF, et al. Infected (mycotic) aneurysms: spectrum of imaging appearances and management. Radiographics 2008;28(7):1853–68.
26. Hsu RB, Lin FY. Infected aneurysm of the thoracic aorta. J Vasc Surg 2008;47(2): 270–6.
27. Peterss S, Mansour AM, Ross JA, et al. Changing pathology of the thoracic aorta from acute to chronic dissection: literature review and insights. J Am Coll Cardiol 2016;68(10):1054–65.
28. Gouveia EMR, Silva Duarte G, Lopes A, et al. Incidence and prevalence of thoracic aortic aneurysms: a systematic review and meta-analysis of population-based studies. Semin Thorac Cardiovasc Surg 2021;. https://www.acc.org/latest-in-cardiology/articles/2018/05/02/12/52/the-genetics-of-aortic-aneurysms.
29. Bickerstaff LK, Pairolero PC, Hollier LH, et al. Thoracic aortic aneurysms: a population-based study. Surgery 1982;92(6):1103–8.

30. Svensjö S, Bengtsson H, Bergqvist D. Thoracic and thoracoabdominal aortic aneurysm and dissection: an investigation based on autopsy. Br J Surg 1996; 83(1):68–71.
31. Elefteriades JA. Natural history of thoracic aortic aneurysms: indications for surgery, and surgical versus nonsurgical risks. Ann Thorac Surg 2002;74(5): S1877–80 [discussion: S1892-1878].
32. Zafar MA, Chen JF, Wu J, et al. Natural history of descending thoracic and thoracoabdominal aortic aneurysms. J Thorac Cardiovasc Surg 2021;161(2): 498–511.e491.
33. Coady MA, Rizzo JA, Hammond GL, et al. What is the appropriate size criterion for resection of thoracic aortic aneurysms? J Thorac Cardiovasc Surg 1997; 113(3):476–91 [discussion: 489-491].
34. Oladokun D, Patterson BO, Sobocinski J, et al. Systematic review of the growth rates and influencing factors in thoracic aortic aneurysms. Eur J Vasc Endovasc Surg 2016;51(5):674–81.
35. Tsai TT, Nienaber CA, Eagle KA. Acute aortic syndromes. Circulation 2005; 112(24):3802–13.
36. Lombardi JV, Hughes GC, Appoo JJ, et al. Society for Vascular Surgery (SVS) and Society of Thoracic Surgeons (STS) reporting standards for type B aortic dissections. J Vasc Surg 2020;71(3):723–47.
37. Hagan PG, Nienaber CA, Isselbacher EM, et al. The international registry of acute aortic dissection (IRAD): new insights into an old disease. JAMA 2000;283(7): 897–903.
38. Kuzmik GA, Sang AX, Elefteriades JA. Natural history of thoracic aortic aneurysms. J Vasc Surg 2012;56(2):565–71.

Aortic Dissection

D. Keegan Stombaugh, MD[a,b], Venkat Reddy Mangunta, MD[a,b,*]

KEYWORDS

- Aortic dissection • Anesthetic management of aortic dissection
- Echocardiography in aortic dissection • Operative management of aortic dissection
- Hemodynamic monitoring in aortic dissection
- Hemodynamic management in aortic dissection • Cardiovascular anesthesiology

KEY POINTS

- Intraoperative management of a patient with aortic dissection requires rapid and coordinated care by cardiovascular surgeons, cardiovascular anesthesiologists, nurses, and perfusionists.
- Surgical management of acute Stanford type A dissections can vary in approach, but general consensus exists with regard to the replacement of the ascending aorta and at least part of the aortic arch.
- Initial medical management of acute Stanford type B dissections has been the standard. However, more recent data show approximately 50% mortality at 5 years with this approach.
- Before induction of anesthesia, a careful assessment for clinical signs of cardiac tamponade and review of any available imaging, including echocardiography, is critical.
- Decisions on location of invasive monitors and targets for goal-directed resuscitation require a detailed understanding of the anatomy of the dissection and surgical technique.

EPIDEMIOLOGY

Acute thoracic aortic dissection (ATAD) is the most common disastrous event to affect the aorta, with Stanford Type A dissection remaining the most frequently transferred emergency through regional rapid transport systems.[1] Stanford type A dissections account for two-thirds of ATADs, half of these are classified as DeBakey type I.[2–4]

a Department of Anesthesiology, Division of Cardiovascular Anesthesia, University of Virginia, School of Medicine, University of Virginia Health System, PO Box 800710, Charlottesville, VA 22908, USA; b Department of Anesthesiology, Division of Critical Care Medicine, University of Virginia, School of Medicine, University of Virginia Health System, PO Box 800710, Charlottesville, VA 22908, USA
* Corresponding author. Department of Anesthesiology, Division of Cardiovascular Anesthesia, University of Virginia, School of Medicine, University of Virginia Health System, PO Box 800710, Charlottesville, VA 22908.
E-mail address: JWV6BH@hscmail.mcc.virginia.edu

Anesthesiology Clin 40 (2022) 685–703
https://doi.org/10.1016/j.anclin.2022.08.012   anesthesiology.theclinics.com
1932-2275/22/© 2022 Elsevier Inc. All rights reserved.

Approximately 37% of ATADs are classified as Stanford Type B/Debakey Type III dissections.[2,3,5] Rupture is the most common cause of death.[3]

There is limited information regarding the geographic, racial, and ethnic distribution of ATAD. The estimated incidence of ATADs is three to four cases per 100,000 person-years.[1–3,6] Among White Americans between the years 1980–1994 the incidence is reported to be 3.4 per 100,000 person-years based on 1990 census numbers.[2] Sen and colleagues[6] report an ATAD incidence of 4.4 per 100,000 person-years from 1995 to 2015 in the same population, indicating a stable incidence of disease over the last 30 years. Despite this, some studies have shown an increased incidence in ascending aortic syndromes that include ATAD, intramural hematoma, and penetrating aortic ulcer.[2,3,6,7] The International Registry of Acute Aortic Dissection Interventional Cohort Database (IRAD) shows that African Americans are more likely to present with ATAD at a younger age, with a higher incidence of hypertension, and diabetes compared with White Americans.[1,8,9] However, mortality is similar between both groups.[8] It should be noted that the aforementioned data may not be comprehensive, however, as a substantial proportion of individuals with ATAD die before reaching a hospital, or the diagnosis is made and not counted unless an autopsy is performed.[3] Data from Sweden, where an autopsy is mandatory for an unexplained death, show that 22% of ATADs were diagnosed only upon autopsy.[3,7]

Clinical associations among patients with ATAD are hypertension, aortic dilation, smoking, iatrogenic injuries (cardiac catheterization and cardiac surgery), aortitis, bicuspid aortic valve, and connective tissue disorders. Men are at a higher risk of developing ATAD compared to women (5.2 per 100,000 per year vs 2.2 per 100,000 per year) with sex distribution being consistent for both Stanford type A and type B dissections.[2,3] The average age of onset for type A ATAD is 61 years, and 66 years for type B ATAD.[2,3,10] The exception to these data are younger patients with connective tissue disorders. Patients <40 years of age were more likely to have a connective tissue disorder or bicuspid aortic valve.[3,11] Unclear correlations with ATAD include pregnancy, trauma, cocaine use (especially crack cocaine), diabetes, and atherosclerosis.[2,3,10]

PATHOPHYSIOLOGY

An acute aortic dissection occurs when blood suddenly leaves the aortic lumen through a tear or defect in the tunica intima and rapidly dissects the layers of the tunica media producing a false lumen. Although a dissection can occur without evidence of an intimal tear, this is uncommon.[12] A patient is considered to have an acute dissection if the dissection occurred within the past 14 days.[12] Although arbitrary, the 14-day mark derives from the International Registry of Acute Aortic Dissection (IRAD) data that suggest the total mortality of type A and B dissections treated medically plateau at 14 days.[2,13] Connective tissue disorders such as Loeys-Dietz, Marfans, and Ehlers Danlos are well characterized. Recently, investigations into nonsyndromic familial aortic aneurysms and dissections have led to the discovery of other genes which confer defects in cell signaling pathways and assembly of the vascular smooth muscle contractile proteins. Importantly, transforming growth factor β receptor 2 (TGFBR2) mutations that are different from those seen in Loey's-Dietz syndrome result in cell signaling defects.[13] These defects affect the synthesis of key proteins involved in the contractile nature of vascular smooth muscle and can lead to aneurysms and dissection in people with aortic diameters of less than 5 cm.[13]

Disruption and degeneration of the aortic media are hallmarks of patients with acute aortic dissections. In younger patients with connective tissue diseases, the elastic elements of the media are disorganized and disrupted.[13] In older patients, the vascular smooth muscle of the media often displays signs of degeneration due to long-standing hypertension as well as aging. Age and hypertension-related changes are the result of repeated injury and repair of the aortic wall.[13] These observations have led to the suggestion that aortic dissection is considered the result of either changes to the elastic fibers of the media in younger patients or changes and degeneration of the smooth muscle cells of the media in older patients.[13] A hallmark of patients with connective tissue disease involves loss of the elastic lamellae of the media and replacement with mucoid material.[13] In postmortem analysis, the media of aortic dissection patients show evidence of activated T lymphocytes, macrophages, and evidence of vascular smooth muscle apoptosis.[13] In addition, increase in collagen types I and III as well as connective tissue growth factors are implicated in the decreased elasticity and increased stiffness of the aortic wall in patients with aortic dissection.[13] Similarly, excessive activity of matrix metalloproteinases, zinc-dependent enzymes, have been implicated in patients with increased risk of aortic dissection.[13]

In the vast majority of aortic dissections, a tear in the tunica intima, the innermost layer of the aortic wall, is the precipitating event. As a result of this intimal tear, high-pressure blood enters the tunica media from the aortic lumen separating the layers of circumferential smooth muscle and elastic fibers (**Fig. 1**).[13,14] The blood then propagates through the media creating a dissecting hematoma (**Fig. 2**). Intimal disruption occurs at points in the thoracic aorta where wall stress is extremely high.[13] Intimal tears usually involve half to two-thirds of the circumference of the aorta and lie in transverse fashion. In Stanford type A dissections, 60% to 70% of the intimal tears are located in the proximal ascending aorta (**Fig. 3**), immediately distal to the sinotubular junction.[13] In 10% to 20% of cases, the intimal tear is in the aortic arch along the lesser curvature of the aorta. In a small minority of dissections, the intimal tear is located in the proximal descending thoracic aorta or the abdominal aorta with retrograde propagation to the ascending aorta.[13] Dissections typically propagate

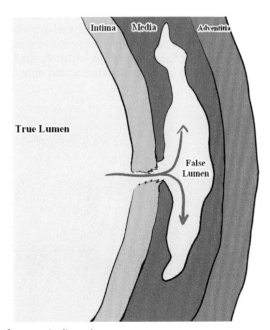

Fig. 1. Anatomy of an aortic dissection.

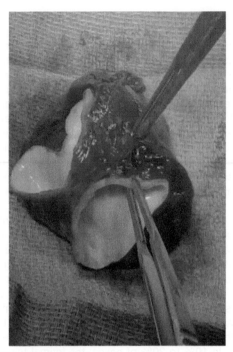

Fig. 2. Medial separation with hematoma.

antegrade from the intimal tear in a spiral configuration.[13] Factors that determine how the dissection propagates include aortic dP/dt (rate of aortic pressure rise), aortic diastolic elastic recoil, aortic wall stiffness, and aortic peak and mean pressures.[13] It is rare for a Stanford type A dissection to remain confined to the ascending aorta (DeBakey type II). Rather, barring significant atherosclerotic disease or other impediments to propagation, dissections usually progress along the length of the aorta and frequently involve branching vessels.[13] The true aortic lumen is usually smaller than the false lumen. In addition, the false lumen is usually located on the right anterior side in the

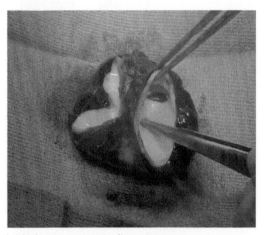

Fig. 3. Intimal tear initiating acute aortic dissection.

ascending aorta and along the greater curvature of the aortic arch, frequently involving the great vessels.[13] Over time, the false lumen can thrombose. However, if multiple points of reentry exist in the distal aorta, constant blood flow into the false lumen can maintain patency over time.[13] In fact, a distal patent false lumen is seen in approximately 90% of patients after surgical repair of an ascending aortic dissection, leading to poor long-term prognosis.[13] In contrast to acute dissections, intramural hematomas (IMH) are thought to originate from the rupture of the vasa vasorum that lies in the outer aspect of the tunica media. Traditionally, in an IMH, an intimal tear is not found, giving rise to the theory that the extravasated blood in the media arises from the vasa vasorum.[13,15] The rupture of the vasa vasorum results in the accumulation of blood in the outer aspect of the tunica media. Traditionally, in IMH, there is no contact between the aortic lumen and the hematoma. However, in up to one-third of cases, IMH can evolve into a dissection.[15] The natural history of IMH is similar to that of an acute aortic dissection and requires emergent treatment.[13]

CLINICAL PRESENTATION

Although exceptionally difficult to verify without accurate autopsy data, it is postulated that death occurs immediately in approximately 40% of patients with ATAD.[1,16] Mortality most often results from cardiogenic shock secondary to pericardial tamponade after rupture, severe aortic insufficiency (AI), or coronary dissection. According to IRAD, approximately 85% of patients with Stanford type A dissections experience classic retrosternal tearing chest pain.[10] Additional signs and symptoms can vary depending on the extent of the dissection and compromised anatomic structures. Additional signs and symptoms may include hypertension due to pain and catecholamine surge, syncope secondary to rupture, cerebrovascular accident, altered sensorium, diastolic murmur due to AI, neurologic deficits due to spinal cord ischemia, general end organ, and limb ischemia, and shock due to aortic rupture, pericardial tamponade, or coronary artery dissection.[1,6,10] Recurrent pain or refractory hypertension can be signs of extending dissection or impending rupture. Multiple logistic regression analyses of IRAD data showed that refractory pain or hypertension was an independent predictor of in-hospital mortality (odds ratio 3.3). Age of 70 years or older and absence of chest pain on admission were also predictors of death, with aortic rupture as the most common cause.[17] 33% of patients with type A dissections will present with signs and symptoms of end-organ ischemia.[10] The Penn classification of type A dissection ischemic profiles can determine mortality and influence management options (**Table 1,**[18] **Fig. 4**[19]). Amongst type A dissections at the University of Pennsylvania ($N = 221$: 1993–2004), hospital mortality was 3.1% for class a, 25.6% for class b, 17.6% for class c, and 40% for class bc.[18] The IRAD database shows independent predictors of mortality include hypotension on presentation (OR 3.23; 95% confidence interval (CI) 1.95–5.37), myocardial ischemia on presentation (odds ratio [OR] 1.76; 95% CI 1.02–3.03), any pulse deficit on presentation (OR 1.75; 95% CI 1.06–2.88), and renal failure on presentation (OR 4.77; 95% CI 1.80–12.6).[18,20] In addition, the presence of pericardial tamponade more than doubled mortality.[21] Several studies, including a 17-year study from IRAD, indicated no significant difference in clinical presentation between Stanford type A and Stanford type B dissections.[6,22,23] However, the clinical presentation can differ based on age. Reports from IRAD indicate patients aged ≥70 years are more likely to present with abnormal blood pressure, pleural effusion, and thrombosed false lumen. They are less likely to experience an abrupt onset of pain and pulse deficits than younger patients with ATAD.[3,11,24] Delay in ATAD diagnosis is more likely in patients without the abrupt onset of pain, minimal

Table 1
Aortic dissection classification systems

Classification	Subtype	Origin of Intimal Tear
Stanford	Type A	Ascending aorta.
DeBakey	I	Type A dissection with involvement of the descending aorta.
DeBakey	II	Type A dissection with NO involvement of the descending thoracic aorta.
Penn	Class a	Type A dissection with absence of branch vessel malperfusion or circulatory collapse.
	Class b	Type A dissection with branch vessel malperfusion with ischemia.
	Class c	Type A dissection with circulatory collapse with or without cardiac involvement.
	Class bc	Type A dissection with both branch vessel malperfusion and circulatory collapse.
Stanford	Type B	Descending aorta.
Debakey	IIIa	Dissection tear only in the descending aorta.
Debakey	IIIb	Dissection tear extending below the diaphragm.

pain, lack of pulse deficit, normotension, and patients who initially presented to a non-tertiary care hospital.[25,26]

Medical and Surgical Management

Early mortality with Stanford type A ATAD remains high at an overall in-hospital mortality of 30%.[1,27] For unrepaired acute Stanford type A ATAD, mortality increases by as much as 1% to 2% per hour in the early phase after symptom onset with 24 h unrepaired mortality of 20%, 30% at 48 h, and 50% at 2 weeks.[1,28] The majority of deaths are caused by aortic rupture.[3,6] Traditionally, surgical repair of ATAD carries an in-hospital mortality of 18% to 23%, with medically managed cases incurring a mortality of 59%.[3,28,29] However, recent IRAD data have shown a steady decline in operative mortality starting in the early 2000s. IRAD data between 2010 and 2016 show an in-hospital mortality after surgical repair of 12% with postoperative mortality correlated with age >70, chronic renal insufficiency, renal failure, and need for concomitant coronary artery bypass grafting as predictors of mortality.[28] The etiology of this mortality decline is unclear. It is postulated that improved perfusion strategies, improved organ protection, strict IRAD center diagnostic criteria, experienced physicians at IRAD centers, and increasing surgical experience have led to a significant mortality decline.[28,30] This mortality decline may not apply to non-IRAD centers. Overall in-hospital mortality associated with acute Stanford type B ATAD is 13%, with aortic rupture responsible for 39% of deaths.[3,31] Acute operative repair of type B ATAD is usually reserved for life-threatening complications. According to IRAD, in-hospital mortality of surgical repair of type B ATAD is 20%. In comparison, in-hospital mortality for endovascular repair or medical treatment is 10% to 20% and 10%, respectively.[5,31] Both type A and type B ATAD have survival rates of 96% at 1 year, and 91% vs 83% respectively at 3 years after hospital discharge.[3,20,27]

STANFORD TYPE A DISSECTION

As the initial mortality of type A dissections is so high and increasing by the hour during the acute phase, expedient evaluation is of the utmost importance. Important goals of

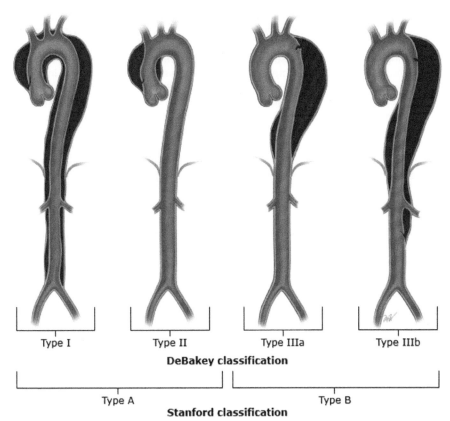

Type I   Type II   Type IIIa   Type IIIb

DeBakey classification

Type A   Type B

Stanford classification

Fig. 4. Figure depicting Stanford Type A, Stanford type B, and DeBakey type I–IIIb dissection tear origins. (*From* UpToDate, with permission.)

imaging the aorta include diagnosis confirmation, dissection classification, localization of tears, and assessment of secondary pathology such as hemopericardium. Currently, the most expeditious and widely available imaging modality is contrast-enhanced computed tomography (CT) angiography.[1,17,32] Transesophageal echocardiography (TEE) and MRI show similar pooled sensitivities and specificities to CT angiography, but require more time and skilled personnel as compared with CT angiography.[17,33] Transthoracic echocardiography is insensitive owing to inadequate imaging windows for the ascending aorta.[34] Additional cardiac biomarkers, baseline labs, and an electrocardiogram should be obtained. D-dimer and smooth muscle cell myosin heavy chain elevation can be useful in differentiating ATAD from the acute coronary syndrome.[17,34]

The gold standard for treatment of acute Stanford type A dissection is the emergency open replacement of the ascending aorta with extension to the aortic root and arch as indicated. Excellent short and long-term outcomes have been associated with this approach.[1,6,17,18,28,35] Type of surgical repair depends on the involvement of the aortic root, aortic valve pathology and degree of insufficiency, and involvement of the aortic arch. Patients requiring a combined aortic valve and aortic root pathology may require a Bentall procedure with replacement of the aortic valve, root, and ascending aorta in a composite graft. The Yacoub and David procedures can be used to replace the aortic root without replacement of the aortic valve, and require reimplantation of the coronary buttons.[36] Significant changes in the surgical management of type A dissections at IRAD centers from the time period of 1996–2003 compared with 2010–2016 include the following: increase in the use of biologic aortic valves when valve replacement was required (35.6% vs 52%), increase in the use of valve-sparing procedures including Yacoub remodeling or David reimplantation (3.9% vs 26.7%), decline in the use of surgical glue (74.4% vs 45%), increase in right axillary artery cannulation for inflow (18% vs 55.7%), decrease in femoral artery cannulation for inflow (76% vs 30.1%), increased hemiarch replacement (27% vs 51.7%), use of hypothermic circulatory arrest (HCA) only decreased over time (27.8% vs 8.6%), and HCA with antegrade cerebral perfusion (ACP) increased over time (22.0% vs 50.8%) with an unclear trend in HCA with retrograde cerebral perfusion (RCP). HCA only median temperature was 18.0 °C, HCA with ACP median temperature was 24.7°C, and HCA with RCP 18.0°C.[28] Hemiarch replacement and use of ACP were negative predictors of mortality.[28] Coselli and colleagues[15] often use bilateral ACP given the ease at which this can be done. The use of ACP has allowed many centers to tolerate warmer temperatures during HCA.[15] Once the distal anastomosis is complete, the tourniquet is removed from the innominate artery and a clamp is placed across the graft allowing full cardiopulmonary bypass (CPB) flow to be reestablished, perfusing everything distal to the ascending aorta with active rewarming.[15] The aortic valve is then assessed. If the valve is intact, it is resuspended and the proximal anastomosis is completed (**Fig. 5**). If any part of it is not intact, it is replaced. If the patient has a known connective tissue disease, the root is replaced by a modified Bentall procedure.[15] Coselli and colleagues[15] avoid replacing the aortic root if the sinuses are intact. Aortic valve-sparing root replacements are usually done on patients who are hemodynamically stable with disease confined to the ascending aorta (DeBakey type II, see **Fig. 4**)[19].[15]

The distal extent of the type A dissection remains a major risk factor for poor long-term outcomes after open surgical repair due to concern for the patency of the false lumen in the descending aorta. Endovascular technology has become integrated with the open approach to repairing type A dissection with success in improving long-term distal aortic remodeling.[6,17,18] Deployment of an antegrade stent in the descending thoracic aorta during the time of open repair in the form of the frozen elephant trunk can help obliterate the distal false lumen and decrease the need for reoperation and complications arising from false lumen patency.[6,18,35] This technique promotes aortic remodeling, leading to less risk of chronic dissecting aneurysm formation eventually potentially requiring further surgery, and resolves visceral malperfusion issues.[15] Approximately 10% of patients who present with type A ATAD are deemed unfit for open surgical procedures due to high or prohibitive risk.[26,37,38] Ahmed and colleagues[37] recently published a literature review of 31 articles describing a total of 92 patients undergoing endovascular repair with type A dissection in patients deemed too high risk for open surgery and reported a 9% 30-day mortality.[37] Further research regarding feasibility and outcomes of this method is warranted. In an elegant review published in 2016, Coselli and colleagues[15] summarize the North American surgical experience with ATAD:

1. Most North American centers tend to replace the ascending aorta and proximal arch (hemiarch) and only embark on more extensive total arch replacement if the intimal tear involves the distal arch or if the arch is larger than 4.5 to 5.0 cm in diameter.[15]
2. Operative mortality in North American centers varies from 5% to 17%, with centers that develop protocolized, dedicated, thoracic aortic teams, likely having lower mortality.[15]

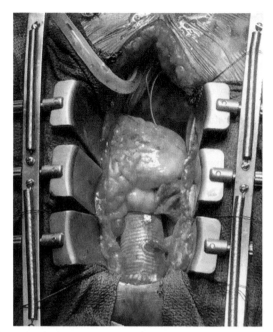

Fig. 5. Distal and proximal anastamoses complete.

3. Mortality rates related to iatrogenic type A dissections are higher (27% for open repair of iatrogenic dissection and 33% to 50% after TEVAR) and this is due to the complexity of repair, older patient population, or the possible need to revise the original repair.[15]
4. With increasing recognition for the downstream complications of false lumen thrombosis when the dissection extends to the descending aorta, many centers are advocating for simultaneous arch or hemiarch repair with placement of an antegrade or retrograde stent graft in the descending aorta. This technique promotes aortic remodeling, leading to less risk of chronic dissecting aneurysm formation and resolution of visceral malperfusion issues.[15]

ATAD may present with a variety of hemodynamic scenarios ranging from shock to hypertensive emergency. Invasive hemodynamic monitoring is essential.[34] Bilateral upper extremity arterial lines may be indicated depending on the degree of vascular compromise and surgical plan. Hemodynamic goals should be focused on decreasing shear stress to the aortic wall by decreasing change in pressure over time (dP/dt). Recommended hemodynamic goals include a target systolic blood pressure between 90 and 120 mm Hg, mean arterial blood pressure of approximately 60 mm Hg, and a heart rate of 60–80 beats per minute.[5,17,39] Intravenous (IV) antihypertensive and anti-chronotropic therapy should be initiated as necessary in order to achieve these parameters, being simultaneously cognizant of the effects of induction of general anesthesia in determining their necessity. IV β-adrenergic blockers, vasodilators, and calcium channel blockers can be used as mono agents or in conjunction. Labetalol, esmolol, clevidipine, nicardipine, sodium nitroprusside, and nitroglycerin are potential pharmacologic agents that can be employed. Although controversial, use of β-adrenergic agents in patients with a history of cocaine abuse may cause unopposed α-adrenergic activity leading to significant hypertension.[40] These patients may be best managed with a combination of benzodiazepines, calcium channel blockers, nitroglycerin, and α-2 agonists such as dexmedetomidine.[36,40] Analgesics should be administered if needed for pain relief and to assist with blood pressure control. Depending on the pathology associated with type A dissection, patients may not always present with elevated blood pressure and heart rate. Presence of pericardial tamponade, acute coronary syndrome, hemorrhagic shock, and severe AI may necessitate IV fluid administration, blood transfusion, vasopressor, and inotropic support. Unstable patients may inevitably require urgent intubation and mechanical ventilation. However, intubation should be delayed until the patient reaches the operating room if clinically reasonable due to potential for hemodynamic collapse with anesthetic induction and initiation of mechanical ventilation. A transthoracic echocardiogram performed by the cardiovascular anesthesiologist in the operating room is helpful to rule out a large pericardial effusion before induction. Adequate venous access and a right radial arterial line are essential.

STANFORD TYPE B DISSECTION

Stanford type B dissections, or aortic dissections involving only the descending thoracoabdominal aorta, can be characterized as uncomplicated or complicated. Uncomplicated type B dissections may be medically managed with targeted blood pressure control and treatment aimed at risk reduction. Complicated type B dissections, which characterize 15% to 20% of type B dissections, involve dissections associated with rupture, visceral malperfusion, or refractory pain and hypertension and often require endovascular intervention to decrease morbidity and mortality.[41]

Although endovascular treatment with TEVAR (thoracic endovascular aortic repair) of type B dissections is still an evolving field, the benefits of early stent graft placement include restoration of flow through the true lumen and prevention of aneurysmal degeneration of the false lumen.[41] Often, restoration of antegrade flow is insufficient in the setting of visceral malperfusion and branch stents or surgical bypass is required to restore adequate flow.[41]

The mainstay of medical therapy is anti-impulse therapy and prompt institution of this therapy has led to in-hospital mortality of less than 10%.[41] However, long-term data are not as clear with IRAD data suggesting that 3-year survival of medically managed acute type B dissections as 78%. Although much of this mortality has been attributed to patient-specific comorbidities, 25% to 50% of these patients do develop late aortic-related complications, such as aneurysmal degeneration of the false lumen.[41] Unfortunately, only two randomized controlled trials on endovascular treatment of acute Stanford type B dissections exist, the Acute Dissection Stent Grafting or Best Medical Treatment (ADSORB) trial and the Investigation of Stent-grafts in patients with type B Aortic Dissections (INSTEAD) trial.[41] Both trials showed improved aortic remodeling (true lumen patency with progressive thrombosis of the false lumen); however, INSTEAD showed that in low risk, subacute type B dissection, this did not lead to better survival secondary to a high rate or periprocedural complications in the intervention group.[41,42] Although most evidence points to improved outcomes with endovascular treatment of complicated acute Stanford type B dissections (TEVAR), the role of endovascular treatment of uncomplicated type B dissections will require further study.[41]

Medical management of acute Stanford type B dissections generally involves anti-impulse therapy with heart rate control agents and antihypertensives such as beta-blockers, calcium channel blockers, and angiotensin-converting enzyme inhibitors (ACEI). Although AHA guidelines focus on a target heart rate of 60 as optimal, this is mostly based on expert opinion and there is a lack of strong evidence to guide therapeutic targets.[42] Blood pressure management is of utmost importance and results of the ADSORB and INSTEAD studies reveal that many conservatively treated patients required at least three antihypertensive agents.[42] Unfortunately, patients may be poorly adherent to antihypertensive therapy and indeed, the results of conservative medical management are not ideal. In fact, registry data show that 12% of patients receiving "optimal medical therapy," had complications such as malperfusion or rupture in the first 30 days.[31,42–44] The intervention-free survival rate was 40% in the medically managed group with some series demonstrating 5-year survival rates of 50%.[31,42–44] As is clear from the downstream mortality rates for medically managed patients with acute type B dissection, more studies are needed that can elucidate therapeutic targets focused on increasing survival.

Anesthetic Management

Stanford type A dissection

Obtaining arterial pressure monitoring before induction is essential as induction, airway management, and initiation of positive pressure ventilation can drastically alter hemodynamics depending on the nature and extent of the type A dissection. Arterial pressure monitoring location will depend on the pathophysiology of the dissection and the surgical plan for HCA. If HCA is planned with ACP, a combination of right upper extremity and either left upper extremity or femoral artery monitoring is necessary to monitor pressures during ACP and CPB.[36,45] If RCP is planned, placement of internal jugular or subclavian central venous access is warranted to allow for pressure monitoring. Anesthetic induction for a type A dissection shares similar hemodynamic goals and considerations as preoperative management. Prebypass hemodynamic goals should aim to decrease aortic dp/dt and aortic wall shear stress, preventing further dissection or rupture. If the patient's clinical status has deteriorated further before induction, transthoracic echocardiography can be useful in determining if pericardial tamponade, myocardial infarction, or AI is present. Continuation or cessation of antihypertensive agents, antichronotropic agents, vasopressors, and inotropes before induction should be based on the patient's clinical status.

Echocardiography

TEE is essential for surgical repair of type A dissection. TEE examination should be undertaken immediately after induction to confirm the presence of aortic dissection before proceeding with surgery. A focused TEE exam should include an assessment of aortic valve integrity, dimensions of aortic anatomic structures from the annulus to descending aorta, location and extent of entry tear, presence of pericardial tamponade, determination of false versus true lumens, presence of regional wall motion abnormalities, and aortic arch branch imaging to evaluate flow and extent of the dissection flap.[36] The latter is difficult to image secondary to tracheal obstruction of the upper esophageal views.[46] If TEE imaging of the aortic arch is difficult, initial CT angiography or epiaortic imaging may assist surgical planning regarding arch branch vessels.[36,47] Distinguishing the true lumen from the false lumen has important implications in the placement of the CPB aortic cannula. Luminal expansion during systole and lack of hematoma formation are characteristics that help distinguish the true lumen from the false lumen (**Figs. 6–9**).[46] M-mode can be used to assess true lumen expansion during systole. If aortic cannula pressures are high, cannula position should be immediately reassessed, as inadvertent false lumen cannulation may cause the dissection to progress or rupture. TEE should be used in the post-CPB period to ensure aortic valve competency, elimination of any entry tears, exclusion of the false

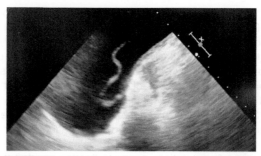

Fig. 6. -TEE–dissection flap in distal ascending aorta and proximal arch.

lumen, lack of ventricular regional wall motion abnormalities, and if possible, evaluation of aortic arch branch vessel patency.

Neuromonitoring and cerebral perfusion

Cerebral monitoring can be accomplished with electroencephalography (EEG), near-infrared spectroscopy (NIRS), and bispectral index (BIS). Owing to complex training, setup, and monitor interpretation, EEG is used with less frequency than BIS. However, BIS is liable to error in the setting of progressive hypothermia, high-dose opioids, N-methyl-D-aspartate (NMDA) receptor antagonists, neuromuscular blocking agents, and forced-air warming devices.[48] NIRS allows for the monitoring of cerebral oxygen saturation but is limited to the frontal cortex, and measurements can be affected by hemodilution, elevated bilirubin, and pathologic alterations in cerebral autoregulation.[36,49,50] Minimal evidence exists linking BIS and NIRS-based management of cerebral oxygenation to improved outcomes in type A repair. However, NIRS can be useful in determining if appropriate cerebral protection is being delivered and can assist in troubleshooting cerebral protection cannulation strategies. For instance, once hypothermia has been achieved, and cardiopulmonary bypass flows are dropped to 10 to 15 mL/kg/min, the innominate artery is clamped, and ACP is started via the right axillary arterial inflow graft. If left-sided NIRS drop significantly, a balloon-tipped catheter can be placed in the left common carotid artery for bilateral ACP.[15]

Surgery involving the aortic arch usually requires the institution of HCA. As stated previously, there has been a shift from deep HCA (14°C to 20°C) to more modest degrees of systemic cooling with equivalent or improved neurologic outcomes.[36,51] Mitigation of neurologic injury is accomplished with selective cerebral perfusion. ACP and

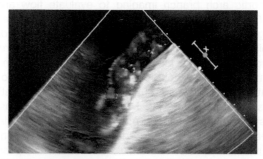

Fig. 7. TEE -Color Doppler demonstrating flow through the true lumen in the aortic arch.

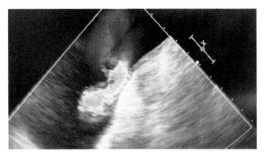

Fig. 8. TEE–Color Doppler demonstrating flow through the true lumen during peak systole in the aortic arch.

RCP are the most common strategies. ACP flow is administered by a right axillary artery cannula with targeted cerebral blood flows of 10 cc/kg/min used most frequently.[36,52] Optimal perfusion pressure is unknown, but equivalent neurologic outcomes have been shown in patients managed with pressures ranging from 50 mm Hg–80 mm Hg.[36,53] NIRS can help determine if bilateral ACP is required.[54,55] RCP blood is directed retrograde through the internal jugular veins with typical pressure ranging from 15 to 25 mm Hg monitored by pressure transduction of internal jugular or subclavian venous access.[36,56] The technique provides bilateral perfusion through the cerebral venous sinuses and promotes flushing of embolic material from cerebral vasculature, but concerns regarding cerebral edema and inadequate neuroprotection due to decreased overall cerebral blood flow remain.[36,57,58] The superiority of either method has yet to be determined.[36] It is unclear if the use of steroids, barbiturates, propofol, mannitol, or packing the head with ice offers any meaningful degree of cerebral protection during HCA, especially with frequent use of selective cerebral perfusion.[36,59,60]

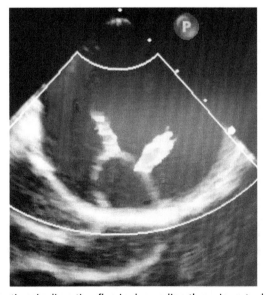

Fig. 9. TEE–Fenestrations in dissection flap in descending thoracic aorta demonstrating flow from true lumen (smaller lumen) into the false lumen.

Post-cardiopulmonary bypass management

Aortic dissection leads to intense fibrinolysis, platelet activation, and clotting factor consumption that is only amplified by HCA and exposure to CPB.[36,61,62] There is scant evidence regarding coagulopathy management after type A repair. Goal-directed transfusion therapy focused on platelet, clotting factor, and fibrinogen repletion should be undertaken based on point of care labs and thromboelastography. Antifibrinolytic therapy administration during cardiac surgery has been shown to decrease perioperative transfusion requirements and is recommended for routine use in current guidelines.[63,64] Clotting factors and fibrinogen can be more impaired than platelet function after type A dissection repair, and transfusion therapy should focus on clotting factors and fibrinogen as opposed to prioritizing platelet function.[65] Use of prothrombin complex concentrates (PCCs) has been shown to correct postoperative coagulopathy after cardiac surgery with an associated decrease in postoperative bleeding, massive transfusion, and surgical re-exploration.[36,66–68] Activated factor seven has been used as salvage therapy for persistent coagulopathy, yet concerns regarding thrombotic complications persist.[36,69,70]

FUTURE DIRECTIONS

Currently, no approved endografts for the ascending aorta or aortic arch exist in the United States. Two vascular grafts placed surgically with a distal stent graft then deployed endovascularly are available in Europe that allows for the repair of the entire ascending aorta and total arch. Clinical trials, such as Endovascular Treatment of Thoracic Aortic Disease or EVOLVE Aorta, are underway, and they may pave the way for future endovascular treatment of ascending aortic aneurysms and dissections.[15,71]

CLINICS CARE POINTS

- Approximately 85% of patients with Stanford type A dissections experience classic retrosternal tearing chest pain.

- Additional signs and symptoms can include hypertension due to pain and catecholamine surge, syncope secondary to rupture, cerebrovascular accident, altered sensorium, diastolic murmur due to aortic insufficiency, neurologic deficits due to spinal cord ischemia, general end organ and limb ischemia, and shock due to aortic rupture, pericardial tamponade, or coronary artery dissection.

- Obtaining arterial pressure monitoring before induction of anesthesia is highly recommended in patients presenting with acute aortic dissection given the propensity for large swings in systemic pressure and heart rate which can affect aortic dP/dt.

- If the surgeon plans for hypothermic circulatory arrest (HCA) with antegrade cerebral perfusion (ACP), a right radial arterial line will allow for continuous pressure monitoring after right axillary graft placement/cannulation for arterial inflow and clamping of the innominate artery for circulatory arrest. A second left radial or femoral arterial line should be placed for arterial pressure monitoring during cardiopulmonary bypass.

- Prebypass hemodynamic goals should aim to decrease aortic dP/dt and aortic wall shear stress, preventing further dissection or rupture.

- Recommended hemodynamic goals include a target systolic blood pressure between 90 and 120 mm Hg, mean arterial blood pressure of approximately 60 mm Hg, and a heart rate of 60 to 80 beats per minute.

- Antihypertensive agents with rapid onset and short half-life are preferred. Antihypertensive/ Beta Blocking agents such as sodium nitroprusside, esmolol, and clevidipine are ideal given their pharmacokinetic properties.
- If the patient's clinical status has further deteriorated upon arrival to the operating room, transthoracic echocardiography should be used before induction to assess for presence of new pericardial effusion, myocardial infarction, or AI.
- After induction of anesthesia, a focused TEE exam should include an assessment of aortic valve integrity, dimensions of aortic anatomic structures ranging from annulus to descending aorta, location and extent of entry tear, presence of pericardial effusion, presence of regional wall motion abnormalities, and aortic arch branch imaging to evaluate flow and extent of the dissection flap.
- Distinguishing the true lumen from the false lumen on TEE has important implications in the placement of the CPB aortic cannula. Luminal expansion during systole and lack of hematoma formation are characteristics that help distinguish the true lumen from the false lumen.
- Despite the paucity of evidence linking near-infrared spectroscopy (NIRS) based management of cerebral oxygenation to improved outcomes in type A repair, it can be useful in determining if appropriate cerebral protection is being delivered and can assist in troubleshooting cerebral protection cannulation strategies. A drop in NIRS values may indicate a need for bilateral ACP.

ACKNOWLEDGEMENTS

Nirav Mathur, MD, *Anatomy of an Aortic Dissection* (see **Fig. 1**).

DISCLOSURE

The authors have nothing to disclose.

REFERENCES

1. Elsayed RS, Cohen RG, Fleischman F, et al. Acute type A aortic dissection. Cardiol Clin 2017;35(3):331–45.
2. Clouse WD, Hallett JW Jr, Schaff HV, et al. Acute aortic dissection: population-based incidence compared with degenerative aortic aneurysm rupture. Mayo Clin Proc 2004;79:176e80.
3. LeMaire SA, Russell L. Epidemiology of thoracic aortic dissection. Nat Rev Cardiol 2011;8(2):103–13. https://doi.org/10.1038/nrcardio.2010.187. Epub 2010 Dec 21. PMID: 21173794.
4. Lombardi JV, Hughes GC, Appoo JJ, et al. Society for Vascular Surgery (SVS) and Society of Thoracic Surgeons (STS) reporting standards for type B aortic dissections. J Vasc Surg 2020;71:723e47.
5.. Nienaber CA, Fattori R, Mehta RH, et al. Gender-related differences in acute aortic dissection. Circulation 2004;109:3014–21.
6. Sen I, Erben YM, Franco-Mesa C, et al. Epidemiology of aortic dissection. Semin Vasc Surg 2021;34(1):10–7.
7. Olsson C, Thelin S, Sta hle E, et al. Thoracic aortic aneurysm and dissection: increasing prevalence and improved outcomes reported in a nationwide population-based study of more than 14,000 cases from 1987 to 2002. Circulation 2006;114:2611e8.

8. Bossone E, Pyeritz RE, O'Gara P, et al. Acute aortic dissection in blacks: insights from the International Registry of Acute Aortic Dissection. Am J Med 2013;126: 909e15.

9. Howard DPJ, Sideso E, Handa A, et al. Incidence, risk factors, outcome and projected future burden of acute aortic dissection. Ann Cardiothorac Surg 2014;3: 278e84.

10.. Hagan PG, Nienaber CA, Isselbacher EM, et al. The international registry of acute aortic dissection (iRAD): new insights into an old disease. JAMA 2000; 283:897–903.

11. Januzzi JL, et al. Characterizing the young patient with aortic dissection: results from the international Registry of Aortic Dissection (iRAD). J Am Coll Cardiol 2004;43:665–9.

12.. Kirklin J, Kouchoukos N, Blackstone EH, et al. Acute aortic dissection. In: Kirklin J, Kouchoukos N, Blackstone EH, Hanley FL, editors. Kirklin/barratt-boyes cardiac surgery. 4th edition. Philadelphia: Elsevier/Saunders; 2013. p. 1509–61.

13.. Demers P, Miller CD. Type A Aortic Dissection. In: Sellke FW, del Nido PJ, Swanson SJ, editors. Sabiston & spencer surgery of the chest, vol 2, 9th edition. Philadelphia: Elsevier; 2016. p. 1227–33.

14. Mathur N. Anatomy of an Aortic Dissection.

15. Preventza O, Coselli JS. Differential aspects of ascending thoracic aortic dissection and its treatment: the North American experience. Ann Cardiothorac Surg 2016;5(4):352–9.

16. Demers P, Miller DC. Chapter 70-type A aortic dissection. 9th Edition. Philadelphia: Elsevier Inc.; 2016. p. 1214–43.

17. Nienaber CA, Clough RE. Management of acute aortic dissection. Lancet 2015; 385(9970):800–11.

18. Augoustides JG, Szeto WY, Desai ND, et al. Classification of acute type A dissection: focus on clinical presentation and extent. Eur J Cardiothorac Surg 2011; 39(4):519–22.

19. Figure depicting Stanford Type A, Stanford Type B, and DeBakey Type I-IIIb dissection tear origins. Copyright © 2022 UpToDate, Inc. and its affiliates and/ or licensors. All rights reserved.

20. Tsai TT, Trimarchi S, Nienaber CA. Acute aortic dissection: perspectives from the International Registry of Acute Aortic Dissection (IRAD). Eur J Vasc Endovasc Surg 2009;37:149–59.

21. Gilon D, Mehta RH, oh JK, et al, International Registry of Acute Aortic Dissection Group. Characteristics and in-hospital outcomes of patients with cardiac tamponade complicating type A acute aortic dissection. Am J Cardiol 2009;103: 1029–31.

22. van Bogerijen GH, Tolenaar JL, Rampoldi V, et al. Predictors of aortic growth in uncomplicated type B aortic dissection. J Vasc Surg 2014;59:1134e43.

23. Pape LA, Awais M, Woznicki EM, et al. Presentation, diagnosis, and outcomes of acute aortic dissection: 17-year trends from the international registry of acute aortic dissection. J Am Coll Cardiol 2015;66(4):350–8.

24.. Mehta RH, Bossone E, Evangelista A, et al. Acute type B aortic dissection in elderly patients: clinical features, outcomes, and simple risk stratification rule. Ann Thorac Surg 2004;77:1622–8.

25. Harris KM, Strauss CE, Eagle KA, et al. Correlates of delayed recognition and treatment of acute type A aortic dissection: the International Registry of Acute Aortic Dissection (IRAD). Circulation 2011;124:1911–8.

26. Berretta P, Patel HJ, Gleason TG, et al. IRAD experience on surgical type A acute dissection patients: results and predictors of mortality. Ann Cardiothorac Surg 2016;5(4):346–51.

27.. Tsai TT, Evangelista A, Nienaber CA, et al. Long-term survival in patients presenting with type A acute aortic dissection: insights from the international Registry of Acute Aortic Dissection (iRAD). Circulation 2006;114(1 Suppl):i350–6.

28. Parikh N, Trimarchi S, Gleason TG, et al. Changes in operative strategy for patients enrolled in the International Registry of Acute Aortic Dissection interventional cohort program. J Thorac Cardiovasc Surg 2017;153(4):S74–9.

29.. Trimarchi S, Eagle KA, Nienaber CA, et al. Role of age in acute type A aortic dissection outcome: report from the international Registry of Acute Aortic Dissection (iRAD). J Thorac Cardiovasc Surg 2010;140:784–9.

30. Knipp BS, Deeb GM, Prager RL, et al. A contemporary analysis of outcomes for operative repair of type A aortic dissection in the United States. Surgery 2007; 142:524–8 [discussion: 528.e1].

31.. Tsai TT, Fattori R, Trimarchi S, et al. Long-term survival in patients presenting with type B acute aortic dissection: insights from the international Registry of Acute Aortic Dissection. Circulation 2006;114:2226–31.

32. Gudbjartsson T, Ahlsson A, Geirsson A, et al. Acute type A aortic dissection - a review. Scand Cardiovasc J 2020;54(1):1–13.

33. Shiga T, Wajima Z, Apfel CC, et al. Diagnostic accuracy of transesophageal echocardiography, helical computed tomography, and magnetic resonance imaging for suspected thoracic aortic dissection: systematic review and meta-analysis. Arch Intern Med 2006;166:1350–6.

34. Krüger T, Conzelmann LO, Bonser RS, et al. Acute aortic dissection type A. Br J Surg 2012;99(10):1331–44.

35. Saw LJ, Lim-Cooke MS, Woodward B, et al. The surgical management of acute type A aortic dissection: Current options and future trends. J Cardiovasc Surg 2020;35(9):2286–96.

36. Gregory SH, Yalamuri SM, Bishawi M, et al. The Perioperative management of ascending aortic dissection. Anesth Analg 2018;127(6):1302–13.

37. Ahmed Y, Houben IB, Figueroa CA, et al. Endovascular ascending aortic repair in type A dissection: a systematic review. J Card Surg 2021;36(1):268–79.

38. Conzelmann LO, Weigang E, Mehlhorn U, et al. Mortality in patients with acute aortic dissection type A: analysis of pre- and intraoperative risk factors from the German Registry for Acute Aortic Dissection Type A (GERAADA). Eur J Cardiothorac Surg 2016;49(2):e44–52.

39. Carl M, Alms A, Braun J, et al. S3 guidelines for intensive care in cardiac surgery patients: hemodynamic monitoring and cardiocirculary system. Ger Med Sci 2010;8:Doc12.

40. Javed F, Benjo AM, Reddy K, et al. Dexmedetomidine use in the setting of cocaine-induced hypertensive emergency and aortic dissection: a novel indication. Case Rep Med 2011;2011:174132.

41. Hughes GC, Andersen ND, McCann RL. Management of acute type B aortic dissection. J Thorac Cardiovasc Surg 2013;145(3 Suppl):S202–7.

42. Yuan X, Mitsis A, Ghonem M, et al. Conservative management versus endovascular or open surgery in the spectrum of type B aortic dissection. J Vis Surg 2018; 4:59.

43. Durham CA, Cambria RP, Wang LJ, et al. The natural history of medically managed acute type B aortic dissection. J Vasc Surg 2015;61:1192–8.

44. Coady MA, Ikonomidis JS, Cheung AT, et al. Surgical management of descending thoracic aortic disease: Open and endovascular approaches: a scientific statement from the American Heart Association. Circulation 2010;121:2780–804.

45. Svyatets M, Tolani K, Zhang M, et al. Perioperative management of deep hypothermic circulatory arrest. J Cardiothorac Vasc Anesth 2010;24:644–55.

46. Tan CN, Fraser AG. Perioperative transesophageal echocardiography for aortic dissection. Can J Anaesth 2014;61:362–78.

47. Assaad S, Geirsson A, Rousou L, et al. The dual modality use of epiaortic ultrasound and transesophageal echocardiography in the diagnosis of intraoperative iatrogenic type-A aortic dissection. J Cardiothorac Vasc Anesth 2013;27:326–8.

48. Kertai MD, Whitlock EL, Avidan MS. Brain monitoring with electroencephalography and the electroencephalogram derived bispectral index during cardiac surgery. Anesth Analg 2012;114:533–46.

49. Murkin JM, Arango M. Near-infrared spectroscopy as an index of brain and tissue oxygenation. Br J Anaesth 2009;103(suppl 1):i3–13.

50. Heringlake M, Garbers C, K bler JH, et al. Preoperative cerebral oxygen saturation and clinical outcomes in cardiac surgery. Anesthesiology 2011;114:58–69.

51. Tian DH, Wan B, Bannon PG, et al. A meta-analysis of deep hypothermic circulatory arrest versus moderate hypothermic circulatory arrest with selective antegrade cerebral perfusion. Ann Cardiothorac Surg 2013;2:148–58.

52. Spielvogel D, Tang GH. Selective cerebral perfusion for cerebral protection: what we do know. Ann Cardiothorac Surg 2013;2:326–30.

53. Li Y, Siemeni T, Optenhoefel J, et al. Pressure level required during prolonged cerebral perfusion time has no impact on neurological outcome: a propensity score analysis of 800 patients undergoing selective antegrade cerebral perfusion. Interact Cardiovasc Thorac Surg 2016;23:616–22.

54. Higami T, Kozawa S, Asada T, et al. Retrograde cerebral perfusion versus selective cerebral perfusion as evaluated by cerebral oxygen saturation during aortic arch reconstruction. Ann Thorac Surg 1999;67:1091–6.

55. Harrer M, Waldenberger FR, Weiss G, et al. Aortic arch surgery using bilateral antegrade selective cerebral perfusion in combination with near-infrared spectroscopy. Eur J Cardiothorac Surg 2010;38:561–7.

56. Reich DL, Uysal S, Ergin MA, et al. Retrograde cerebral perfusion as a method of neuroprotection during thoracic aortic surgery. Ann Thorac Surg 2001;72: 1774–82.

57. Apostolakis E, Shuhaiber JH. Antegrade or retrograde cerebral perfusion as an adjunct during hypothermic circulatory arrest for aortic arch surgery. Expert Rev Cardiovasc Ther 2007;5:1147–61.

58. Misfeld M, Mohr FW, Etz CD. Best strategy for cerebral protection in arch surgery - antegrade selective cerebral perfusion and adequate hypothermia. Ann Cardiothorac Surg 2013;2:331–8.

59. Kruger T, Hoffmann I, Blettner M, et al, GERAADA Investigators. Intraoperative neuroprotective drugs without beneficial effects? Results of the German Registry for Acute Aortic Dissection Type A (GERAADA). Eur J Cardiothorac Surg 2013; 44:939–46.

60. Roach GW, Newman MF, Murkin JM, et al. Ineffectiveness of burst suppression therapy in mitigating perioperative cerebrovascular dysfunction: Multicenter Study of Perioperative Ischemia (McSPI) research group. Anesthesiology 1999; 90:1255–64.

61. Guan XL, Wang XL, Liu YY, et al. Changes in the hemostatic system of patients with acute aortic dissection undergoing aortic arch surgery. Ann Thorac Surg 2016;101:945–51.
62. Paparella D, Rotunno C, Guida P, et al. Hemostasis alterations in patients with acute aortic dissection. Ann Thorac Surg 2011;91:1364–9.
63. Myles PS, Smith JA, Forbes A, et al. ATACAS Investigators of the ANZCA Clinical Trials Network. Tranexamic acid in patients undergoing coronary-artery surgery. N Engl J Med 2017;376:136–48.
64. Koster A, Faraoni D, Levy JH. Antifibrinolytic therapy for cardiac surgery: an update. Anesthesiology 2015;123:214–21.
65. Liu Y, Han L, Li J, et al. Consumption coagulopathy in acute aortic dissection: principles of management. J Cardiothorac Surg 2017;12(1):50.
66. Cappabianca G, Mariscalco G, Biancari F, et al. Safety and efficacy of prothrombin complex concentrate as first-line treatment in bleeding after cardiac surgery. Crit Care 2016;20:5.
67. Fitzgerald J, Lenihan M, Callum J, et al. Use of prothrombin complex concentrate for management of coagulopathy after cardiac surgery: a propensity score matched comparison to plasma. Br J Anaesth 2018;120:928–34.
68. Gorlinger K, Dirkmann D, Hanke AA, et al. First-line therapy with coagulation factor concentrates combined with point-of-care coagulation testing is associated with decreased allogeneic blood transfusion in cardiovascular surgery: a retrospective, single-center cohort study. Anesthesiology 2011;115:1179–91.
69. Grubitzsch H, Vargas-Hein O, Von Heymann C, et al. Recombinant activated factor VII for treatment of refractory hemorrhage after surgery for acute aortic dissection. J Cardiovasc Surg (Torino) 2009;50:531–4.
70. Lehr EJ, Alford TJ, Wang SH. Recombinant activated factor VII for postoperative hemorrhage following repair of acute type A aortic dissection. Heart Surg Forum 2010;13:E275–9.
71.. Eagleton M. Endovascular Treatment of Thoracic Aortic Disease (EVOLVE Aorta). NIH US National Library of Medicine. 2022. https://clinicaltrials.gov/ct2/show/NCT00583817.

Anesthetic Management for Open Thoracoabdominal and Abdominal Aortic Aneurysm Repair

Laeben Chola Lester, MD, Megan P. Kostibas, MD*

KEYWORDS

- Open thoracoabdominal • Abdominal • Aortic aneurysm • Distal Perfusion
- Extracorporeal support • Cerebroshpinal fluid drainage • Organ protection

KEY POINTS

- Open thoracoabdominal and abdominal aortic aneurysm repairs are some of the most challenging cases for anesthesiologists.
- The extent of the aneurysm also dictates the extent of the repair and correlates with the risk of paralysis, organ failure, and even death.
- Patient outcomes in aortic surgery correlate with the degree of organ protection, and the amount of time organs are ischemic.
- Strategies to decrease the chances of paraplegia include cerebrospinal fluid drainage, maintaining mean arterial pressure, left heart bypass, cooling, and the reimplantation of intercostal/radicular arteries.

Abbreviations	
ICU	intensive care unit
LOE	level of evidence
IL	interleukin
PTT	partial thromboplastin time
PT	prothrombin time
INR	international normalized ratio
FFP	fresh frozen plasma

INTRODUCTION: HISTORY AND INCIDENCE

Although the number of open repairs of descending thoracic, thoracoabdominal (TAAA), and abdominal aortic aneurysms (AAA) has declined with advancements in endovascular options, open repairs are still the preferred method in some patient

Department of Anesthesiology and Critical Care Medicine, Johns Hopkins School of Medicine, Zayed 6212, 1800 Orleans Street, Baltimore, MD 21287, USA
* Corresponding author.
E-mail address: mkostib1@jhmi.edu

Anesthesiology Clin 40 (2022) 705–718
https://doi.org/10.1016/j.anclin.2022.08.013
1932-2275/22/© 2022 Elsevier Inc. All rights reserved.
anesthesiology.theclinics.com

populations and disease processes. In this article, management of open repairs will be discussed. Medial degeneration and dissection make up the majority of cases presenting for open surgical repair.[1] Open TAAA and AAA repairs are some of the most challenging cases for anesthesiologists because of the potential for rapid blood loss combined with clamping and reperfusion, potential use of left heart bypass (LHB), the potential need for lung isolation, and potential placement and management of a spinal drain. In addition, patients often present with other significant comorbidities and a detailed understanding of the disease process, the complex physiology throughout the case, and the intricacies of organ protection are critical.

Extent of Repair

There are four main types of thoracoabdominal aneurysms according to the Crawford classification[2] (eg, **Fig. 1**). The extent of the aneurysm also dictates the extent of the repair and correlates with the risk of paralysis, organ failure, and even death. Type I aneurysms consist of repair that extends from the proximal descending aorta at the origin of the left subclavian (above T6) to the suprarenal abdominal aorta. Type II extends from the proximal descending aorta at the left subclavian (above T6) to the aortoiliac bifurcation. This type of repair has the most inherent complications both intraoperatively and postoperatively. Type III repair extends from the distal thoracic, descending aorta below T6 to below the diaphragm. Finally, Type IV extends from the diaphragm and progresses distally to the bifurcation.

Anesthetic Goals

Premedication

Premedications for analgesia can be considered, and an Enhanced Recovery after Surgery (ERAS) pathway is frequently tailored to these operations. Premedications can include acetaminophen 1 g by mouth and gabapentin 300 to 600 mg by mouth. Additional discussion regarding the ERAS pathway is discussed later in this article.

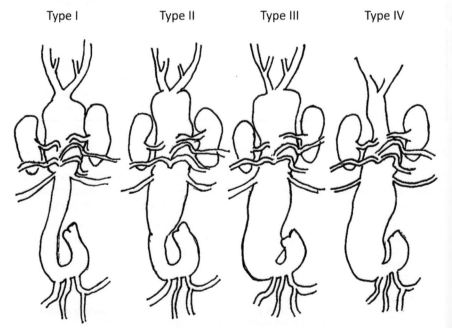

Type I   Type II   Type III   Type IV

Fig. 1. Crawford classification of thoracoabdominal aortic aneurysms.

Induction
In elective or urgent cases presenting before rupture has occurred, limiting aortic wall stress to avoid rupture is of central importance during the induction of anesthesia. A careful, slow, and controlled induction is paramount to maintaining safety and avoiding sudden increased stress on the aneurysm caused by stimulation during intubation that can be catastrophic. Hypertension and tachycardia cause increased wall stress and must be prevented by ensuring adequate depth of anesthesia and analgesia before intubation or other stimulating procedures. Short acting beta blockers such as esmolol and vasodilators, such as nitroglycerin, are very useful and should be readily available. Propofol and inhaled anesthetics can be used to ensure adequate depth of anesthesia, decrease the systemic vascular resistance and, along with opioids, help to blunt sympathetic stimulation. Placement of an awake arterial line for close continuous monitoring of arterial blood pressure during induction of anesthesia can be considered, especially in high-risk patients with other cardiovascular comorbidities.

In patients presenting with an emergent case, balancing the risk of hypotension and malperfusion from bleeding, such as in a ruptured AAA, with the need to avoid hypertension, as in a contained rupture, makes induction more challenging.[3] Preinduction placement of an arterial line can be very useful in these patients if their condition allows for it. In general, rapid sequence intubation is recommended if the patient has not adequately fasted, but must be balanced with the hemodynamic requirements of the patient. Hemodynamic collapse can occur after induction due to the relaxation of abdominal vasculature, thereby lessening tamponade effect, positive pressure decreasing venous return, and a reduction in sympathetic tone in patients in extremis. Therefore, surgeons and resources should be readily available in the room before induction.

Airway
Open thoracic and thoracoabdominal aneurysms require lung isolation for visualization. Lung isolation can be accomplished with double-lumen tube (DLT) or a bronchial blocker. Given the complexity of the case, including correction of shock and coagulopathy and concern for potential pulmonary edema, patients are often taken to the intensive care unit (ICU) postoperatively, remaining intubated and requiring mechanical ventilation. Using a bronchial blocker in this situation obviates the need to change out the DLT at the end of the case. Many studies have looked at the quality of lung isolation and frequency of dislodgement during isolation between DLT and bronchial blockers. Overall, the quality of isolation and frequency of dislodgement are thought to be similar if not improved.[4,5] However, if is thought that the chance of intrapulmonary bleed is increased, a DLT has its advantages for clot evacuation and protecting the opposite lung while continuing lung isolation. Appropriate endotracheal placement should always be confirmed with bronchoscopy. Another consideration when assessing the airway and planning for intubation is that large thoracic aneurysms might displace or compress the airway, most frequently the left bronchus.[5,6] This can make left-sided DLTs difficult to impossible to place. A right-sided DLT might be required in this instance. Review of chest x-ray and/or computed topography should be evaluated to understand the size and location of the aneurysm in relation to the left bronchus.

Access
Central venous access (8.5 or 9 French introducer) and large bore peripheral access (8.5-French rapid infusion catheter or 14-gauge catheter) should be obtained for rapid resuscitation and medication delivery. It has been reported that open TAAA repairs have a minimal blood loss of 2.5 L up to approximately 12 L of blood, with median range about 5 L.[7] This blood loss can also happen very acutely with transitions of

clamping/unclamping. Frequently, multiple central lines in the neck are placed as well as peripheral rapid infusion catheters. Once placed, the rate of flow should be confirmed both before and after positioning. Frequently, during these cases, a rapid infuser pump is used to ensure rapid and warm resuscitation. New models, such as the Belmont® Rapid Infuser and the ThermaCor® Rapid Infuser can flow more than 1 L per minute and can detect exact flow rates in milliliters (mL) per minute.

Pulmonary artery catheters (PACs) can be considered if the expertise is available. However, the literature does not specifically address the use of these in aortic surgeries. In a recent publication, over 4600 patients undergoing bypass or valve surgery requiring cardiopulmonary bypass with the use of PACs were compared with propensity-matched patients undergoing similar surgery without pulmonary catheters.[8] This study did not find an improved mortality in the catheter group, and no statistically significant change in stroke, sepsis, and new renal failure. Those with PACs were found to have longer ICU stays and more red blood cell transfusions ($P < 0.001$). Even though PACs have not been shown to lead to a reduced mortality in clinical trials, consideration can be considered in high-risk patients with high-risk procedures in centers where expertise is available. For instance, one might consider a PAC in those with low ejection fraction, right heart dysfunction, pulmonary hypertension or end-stage renal disease.

At least one arterial line should be obtained for the procedure and consideration should be made to placing this before induction as mentioned earlier. During induction, it is critically important to maintain tight blood pressure control to avoid shear wall stress on the aorta, minimizing chances of rupture and/or worsening dissection. Right radial access is preferred compared with left radial access in the event that the aortic cross-clamp is placed proximal to the left subclavian artery.[8,9] A left radial arterial line would be inaccurate in this setting, whereas right radial will reflect perfusion in the carotid and coronary arteries during periods of cross-clamp proximal to the left subclavian artery. Simultaneous femoral arterial cannulation can also be useful in these cases to assess perfusion distal to the cross-clamp. Femoral arterial access is especially useful in cases with higher cross-clamps, such as supraceliac. Perfusion will decrease distal to the cross-clamp and titration of LHB or extracorporeal support is partially guided by the pressure seen on the femoral arterial line.

Distal Perfusion Techniques and Extracorporeal Support

Patient outcomes in aortic surgery correlate with the degree of organ protection and the amount of time organs are ischemic. There are two main ways of ensuring distal perfusion during aortic-cross clamping. The first is passive aortic shunting and the second is LHB or partial bypass. Today, LHB is the most frequently used approach. Although less common, full cardiopulmonary bypass can also be used, but requires higher heparinization levels. There are also more organ-targeted methods such as selective renal protection (SRP) or selective visceral protection (SVP) (eg, **Fig. 2**).[10] Both SRP and SVP will be discussed later when addressing renal and visceral protection of the respected organs.

There are three main benefits of distal perfusion with LHB. The first is more obvious—perfusion of oxygenated blood to the tissue distal to the clamp. The second benefit of distal perfusion is less obvious—to limit the degree of proximal hypertension that can be seen once the cross-clamp is placed by reducing left atrial preload and left ventricular cardiac output. In addition, one of the most important benefits of LHB is that it reduces the rates of paraplegia. In one study looking at patients undergoing repair for type II TAAA, LHB was shown to decrease the incidence of paraplegia from 13.1% to 4.8%.[11] Additional benefits of distal perfusion techniques include reduction in visceral and renal ischemia, reduction in acidosis, ability to cool/warm

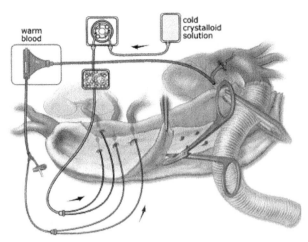

Fig. 2. Left heart bypass with normothermic blood visceral perfusion and selective renal protection with cold crystalloid renal perfusion. (*From* Köksoy[10]; with permission.)

patients, reduction in disseminated intravascular coagulation (DIC) incidence, and supplemental oxygenation via the extracorporeal circuit. Potential drawbacks include injury with cannula placement, embolus from thrombus, plaque or air, increased operative time, and the potential for bleeding at cannula sites.[12]

Typically, an LHB circuit includes an extracorporeal pump and an inflow and outflow cannula. The inflow cannula is usually placed in the left atrium via a left-sided pulmonary vein, although an inflow cannula can also be placed in the thoracic aorta after heparinization. Goal activated clotting time should be above 200 seconds and checked every 30 minutes. The outflow cannula is usually placed in the left femoral artery but is sometimes placed in the distal descending aorta. Although the outflow cannula can be placed directly into the femoral artery, placement through a short graft sewn end-to-end onto the femoral artery may be preferred as direct cannulation in the artery has been associated with leg ischemia, myoglobin release, and increased incidence of renal failure in the postoperative period.[13] Miller and colleagues found that using this sidearm, an end-to-end approach led to a 15% to 20% decrease in postoperative renal complications in those with GFR less than 60.[13] Before aortic cross-clamping the flow on the pump is usually around 500 mL per minute, but this is increased to 1 to 2.5 L per minute once the cross-clamp is in place. Adequate mean arterial pressure (MAP) should be evaluated by a lower extremity (femoral) arterial line. If proximal blood pressures remain elevated, options include increasing flows in the LHB circuit or intravenous titration of systemic vasodilators.[1] However, one must be mindful that while an increase in flow via the LHB circuit, you are simultaneously decreasing flow, and therefore perfusion, to those organs above the cross-clamp. Careful assessments of pressure on all arterial lines are critical to balance flow and perfusion to all tissues of the body.

Transesophageal Echocardiography

If expertise and equipment allow, intraoperative transesophageal echocardiography (TEE) should be considered. According to the American Society of Anesthesiology (ASA), unless there is a contraindication, "For adult patients without contraindications, TEE should be used in all . . . thoracic aortic surgical procedures."[14] Although the ASAs recommendation for TEE during open abdominal procedures is equivocal, they do recommend, "TEE may be used when the nature of the planned surgery or the patient's known or suspected cardiovascular pathology might result in severe hemodynamic, pulmonary, or neurologic compromise." TEE will help to assess volume status, monitor for antegrade dissection, evaluate for regional wall motion abnormalities in the setting of coronary ischemia and potentially aid is cannulation for LHB. Also, TEE is nearly indispensable for positioning of the left atrial cannula to ensure proper positioning and adequate flow during LHB without the administration of excessive volume.

Temperature Management

Both esophageal and bladder temperature probes should be used to assess core and visceral temperatures, as both hypothermia and hyperthermia can lead to deleterious outcomes. Hyperthermia will lead to increased metabolic rate, predisposing organs to worsening ischemia.[15] Hypothermia is associated with higher infectious complications and coagulopathy. However, hypothermia is also important for neurologic protection. Oxygen requirements are reduced by approximately 5% to 7% for every degree centigrade decrease in temperature.[16] Additional benefits of mild to moderate hypothermia included decreased excitatory neurotransmitter release, decreased oxygen free radical release, and decreased postischemic edema.[9] Passive hypothermia is allowed in which temperatures will decrease to 32° to 35°C and is usually easily obtained with a cool operating room, large incision, and use of extracorporeal (LHB) circuit. Full cardiopulmonary bypass allows for deep hypothermic circulatory arrest with temperatures at 15°C to 18°C. This is more ideal for longer cross-clamp times up to 45 minutes.

At the cessation of the case, the patient should be warmed to 36°C or greater to minimize or eliminate temperature-related coagulopathy. Consideration should be made to not warm the lower extremities/body during cross-clamping as this portion of the body already has increased metabolic rate. After cross-clamps are released, forced air or other warmers can be used. Rewarming in thoracoabdominal cases without LHB can be especially challenging as there is minimal upper body surface area to place warmers.

Positioning and Incision

Positioning for open thoracoabdominal repair is corkscrew, modified right lateral decubitus position, with shoulders and hips at 60° and 30° horizontally. A beanbag is used to maintain this position. To minimize the chances of brachial plexus injury, an axillary role should be used, and all pressure points padded. The left arm should be extended superiorly and both arms supported with slings. Usually, the table is also flexed. After positioning, the endotracheal tube and all venous access lines should be checked to confirm position and functionality. The left chest, left flank, and groins are prepped in the field.[9,17]

Organ Protection

Lungs

Type I, II, III repairs have a high risk of post-op pulmonary complications. Owing to the degree of retraction required for visualization, the left lung can sustain trauma. High volume resuscitation and transfusions, diaphragmatic dysfunction, phrenic and recurrent laryngeal nerve damage are all additional factors increasing the risk of pulmonary dysfunction. Lung-protective ventilation should be used throughout the procedure.[9]

Clamping

The degree of hemodynamic effects of aortic cross-clamping depends on the level of cross-clamp, with the most pronounced changes following supraceliac clamping. No matter the level of cross-clamp, there will be an increase in systemic vascular resistance, with more increase at higher clamp levels. Supraceliac clamping will cause a dramatic increase in afterload, thereby increasing the MAP, left ventricle end-systolic wall stress and myocardial oxygen requirements and decreasing cardiac output.[18] MAP can increase up to 40%.[18,19] There is also an increase in preload thought to be due to volume distribution from veins distal to the aortic occlusion, and a resultant increased central venous pressure and pulmonary artery occlusion pressure.[12] These changes are much less obvious or even noticed in infrarenal clamping. Roizen and colleagues used TEE in 24 patients undergoing open aortic reconstruction and evaluated changes in left ventricular end-systolic and end-diastolic areas, ejection fraction, and wall motion abnormalities during cross-clamping at various levels.[20] In patients undergoing supraceliac cross-clamp, the proximal MAP increased by more than 50%, filling pressures by 40%, and end-diastolic and end-systolic areas by 28% and 70%, respectively, while ejection fraction decreased by almost 40%. Remarkably, 92% had wall motion abnormalities. In patients with infrarenal cross-clamp, no regional wall motion abnormalities were noted, and other changes were minimal compared with the supraceliac patients.

Because aortic cross-clamp leads to an increase in oxygen demand, the response of the coronary vasculature is to appropriately increase supply, and studies have shown up to a 65% increase in coronary blood flow after aortic cross-clamp is placed.[21] The "Anrep effect" also plays a role in this setting.[18] This principle states that a sudden increase in aortic pressure will cause an increase in left ventricular end-diastolic volume, thereby increasing demand and coronary blood flow, which will result in a positive inotropic effect leading to the end-diastolic volume returning to normal. However, this autoregulation is impaired in patients with coronary disease, resulting in ventricular failure. There is limited ability for a heart with coronary disease to increase coronary blood flow, also leading to an inability to generate the Anrep effect. In an effort to attenuate the increased MAP, left ventricle end-systolic wall stress, and oxygen demand, afterload reducers can be used such as nitroprusside, nitroglycerin, or nicardipine. These agents work mainly by decreasing the increased systemic vascular resistance, thereby increasing cardiac output. Beta blockers can also be used to decrease shear wall stress, with short-acting esmolol the preferred agent given the potential for hypotension during these cases.

As cross-clamp time increases, systemic vascular resistance increases, whereas cardiac output will decrease. The reasons for this are thought to be due to the transcapillary pressure increase which results in increased interstitial edema and therefore less circulating blood volume with increased vascular resistance.[18]

Distal to the cross-clamping, reduction in MAP can result in ischemia of the viscera, liver, kidneys, and spinal cord. With clamping, blood flow below the clamp can be reduced up to 80% of preceding values.[19] Using the femoral arterial line, one can aim to control for adequate pressure to minimize the degree of ischemia. The perfusion depends on LHB and collaterals.

Reperfusion after the removal of the aortic cross-clamp can cause a dramatic change in hemodynamics. Preparation and communication with the surgeon are paramount to quickly ameliorate the hypotension and avoid catastrophe. This drastic decrease in systemic vascular resistance is due to a sudden release of ischemic and negative ionotropic mediators, including lactate, oxygen-free radicals, and cytokines. Before unclamping, the patient should be optimized to deal with this hemodynamic change. Laboratories such as hemoglobin, pH, base deficit, and lactate should be checked before removal of the clamp to allow for correction and optimization. Adequate preload as evidenced by central venous pressure, pulmonary artery occlusion pressure, TEE volume assessment, and clinical judgment should be achieved. Also, pharmacologic support should be readily available including epinephrine, norepinephrine, vasopressin, phenylephrine, sodium bicarbonate, and calcium chloride. Hyperventilation just before release of the cross-clamp can help compensate for the degree of metabolic acidosis that will accompany clamp release. The clamp can be slowly released to slow the release of the mediators of hypotension and ease the drop systemic vascular resistance. Replacing the clamp can be considered if needed to buy time for further optimization.

Spinal Cord/Neurologic Protection

Cerebrospinal fluid drainage

Paraplegia is a devastating but known complication with TAAA repairs. In the literature, it is reported to happen from 2.7% to 20% of the time.[22] Cerebrospinal fluid (CSF) drainage in the intraoperative and postoperative period can decrease this risk (Class I recommendation, LOE B).[9] Other strategies to decrease the chances of paraplegia include maintaining MAP, LHB, cooling, and the reimplantation of intercostal/radicular arteries. Placement of CSF drainage catheter (spinal drain) is performed sterilely before induction or just after. Some institutions will place the catheter the day before the procedure to allow time for difficult placement and avoid risk of delaying to surgical case. In the event of a bloody tap, placement of the spinal drain the day before allows time for resolution before heparinization. CSF drainage is important because aortic cross-clamping is associated with a rise in venous pressure and a corresponding CSF pressure rise, which causes a decrease in spinal cord perfusion pressure (SCPP). SCPP is estimated as the MAP-CSF pressure. Therefore, measures that increase MAP and decrease CSF pressure result in improved spinal cord perfusion, thereby lessening the risk and degree of ischemia of the spinal cord. Once the CSF catheter is in, it is attached to a drain, transducer, and pressure monitoring line so that SCPP can be calculated. CSF should be drained to maintain a CSF pressure of less than 15 mm Hg, without exceeding a maximal drainage rate of 10 to 15 mL per hour. This can be carefully titrated to allow for more drainage if perfusion pressure drops, but increased drainage has been associated with high risk of subdural hematoma.

As mentioned earlier, hypothermia is beneficial in terms of spinal cord ischemia and shows improved neurologic outcomes after aneurysm surgery (Class IIa, LOE B).[9,23] Spinal cord hyperemia can be seen after ischemia of the spinal cord, which is proportional to the incidence of paraplegia.[9] While not completely known, this is thought to be due to edema, potential compartment syndrome of the spinal cord, and increased oxygen free radicals. Epidural cooling with infusion of lactated Ringer's at 4°C and regional cooling of the spinal cord have been studied. Studies are ongoing at approaches spinal cord cooling and practices mixed.[9,24]

There are also some pharmacologic methods that promote spinal cord protection.[9,25] The most common variable that can be controlled is increasing the MAP to allow for increased SCPP. This can be done with agents such as norepinephrine, epinephrine, vasopressin, or phenylephrine. Steroids, such as methylprednisolone, have been used to reduce neuronal excitotoxicity, stabilize neuronal membranes, reduce edema and have anti-inflammatory effects. Intrathecal papaverine may enhance spinal cord perfusion and provide some neuroprotection in patient undergoing descending thoracic aneurysm repair.[26] Naloxone infusion has been shown to reduce excitatory neurotransmitter release that can exacerbate ischemic injury.[25,27]

Neuromonitoring

Paraplegia is one of the most dreaded complications following TAAA due to anterior cord ischemia. The duration of cross-clamp time is the most important determinate in spinal cord ischemia. According to the 2010 Guidelines for the diagnosis and management of patients with thoracic aortic disease, motor evoked potential (MEP) or somatosensory evoked potential (SSEP) monitoring can be useful when the information will help the surgical and anesthetic team guide therapy with level of evidence: B.[9] SSEPs are less sensitive to anesthetics and paralytics compared with MEPs; however, its use is limited because it only dependes on the lateral and posterior spinal columns.[28] The anterior cord is more likely to suffer from ischemia during aortic aneurysm repair, and this is seen by changes in MEPs. The loss of MEPs during the surgical case is associated with paraplegia. If a change is noted in increased latency or decreased amplitude of the potential, interventions can include moving the cross-clamp to allow better perfusion though the intercostal arteries, reimplantation of critical intercostal artery, increasing drainage of CSF, and increasing the MAP with vasopressor use.[19] Accurate monitoring of MEPs requires minimal paralysis and ongoing discussion with the neuromonitoring team. Although still being studied and utility not well understood, there are some early proponents of using near-infrared spectroscopy along the paravertebral muscles during aortic surgery in an effort to indirectly and noninvasively monitor real-time oxygenation/perfusion of the spine.[29]

Renal Protection

Renal dysfunction after TAAA repairs can occur in up to 28% of patients and requires dialysis in up to 12%.[30] Intraoperative cross-clamp time over 30 minutes and preoperative renal dysfunction are the two most common factors leading to postoperative renal failure. Preoperative renal failure is linked to higher operative mortality and morbidity.[12] In 2017, Girardi and colleagues looked at over 700 patients undergoing open repair of TAAA and descending thoracic aneurysms.[10] They compared patients with normal preoperative renal function with those that were considered to have preoperative renal failure, as defined by a serum creatinine greater than 1.5 gm/dL or on hemodialysis. The analysis found that the operative mortality was seven times higher in the patients with renal failure (14.2% vs 2.2%; $P < 0.001$). The 5-year survival was also significantly lower in the preoperative renal failure patients (45% vs 69.8%; $P < 0.001$).

Historically, renal protection involved shunting.[10] This allowed for antegrade flow from the thoracic aorta to the infrarenal aorta with pulsatile flow. However, this method is not without its limits, and perfusion depends on adequate MAP proximal to the clamp.

In the mid 1990s, partial bypass, or LHB, became popular due to improved morbidity and mortality associated with its use.[10] Full cardiopulmonary bypass can also be, which allows for selective perfusion of the kidneys with cold blood. However, a full cardiopulmonary circuit requires higher heparinization and increased bleeding risk.

Current guidelines recommend the use of SRP with cold crystalloid or blood perfusion as a method for renal protection during TAAA repair (class IIB, level of evidence B).[10] The target temperature with SRP during the ischemic period is 15°or less.[31] When using SRP, a goal perfusion pressure of 60 mm Hg is suggested,[32] whereas some studies will suggest a mean pressure of 85 through the perfusion cannula for those with chronic kidney disease.[13] Dr Crawford was a proponent of this back in the 1980s by using lactated Ringer's solution at 4°C. In the early 2000s, Coselli and colleagues randomized patients undergoing Crawford type II repair with LHB to either receive cold crystalloid perfusion at 4°C to the kidneys versus normothermic blood.[10] After multivariate analysis, cold crystalloid perfusate was found to be protective again postoperative renal dysfunction. Later Coselli randomized patients undergoing type II or III repair to receive either cold crystalloid at 4°C or cold blood at 4°C.[31] There was no significant difference between the two groups in terms of postoperative renal dysfunction, but there was a nonsignificant trend toward less paraplegia in the crystalloid group. In addition, surgeons will often place renal stents preoperatively or intraoperatively or perform renal endarterectomy in patients with significant renal artery stenosis or dissection.[33]

The patient should present to the operation well hydrated. The use of low-dose dopamine, Lasix, and fenoldopam has not been found to be beneficial in preserving renal function in euvolemic patients.[34] Although it is often still used, many randomized control trials have failed to clearly demonstrate a clinical reduction in the incidence of renal failure with mannitol administration.

Protection of the Viscera

Although the viscera may be less prone to ischemia than the kidneys, the liver, pancreas, and bowel can become ischemic during cross-clamping for repair of Crawford Type II, III, IV aneurysms.[32] This results in an increase in lactate, hepatic dysfunction and contributes to coagulopathy. In cases where moderate systemic hypothermia is used (30°C–32°C), the selective perfusion of the celiac and superior mesenteric artery does not seem to be beneficial.[9] Several studies have looked at selective perfusion to supply direct perfusion to the celiac and superior mesenteric artery, whereas the aneurysm is open. This is usually done with isothermic blood, but not routinely in practice due to the lack of clinical studies showing a morbidity and mortality benefit. In a porcine model, Kalder and colleagues found an improved acidosis, microcirculation, and less IL8 production; however, it did not result in less lactate production or mucosal injury. In regard to the SVP effect on the hepatosplenic system, there is still as significant decrease in hepatic venous oxygen saturation and lactate extraction, suggesting that it does not allow for adequate perfusion.[32,35]

Hematologic Considerations

Owing to the extensive surgical repair, long operative times, heparinization, both passive and active cooling, ischemia related to cross-clamping, extracorporeal circuit support and large resuscitation, bleeding due coagulopathy are frequently seen. Heparin is used to prevent thromboembolic complications, and a recommended dose of unfractionated heparin is 50 to 100 units/kilogram allowing for an activated clotting time greater than 200 seconds. The extent of resuscitation, bleeding, and coagulation correlates with how proximal the cross-clamp is placed and how long it is in place, with higher cross-clamps and longer cross-clamp times associated with more bleeding and coagulopathy. Also, underlying DIC can result from organ ischemia and release of endothelin and thromboplastin from the exposed subendothelial tissue of the aorta. According to de Figueiredo and colleagues, "Platelet deficiencies both qualitative and quantitative are the most predictable and consistent disturbance in the hemostatic function and the most common cause of intraoperative and postoperative bleeding."[36] Baseline coagulation laboratories should be taken before the operation and checked at a regular basis throughout the operation to allow for correction. These laboratories include hemoglobin or hematocrit, platelet levels, fibrinogen, PTT, PT, INR, thromboelastogram (TEG), or rotational thromboelastometry (ROTEM).

Blood products including red blood cells (RBCs), plasma, platelets, cryoprecipitate, and even concentrated factors should be readily available. Washed cell salvage and whole blood salvage options are also readily used in these cases to limit transfusions from allogeneic units and have been well documented as being associated with reduced length of stay and red blood cell transfusions.[37] Merkel and colleagues reported on the use of high- and ultra-high utilization of cell salvage in open TAAA and AAA procedures at our institution and showed that administration of up to 12 L of cell salvage did not result in coagulopathy when cell salvage was balanced with FFP, platelets, and cryoprecipitate.[38] In essence, using a 1:1 ratio of RBC to FFP as a guide while counting each 300 mL of cell salvage administration as equivalent of a unit of packed RBC is a very good guide, which can then be fine-tuned with laboratory assessment including TEG or ROTEM, platelet count, fibrinogen concentration, and coagulation studies. The use of cell salvage is especially important given the current shortage of blood products associated with the SARS-COV-2 pandemic.[39]

There are also pharmacologic methods that can be used that have been shown to help limit blood loss, improve coagulation, and promote platelet function. Tranexamic acid (TXA) has been shown to reduce blood loss in general surgery, traumas, and postpartum hemorrhage. Alpha-aminocaproic acid and TXA are both antifibrinolytics that can be used as clot stabilizers. Monaco and colleagues randomized 100 patients undergoing open AAA repair to either receive a bolus dose and continuous infusion of TXA versus no TXA.[40] Although they did not find any statistically significant difference in intraoperative blood loss, the authors found a 33% reduction in postoperative blood loss during the first 24 hours ($P = 0.003$) with a trend toward lower transfusion rate in the TXA group.

Desmopressin (DDAVP) has a potential role in patients undergoing aortic surgery, with a low side-effect profile. It works to increasing plasma von Willebrand factor, factor VIII, and intracellular platelet calcium/sodium ion concentration. It also increases the formation of procoagulant platelets and platelet adhesion to collagen and has been shown to be beneficial in patients with platelet dysfunction. In a systematic review by Desborough and colleagues, they found that DDAVP may be useful in decreasing bleeding and transfusion requirements in patients with platelet dysfunction or on antiplatelets undergoing cardiac surgery.[41] However, Clagett and colleagues did not find that DDAVP decreased bleeding or transfusion requirements in patients randomized control trial of patients undergoing aortic surgery, although only infrarenal aortic aneurysm repair or aortofemoral bypass cases were included.[42]

As mentioned earlier in this article, open aortic repairs can cause blood loss of over 10 L. Therefore, rapid resuscitation methods should be used. Belmont Rapid Infuser and the ThermaCor Rapid Infuser can detect exact flow rates in mL per minute and are designed for the rapid correction of hypovolemia while allowing for warming of the fluid/blood.

Enhanced Recovery after Surgery

The ERAS pathway has been beneficial to many surgical populations. In 2022, the ERAS Society and Society for Vascular Surgery collaborated to form a consensus statement for undergoing vascular surgery including patients with supraceliac, suprarenal, and infrarenal clamp sites, for aortic aneurysm and aortoiliac occlusive disease.[34] The consensus not only addresses intraoperative recommendations but also preadmission, preoperative, and postoperative as well. Intraoperative considerations address appropriate antibiotics, postoperative nausea and vomiting prevention, multimodal analgesia, neuromuscular blockade monitoring, lung protective ventilation, cell salvage, and temperature management.

Epidural analgesia has been found to be beneficial in some patients undergoing aortic surgery, specifically AAA repair. A Cochrane review reported no difference in 30-day mortality after open AAA surgery, but found low to moderate quality evidence of reduced rate of myocardial infarction, time to extubation, length of stay in critical care, and postoperative respiratory failure favoring epidural analgesia. In the ERAS consensus statement with level of evidence B, a T6-9 epidural "is recommended intraoperatively and continued postoperatively as an infusion or patient-controlled analgesia using a combination of local anesthetic and an opioid."[34] The risks of epidural placement in the setting of coagulopathy, heparinization, and possible interference with neurologic examinations have to be discussed and weighed against the benefits.

In summary, anesthetic management of these open repairs requires focused preparation, communication with surgical colleagues, complex monitoring strategies, titrated hemodynamic management, and intense resuscitative strategies to success-fully get these patients through these complex cases while optimizing successfully outcomes and minimizing risks.

CLINICS CARE POINTS

- Open TAAA and AAA repairs have the potential for rapid blood loss and challening hemodynamics due to volume changes along with clamping and reperfusion, and left heart bypass.
- Ensuring distal perfusion during cross clamp period can be done with passive shunting, left heart bypass, and full cardiopulmonary bypass.
- Benefits of distal perfusion include providing oxygenated blood to distal tissues, limiting the degree of proximal hypertension, and decreased rates of paraplegia.

DISCLOSURE

The authors have nothing to disclose.

REFERENCES

1. Anton JM, Herald KJ. Anesthetic management of open thoracoabdominal aortic aneurysm repair. Int anesthesiology Clin 2016;54(2):76–101. Available at: https://www.ncbi.nlm.nih.gov/pubmed/26967803.
2. Crawford ESCJ. Thoracoabdominal aneurysm surgery. Semin Thorac Cardiovasc Surg 1991;3(4):300–22.
3. Leonard A, Thompson J. Anaesthesia for ruptured abdominal aortic aneurysm. Continuing Education Anaesth Crit Care Pain 2008;8(1):11–5.
4. Bussières JS, Somma J, del Castillo, et al. Bronchial blocker versus left double-lumen endotracheal tube in video-assisted thoracoscopic surgery: A randomized-controlled trial examining time and quality of lung deflation. Can J Anesth/j Can Anesth 2016;63(7):818–27. Available at: https://link.springer.com/article/10.1007/s12630-016-0657-3.
5. Mourisse JMJ, Liesveld J, Verhagen AFTM, et al. Efficiency, efficacy, and safety of EZ-blocker compared with left-sided double-lumen tube for one-lung ventilation. Anesthesiology (Philadelphia) 2013;118(3):550–61. Available at: https://www.narcis.nl/publication/RecordID/oai:repository.ubn.ru.nl:2066%2F118367.
6. Kumar A, Dutta V, Negi S, et al. Vascular airway compression management in a case of aortic arch and descending thoracic aortic aneurysm. Ann Card Anaesth 2016;19(3):568–71. Available at: http://www.annals.in/article.asp?issn=0971-9784;year=2016;volume=19;issue=3;spage=568;epage=571;aulast=Kumar;type=0.
7. Pieri M, Nardelli P, De Luca M, et al. Predicting the need for intra-operative large volume blood transfusions during thoraco-abdominal aortic aneurysm repair. Eur J Vasc endovascular Surg 2016;53(3):347–53. Available at: https://www.clinicalkey.es/playcontent/1-s2.0-S1078588416306451.
8. Brown JA, Aranda-Michel E, Kilic A, et al. The impact of pulmonary artery catheter use in cardiac surgery. J Thorac Cardiovasc Surg 2021;S0022-5223(21):00185–9.
9. Hiratzka LF MD, Bakris GL, et al. 2010 ACCF/AHA/AATS/ACR/ASA/SCA/SCAI/SIR/STS/SVM guidelines for the diagnosis and management of patients with thoracic aortic disease. J Am Coll Cardiol 2010;55(14):e27–129. Available at: https://www.clinicalkey.es/playcontent/1-s2.0-S0735109710007151.

10. Köksoy C, LeMaire SA, Curling PE, et al. Renal perfusion during thoracoabdominal aortic operations: Cold crystalloid is superior to normothermic blood. Ann Thorac Surg 2002;73(3):730–8.

11. Coselli JS, LeMaire SA. Left heart bypass reduces paraplegia rates after thoracoabdominal aortic aneurysm repair. Ann Thorac Surg 1999;67(6):1931–4.

12. Goel N, Jain D, Savlania A, et al. Thoracoabdominal aortic aneurysm repair: What should the anaesthetist know? Turkish J Anaesthesiology Reanimation 2019; 47(1):1–11. Available at: https://www.ncbi.nlm.nih.gov/pubmed/31276105.

13. MILLER CC, VILLA MA, ACHOUH P, et al. Intraoperative skeletal muscle ischemia contributes to risk of renal dysfunction following thoracoabdominal aortic repair. discussion. Eur J cardio-thoracic Surg 2008;33(4):691–4.

14. Tyhs D. An updated report by the american society of anesthesiologists and the society of cardiovascular anesthesiologists task force on transesophageal echocardiography; practice guidelines for perioperative transesophageal echocardiography. Anesthesiology 2010;112:1084–96.

15. Crawford F Jr, Sade RM. Spinal cord injury associated with hyperthermia during aortic coarctation repair. J Thorac Cardiovasc Surg 1984;87(4):616–8. Available at: http://jtcs.ctsnetjournals.org/cgi/content/abstract/87/4/616.

16. Omairi AM, Pandey S. Targeted Temperature Management. 2022 Jun 5. In: StatPearls [Internet]. Treasure Island (FL): StatPearls Publishing; 2022 Jan. PMID: 32310584.

17. Black JH. Technique for repair of suprarenal and thoracoabdominal aortic aneurysms. J Vasc Surg 2009;50(4):936–41. Available at: https://www.clinicalkey.es/playcontent/1-s2.0-S0741521409004984.

18. GELMAN S. The pathophysiology of aortic cross-clamping and unclamping. Anesthesiology (Philadelphia) 1995;82(4):1026–60. Available at: https://www.ncbi.nlm.nih.gov/pubmed/7717537.

19. Shine TSJ, Murray MJ. Intraoperative management of aortic aneurysm surgery. Anesthesiol Clin North Am 2004;22(2):289–305.

20. Roizen MF, Beaupre PN, Alpert RA, et al. Monitoring with two-dimensional transesophageal echocardiography: Comparison of myocardial function in patients undergoing supraceliac, suprarenal-infraceliac, or infrarenal aortic occlusion. J Vasc Surg 1984;1(2):300–5.

21. Brusoni B, Colombo A, Merlo L, et al. Hemodynamic and metabolic changes induced by temporary clamping of the thoracic aorta. Eur Surg Res 1978; 10(3):206–16. Available at: https://www.karger.com/Article/FullText/128009.

22. LeMaire SA, Miller CC, Conklin LD, et al. Estimating group mortality and paraplegia rates after thoracoabdominal aortic aneurysm repair. Ann Thorac Surg 2003;75(2):508–13.

23. Svensson LG, Khitin L, Nadolny EM, et al. Systemic temperature and paralysis after thoracoabdominal and descending aortic operations. invited critique. Arch Surg (Chicago. 1960) 2003;138(2):175–80. Available at: https://search.proquest.com/docview/232550198.

24. Moomiaie RMA, Ransden J, Stein J, et al. Cooling catheter for spinal cord preservation in thoracic aortic surgery. J Cardiovasc Surg 2007;48(1):103–8. Available at: https://www.ncbi.nlm.nih.gov/pubmed/17308529.

25. Kemp CM, Feng Z, Aftab M, et al. Preventing spinal cord injury following thoracoabdominal aortic aneurysm repair: The battle to eliminate paraplegia. JTCVS Tech 2021;8:11–5.

26. Lima B MD, Nowicki ER, et al. Spinal cord protective strategies during descending and thoracoabdominal aortic aneurysm repair in the modern era: The role of

intrathecal papaverine. J Thorac Cardiovasc Surg 2012;143(4):945–52.e1. Available at: https://www.clinicalkey.es/playcontent/1-s2.0-S0022522312000554.

27. Kunihara T, Matsuzaki K, Shiiya N, et al. Naloxone lowers cerebrospinal fluid levels of excitatory amino acids after thoracoabdominal aortic surgery. J Vasc Surg 2004;40(4):681–90. https://doi.org/10.1016/j.jvs.2004.07.005.

28. Svensson LG. Paralysis after aortic surgery: In search of lost cord function. Surgeon (Edinburgh) 2005;3(6):396–405.

29. von Aspern K, Haunschild J, Ziemann M, et al. Evaluation of collateral network near-infrared spectroscopy during and after segmental artery occlusion in a chronic large animal model. J Thorac Cardiovasc Surg 2019;158(1):155–64, e5.

30. Aftab M, Coselli JS, et al. Renal and visceral protection in thoracoabdominal aortic surgery. J Thorac Cardiovasc Surg 2014;148(6):2963–6. Available at: https://www.clinicalkey.es/playcontent/1-s2.0-S0022522314008976.

31. LeMaire SA, Jones MM, et al. Randomized comparison of cold blood and cold crystalloid renal perfusion for renal protection during thoracoabdominal aortic aneurysm repair. J Vasc Surg 2009;49(1):11–9. Available at: https://www.clinicalkey.es/playcontent/1-s2.0-S0741521408014018.

32. Waked K, Schepens M. State-of the-art review on the renal and visceral protection during open thoracoabdominal aortic aneurysm repair. J visualized Surg 2018;4:31. Available at: https://www.ncbi.nlm.nih.gov/pubmed/29552513.

33. Agroyannis B, Chatziioannou A, Mourikis D, et al. Abdominal aortic aneurysm and renal artery stenosis: Renal function and blood pressure before and after endovascular treatment. J Hum Hypertens 2002;16(5):367–9. Available at: https://www.ncbi.nlm.nih.gov/pubmed/12082500.

34. McGinigle KL, Spangler EL, Pichel AC, et al. Perioperative care in open aortic vascular surgery: A consensus statement by the enhanced recovery after surgery (ERAS) society and society for vascular surgery. J Vasc Surg 2022;75(6):1796.

35. Kunihara T, Shiiya N, Wakasa S, et al. Assessment of hepatosplanchnic pathophysiology during thoracoabdominal aortic aneurysm repair using visceral perfusion and shunt. Eur J Cardiothorac Surg 2009;35(4):677–83. Available at: http://ejcts.ctsnetjournals.org/cgi/content/abstract/35/4/677.

36. de Figueiredo LF, Coselli JS. Individual strategies of hemostasis for thoracic aortic surgery. J Card Surg 1997;12(2 Suppl):222–8. Available at: https://www.ncbi.nlm.nih.gov/pubmed/9271749.

37. Shantikumar S, Patel S, Handa A. The role of cell salvage autotransfusion in abdominal aortic aneurysm surgery. Eur J Vasc endovascular Surg 2011;42(5):577–84. Available at: https://www.clinicalkey.es/playcontent/1-s2.0-S107858841100222X.

38. Merkel KR, Lin SD, Frank SM, et al. Balancing the blood component transfusion ratio for high- and ultra high-dose cell salvage cases. J Cardiothorac Vasc Anesth 2021;35(4):1060–6.

39. Ngo A, Masel D, Cahill C, et al. Blood banking and transfusion medicine challenges during the COVID-19 pandemic. Clin Lab Med 2020;40(4):587–601.

40. Monaco F, Nardelli P, Pasin L, et al. Tranexamic acid in open aortic aneurysm surgery: A randomised clinical trial. Br J Anaesth : BJA. 2020;124(1):35–43.

41. Desborough MJ, Oakland K, Brierley C, et al. Desmopressin use for minimising perioperative blood transfusion. Cochrane database Syst Rev 2017;2017(7): CD001884. Available at: https://www.cochranelibrary.com/cdsr/doi/10.1002/14651858.CD001884.pub3.

42. Clagett GP, Valentine RJ, Myers SI, et al. Does desmopressin improve hemostasis and reduce blood loss from aortic surgery? A randomized, double-blind study. J Vasc Surg 1995;22(3):223–30.

Anesthetic Management for Endovascular Repair of Thoracic and Abdominal Aortic Aneurysms

Callie Ebeling, MD*, Sreekanth Cheruku, MD, MPH

KEYWORDS

- Aortic aneurysm • Endovascular repair • Endovascular aortic repair (EVAR)
- Thoracic EVAR • Endoleak • Spinal cord injury

KEY POINTS

- Aneurysms of the descending aorta are areas of localized dilation occurring due to degenerative processes resulting from several genetic, metabolic, inflammatory, and infectious conditions.
- Endovascular repair of the aorta (EVAR) is the recommended approach to treating most aneurysms of the descending aorta as well as intramural hematomas and penetrating aortic ulcers.
- Patients undergoing EVAR frequently have comorbid conditions related to their aortic disease including hypertension, coronary artery disease, chronic kidney disease, and chronic obstructive pulmonary disease.
- Anesthetic techniques for EVAR include general anesthesia, neuraxial techniques, and local anesthesia with sedation.
- Complications associated with EVAR include vascular access-related injuries, device-related complications including endoleaks, and ischemic complications including paraplegia.

INTRODUCTION

Aortic aneurysms (abdominal and thoracic) are the 19th leading cause of death in the United States overall and the 15th leading cause of death in people over 55 years of age.[1] Aneurysmal dilation of the aorta is defined as a segmental, full-thickness dilation of the aorta with at least a 50% increase in diameter compared with the expected normal diameter for that segment. The natural history of aneurysms is to grow until they reach a critical size at which point they are likely to rupture or dissect. This necessitates a

Department of Anesthesiology and Pain Management, UT Southwestern Medical Center, Mail Code 9068, 5323 Harry Hines Boulevard, Dallas, TX 75390, USA
* Corresponding author.
E-mail address: Callie.Ebeling@UTSouthwestern.edu

Anesthesiology Clin 40 (2022) 719–735
https://doi.org/10.1016/j.anclin.2022.08.014   anesthesiology.theclinics.com

therapeutic approach in which patients with aneurysmal disease undergo periodic surveillance and surgical treatment before these complications may occur.

The incidence and prevalence of aortic aneurysms can be difficult to characterize because patients are often asymptomatic. Thoracic aortic aneurysms (TAAs) have a lower prevalence but a higher risk of death than abdominal aortic aneurysms (AAAs). The estimated prevalence of TAA is 6 to 10 cases per 100,000 patient-years.[2,3] Prior population-based studies have estimated that the prevalence of AAA in men older than 60 is as high as 3.3%,[4] but current data are unclear because of low screening in the United States, and the fact that most aneurysms are clinically silent until they rupture. Interestingly, the incidence of TAA seems to be increasing, whereas the incidence of AAA is decreasing. The increase in TAA may be related to increased detection on imaging and an aging population, whereas the decrease in AAA is thought to be related to a decrease in smoking prevalence over time.[4] The average age of patients with TAA and AAA is 65 years and 75 years, respectively. Men are more susceptible to aneurysms, especially abdominal aneurysms, with a male to female ratio of 1.7:1 for TAA and 6:1 for AAA.[2]

Both TAA and AAA are degenerative processes associated with shared risk factors including smoking, hypertension, and hyperlipidemia. TAA can also be related to connective tissue disorders such as Marfan and Ehlers–Danlos syndromes, inflammatory disorders, vasculitis, infection, and bicuspid aortic valves. Thoracic aneurysms distal to the ligamentum arteriosum are predominately atherosclerotic, whereas more proximal aneurysms are typically associated with non-atherosclerotic etiologies. There is a strong genetic component to the development of aneurysms—the risk for AAA doubles with family history of AAA in a first-degree relative.[4]

Open surgical repair of the aorta was first performed by Charles Dubost in 1951.[5] Although the open approach was initially associated with significant morbidity, advances in surgical techniques and perioperative management over the following decades resulted in improved outcomes. Successful endovascular repair of both the abdominal and thoracic aorta were reported by the early 1990s. Although the endovascular approach was initially developed for patients who could not tolerate open surgery, it has since become the preferred operative treatment of most thoracic and abdominal aneurysms because of its significantly lower morbidity and mortality.[6,7]

Pathophysiology

Aneurysms result from degeneration of the connective tissue in the tunica media, which weakens the vessel wall and results in progressive dilation.[8] This is a process that is accelerated by genetic factors, inflammation, and diseases that increase biomechanical wall stress such as hypertension. When wall tension increases above a critical threshold, acute aortic events such as dissection and rupture occur. Anatomically, aortic dissection is defined as an intimal tear causing a pressure-induced dissection of the tunica media which creates a false lumen that can extend proximally and distally and lead to impaired perfusion of aortic branches.[9] The most serious and deadly complication is aneurysmal rupture, which can lead to life-threatening bleeding.

Thoracic Aortic Aneurysms

Most TAA are discovered incidentally during imaging for unrelated problems, but surgical intervention is typically indicated if the aneurysm reaches a critical size or dissects. Screening is difficult due to the low sensitivity of transthoracic echocardiography and the high cost and potential radiation exposure associated with computed tomography (CT) imaging. Sixty percent of TAA involve the root or ascending aorta, whereas 40% involve the descending aorta.[8,10] The Crawford classification is used to categorize thoracoabdominal aneurysms by anatomic extent (**Fig. 1**). Ninety-five percent of TAA are asymptomatic before an acute event.[1] In general, the natural history of TAA is slow expansion with a growth rate of approximately 0.1 cm per year.[11] The annual risk of rupture or dissection is 2% for thoracic aneurysms between 4.0 and 4.9 cm and 7% for thoracic aneurysms greater than 6.0 cm[1].

The 2021 Society for Vascular Surgery (SVS) guidelines for thoracic endovascular aortic repair (TEVAR) recommend chest radiograph as an initial evaluation in patients at low or intermediate risk for TAA and urgent CT angiography (CTA) in those at high risk for symptomatic TAA or acute aortic syndrome.[2] Some of the higher risk categories include uncontrolled hypertension, inflammatory vasculitis, and family history of TAA and dissection. TEVAR is the recommended approach for elective repair of descending aortic aneurysms because of reduced morbidity, mortality, and length of stay compared with open procedures.[2] The 2010 American College of Cardiology (ACC) and American Heart Association (AHA) guidelines strongly recommend TEVAR for acute traumatic injury of the descending aorta and acute type B dissection with ischemia. TEVAR is also indicated for TAA greater than 5.5 cm with and without significant comorbidities, uncomplicated Type B dissections, and subacute or chronic dissection.[12] The guidelines do not recommend TEVAR for connective tissue disorders due to problems with endograft landing zones and resultant leaks.

Abdominal Aortic Aneurysms

The associated risk of death with rupture of an AAA is as high as 81%, and larger size is associated with the increased risk of rupture. There is an 11% annual risk of rupture

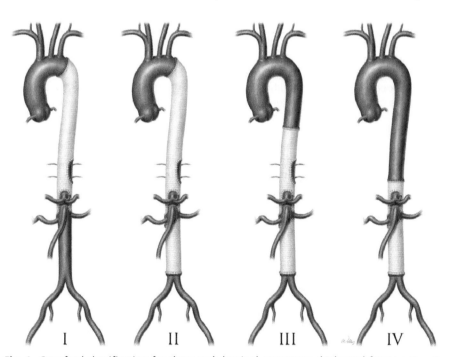

Fig. 1. Crawford classification for thoracoabdominal aneurysms. (*Adapted from* Le Huu A, Green SY, Coselli JS. Thoracoabdominal aortic aneurysm repair: from an era of revolution to an era of evolution. InSeminars in Thoracic and Cardiovascular Surgery 2019 Dec 1 (Vol. 31, No. 4, pp. 703-707); with permission.)

for AAA 5.0 to 5.9 cm in diameter. Both the 2019 US Preventive Services Task Force guidelines and AHA/ACC guidelines recommend one-time ultrasonography screening in men aged 65 to 75 years who have ever smoked.[4,13] Screening with conventional abdominal duplex ultrasonography has high sensitivity and specificity compared with physical examination and avoids potential radiation exposure harm associated with CT. Surgical repair is indicated for AAA 5.5 cm or larger or AAA larger than 4.0 cm with rapid increase in size.[4] Although outcomes for both open and endovascular repair have improved, a significant mortality benefit favors the use of EVAR, which is currently used in 80% of intact AAA repairs and 52% of ruptured repairs in the United States.[4,14] A long-term population-based study of Medicare beneficiaries who underwent aneurysm repair between 2001 and 2004 found that perioperative mortality is significantly lower (1.2% vs 4.8%) after endovascular versus open repair, and that this benefit increases with age.[15] The SVS suggests that elective EVAR procedures should only occur in hospitals that have a mortality and conversion-to-open rate of 2% or less and that perform at least 10 EVAR cases each year.[16]

ENDOVASCULAR PROCEDURE

Endovascular aneurysm repair (EVAR) uses expandable stent-grafts, termed endografts, to exclude aortic pathology. These endografts have an inner metal matrix covered with an impermeable fabric such as synthetic polyester. Before the procedure, CTA with three-dimensional reconstruction is necessary to measure the seal zones for the graft, evaluate aortic and iliac anatomy, and visualize branch vessels. The iliac artery must be wide enough to accommodate the introducer for the endograft, which can have an outer diameter as large as 24 French. Balloon angioplasty or stenting of the iliac vessels may be necessary in patients with stenotic iliac vessels. A 2-cm length of histologically normal aortic tissue is necessary at the proximal and distal landing zones to ensure an adequate endograft seal.[9] Endografts can be branched or fenestrated to perfuse branch vessels arising from the excluded portion of the aorta.

The procedure begins with either percutaneous or surgical cut down access typically to the common femoral artery, the most common conduit for the endograft introducer system. Less commonly, stents can be inserted through the brachial, axillary, and subclavian arteries. Heparin (100–150 IU/kg) is administered to achieve an activated clotting time (ACT) exceeding 250 seconds. Guidewires and catheters used for contrast injection are then advanced into the target section of the aorta under fluoroscopic guidance. A combination of intravascular ultrasound, fluoroscopy, and angiography are used to identify the landing zones.[7] The endograft is then advanced into position and deployed. Balloon dilation of the distal seal zones and any overlaps between grafts is performed to achieve a tight seal. Once the main endograft is deployed, branch vessels can be snared through fenestrations and stented to preserve blood flow.

After the procedure is complete, contrast angiography can be used to confirm proper positioning of the endograft, evaluate for endoleak, and verify branch perfusion. The introducer system is then removed, and the access sites are repaired.

ANESTHETIC CONSIDERATIONS
Preoperative Assessment

Preoperative evaluation for both EVAR and TEVAR should include a comprehensive assessment of medical comorbidities with the understanding that any endovascular procedure could be converted to an open repair. Compared with open repair, endovascular repair avoids exposure of the aorta and aortic cross-clamping and is associated with less blood loss and a shorter recovery period.[15,17–19] The cardiac, pulmonary, and renal systems should be thoroughly evaluated as coronary artery disease, chronic obstructive pulmonary disease, and renal insufficiency are frequently present in patients with aortic aneurysmal disease and are associated with worse outcomes. The 2014 AHA/ACC guidelines for cardiovascular evaluation and management of patients undergoing noncardiac surgery categorize TEVAR and EVAR in the *elevated risk* category, associated with at least a 1% risk of a major adverse cardiac event from the procedure alone.[20] Comorbidities frequently present in vascular surgery patients can further increase this risk.

Cardiac

Cardiac evaluation is imperative as many risk factors for vascular disease also predispose to coronary artery disease. More than 80% of perioperative myocardial ischemic events are asymptomatic and therefore undertreated, which may contribute to increased long-term cardiovascular mortality.[21] Cardiovascular assessment should include an evaluation of functional capacity and a preoperative electrocardiogram (ECG). This ECG will serve as a baseline that can be used if necessary for comparison in the event of ECG changes in the perioperative period. Left ventricular (LV) function should be assessed with transthoracic echocardiography (TTE) in those with dyspnea of unknown origin, worsening functional status, and those with known prior LV or valvular dysfunction if there has been no assessment within 1 year.[20,22] The presence of LV dysfunction along with heart failure symptoms is associated with an increased risk for 30-day cardiovascular events and long-term cardiovascular mortality in patients undergoing endovascular aortic procedures.[23] Preexisting right ventricular dysfunction is also independently associated with postoperative major cardiac complications and a 50% longer length of stay in high-risk patients undergoing both open and endovascular major vascular procedures.[24] More invasive studies like stress testing and coronary angiography should be limited to those with poor functional capacity (<4 metabolic equivalents) or abnormal findings on ECG or TTE[22] (**Fig. 2**). The AHA/ACC guidelines recommend continuation of beta blockers on patients who patients who chronically receive the medication.[20]

Pulmonary

Patients with aortic aneurysms have a higher prevalence of chronic obstructive pulmonary disease (COPD), possibly related to chronic inflammation and hypoxemia that may lead to local hypoperfusion of the aorta.[25] Respiratory complications can be as high as 25% after abdominal aortic surgery, and the presence of COPD exacerbates this risk.[26] Those with thoracic aneurysms may present with respiratory symptoms like dyspnea and cough related to proximity of the aneurysm to the tracheobronchial tree. Preoperative thoracic body imaging should be reviewed to evaluate anatomic relationships, and the patient should be evaluated for the ability to lay flat without experiencing worsening dyspnea. Pulmonary function testing is indicated in those with known or suspected COPD to guide ventilation strategies and postoperative rehabilitation. Patients with significant respiratory disease should be seen by a pulmonary specialist for optimization of inhaled or nebulized medications and consideration for preoperative and postoperative continuous positive airway pressure, especially in patients planned to undergo general endotracheal anesthesia.[26]

Renal

Renal function should be evaluated preoperatively to assess the patient's baseline glomerular filtration rate and electrolyte levels. Physical examination should be used in conjunction with laboratory assessment and imaging to evaluate volume status.

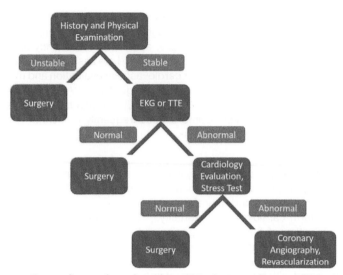

Fig. 2. Preoperative cardiac workup algorithm. EKG, electrocardiogram. (*Adapted from* Ganapathi AM, Englum BR, Schechter MA, et al. Role of cardiac evaluation before thoracic endovascular aortic repair. J Vasc Surg 2014;60(5):1198; with permission.)

Predictors for acute kidney injury (AKI) after TEVAR include preoperative poor renal function, blood transfusions, and the extent of the thoracoabdominal aortic disease.[27] Patients undergoing EVAR and TEVAR are at the risk of developing contrast-induced nephropathy (CIN),[28] and those with preexisting disease who develop acute-on-chronic kidney injury may need temporary or permanent renal replacement therapy in the postoperative period. Patients should be adequately hydrated, and nephrotoxic medications should be stopped before the procedure. The extent and complexity of the aortic disease in relation to the renal arteries may also lead to partial or whole sacrifice of a kidney.

Neurologic
A complete neurologic evaluation of the patient should be performed before surgery to establish a baseline, and any sensory or motor deficits should be noted. Paralysis from spinal cord ischemia (SCI) is a feared and relatively common risk after TEVAR with an incidence ranging from 0.65% to 10% in published studies.[29–33] SCI can have a major impact on quality of life and survival, so awareness and prevention are the key. Patient-related and procedural risk factors for the development of SCI include extensive coverage of the thoracic aorta, prior AAA repair, and coverage of the left subclavian artery.[34] The association of SCI with prior AAA repair is thought to be related to the occlusion of lumbar arteries during the prior repair resulting in reduced total collateral blood supply to the spinal cord.[35]

Intraoperative Management

Anesthetic technique
Both TEVAR and EVAR can be performed using general anesthesia (GA), regional anesthesia (RA), or local anesthesia (LA) with monitored anesthesia care (MAC) (**Table 1**). Important anesthetic goals for both procedures include keeping the patient immobile and comfortable, monitoring hemodynamics, maintaining tight blood pressure control (especially during deployment and positioning of the graft), managing

Table 1 Choice of anesthetic technique for thoracic endovascular aortic repair and endovascular aortic repair	
Anesthesia Type	Advantages
General anesthesia	Immobility Controlled ventilation Controlled hemodynamics Allows cessation of ventilation Facilitates TEE
Regional anesthesia	Decreased myocardial depression Decreased risk of pulmonary complications
Local anesthesia with sedation	Decreased myocardial depression Decreased risk of pulmonary complications Early detection of SCI

Abbreviations: SCI, spinal cord injury; TEE, transesophageal echocardiography.

anticoagulation, achieving adequate hydration to avoid CIN, and monitoring for bleeding and metabolic derangements with serial laboratory assessment and/or arterial blood gas evaluation.

General anesthesia
The benefits of GA include airway protection, controlled ventilation, ability to temporarily pause ventilation, the option to use paralysis to ensure immobility, and facilitation of the use of transesophageal echocardiography (TEE). Some risks of GA include potential hemodynamic instability, changes in pulmonary mechanics, and the need for possible prolonged intubation. Patients who have difficulty lying flat due to preexisting back pain or difficulty breathing will likely require GA. Because of the increased complexity and higher risk of bleeding with TEVAR, these patients most often undergo a general anesthetic.[36] Anesthetic choices for abdominal EVAR cases are more variable. A 2020 meta-analysis by Harky and colleagues that included 12 observational studies with more than 12,000 abdominal EVAR patients found a shorter operative time and shorter length of stay in those who received LA or RA rather than GA, but no mortality difference and no difference in cardiac, renal, or vascular complications in the two groups.[37]

Regional anesthesia
Neuraxial anesthesia for TEVAR or EVAR may include spinal, epidural, or combined spinal–epidural techniques. The advantages of neuraxial anesthesia include decreased myocardial depression and decreased pulmonary complications due to avoidance of mechanical ventilation.[38] Risks with neuraxial techniques include potential hemodynamic instability from sympathetic blockade and development of an epidural or intrathecal hematoma. Effective neuraxial anesthesia should include dermatomal coverage of T6–L3 and last for 3 to 4 hour.[39] Some patients may require supplemental sedation in addition to the neuraxial technique for comfort.

Local anesthesia
Infiltration of the groin with a local anesthetic allows the surgeon to establish femoral or iliac access required for endovascular repair. Most patients will require supplemental sedation with agents such as propofol, dexmedetomidine, or remifentanil. There is some evidence to suggest that LA may have a benefit over GA during EVAR, especially in an emergent setting, but further investigation is needed to determine if the same benefits exist with elective cases.[40] The use of LA also facilitates an early detection

of neurologic complications including SCI. Risks of using LA with MAC include patient movement during critical portions of the case and oversedation that may require intubation.

Hemodynamic monitors

During TEVAR and EVAR, all patients should be monitored with standard ASA monitors including electrocardiography (ECG), blood pressure, pulse oximetry, capnography, and temperature. A 5-lead ECG allows for the detection of rate and rhythm changes as well as ST-segment changes that may be indicative of ischemia. Intra-arterial blood pressure monitoring is required due to the potential for wide hemodynamic swings and the need for titration of vasoactive medications to achieve specific goals during deployment of the graft. Occasionally, arterial pressure monitoring distal to the graft is required and a femoral catheter can be inserted and transduced alongside an upper extremity arterial line. A central venous catheter may be considered in patients undergoing a TEVAR for possible large volume resuscitation, administration of vasoactive infusions, and monitoring of CVP. Abdominal EVAR does not always require central access, but it may be necessary if unable to establish reliable peripheral intravenous access with two large-bore IV catheters or a rapid infusion catheter. A Foley catheter should be used to monitor urine output as a sign of end-organ perfusion and volume status.

Transesophageal echocardiography

TEE is a sensitive imaging modality to evaluate the heart and great vessels. During TEVAR, TEE can be used to directly visualize cardiac function, diagnose aortic pathology, confirm guidewire placement, aid stent graft positioning, and detect endoleaks.[41] Because TAAs and dissections can acutely progress to involve the aortic valve, TEE should be considered for continuous monitoring of the structure and function of the aortic valve. In comparison to angiography or fluoroscopy, TEE provides superior diagnostic accuracy of aortic dissection.[42] In a case series of 42 patients undergoing TEVAR, TEE guidance resulted in decisive changes to the procedure in 16 of 42 patients (38%). These changes included guidewire repositioning in four patients, diagnosis of endoleak in seven patients, and discovery of intimal tears in five patients, none of which were visible with angiography.[42] Although TEE is not routinely used during abdominal EVAR, it can be useful as a diagnostic or rescue tool in the event of cardiovascular collapse.

Neuromonitoring

Intercostal branches from the descending thoracic aorta provide collateral blood flow to the anterior spinal cord via the artery of Adamkiewicz and other radicular branches, and extensive coverage of these branches during TEVAR is a major risk factor for the devastating complication of SCI.[43] Neuromonitoring with motor evoked potentials (MEPs) and somatosensory evoked potentials (SSEPs) is essential in the diagnosis and treatment of SCI that could lead to transient or permanent paraplegia after TEVAR. Risk factors for the development of SCI during TEVAR include prior EVAR or open aortic repair.[43] MEPs are conducted through the anterior corticospinal tract, whereas SSEPs ascend the lateral and posterior columns of the spinal cord. Therefore, monitoring of MEPs and SSEPs together allows for continuous assessment of global spinal cord perfusion. In patients undergoing evoked potential monitoring under GA, the volatile anesthetic concentration should be limited to 0.5 minimum alveolar concentration (MAC), and paralytics should be avoided after intubation. Opioid infusions or propofol, which have milder effects on evoked potential monitoring, can be used to supplement the use of low-dose volatile anesthetic.

Neuromonitoring is generally not used during abdominal EVAR cases because the risk for SCI is low while intervening on the abdominal portion of the aorta.

Near-infrared spectroscopy (NIRS) has been used to monitor tissue oxygenation in the paraspinal muscles as an indirect monitor of spinal cord perfusion.[44,45] This emerging application of NIRS may allow early detection of SCI during the intraoperative and early postoperative period and prompt therapeutic interventions.

Cerebrospinal fluid drainage

Decreased spinal cord perfusion pressure (SCPP) during TEVAR results in hypoperfusion of collateral vessels and subsequent spinal cord injury (SCI). The equation that determines blood supply to the spinal cord is:

SCPP = Mean Arterial Pressure (MAP) – Cerebrospinal Fluid(CSF) pressure.

Therefore, SCPP can be optimized by either increasing MAP or decreasing CSF pressure. Augmenting MAP and improving SCPP through CSF drainage are the most important factors in preventing paraplegia. Lowering CSF pressure is achieved by drainage of cerebrospinal fluid via an intrathecal catheter inserted through a lumbar interspace. The risk for SCI during TEVAR ranges from 0.65% to 10%,[46] and CSF drain placement should be considered in patients with significant risk factors for SCI such as emergent repair, prior aortic repair, left subclavian artery coverage, length of endovascular stent, branched grafts (compared with fenestrated grafts), and perioperative hypotension.[47] Other strategies to reduce the risk of SCI include maintaining adequate hemoglobin, giving supplemental oxygen, minimizing oxygen consumption, and using electrophysiological monitoring.[48] Prophylactic CSF drain placement should be considered in high-risk patients such as those with prior aortic surgery, aortic coverage greater than 205 mm, use of three or more stents, and anticipated massive blood loss.[43] In lower risk patients, it is reasonable to place CSF drains in patients who develop postoperative paraplegia.[49]

Renal protection

During both EVAR and TEVAR, the kidneys are subject to various etiologies for acute injury such as hemodynamic instability, the use of contrast, poor perfusion due to extent of the aneurysm, renally toxic medications, and embolic events. Patients who are hypovolemic when presenting for surgery should be hydrated to reduce the risk of CIN. Renal perfusion pressure should be maintained throughout the procedure to reduce the risk of AKI. Intravenous contrast volume should be limited to the lowest necessary dose; ultrasound may potentially be used as an imaging adjunct in those who have preexisting renal disease or risk factors for acute renal failure.

Induction and maintenance

Anesthetic induction for both EVAR and TEVAR should be performed with special attention to blood pressure control as aneurysms or dissections can progress during an acute hypertensive episode that may occur during sympathetic stimulation with intubation. Standard induction agents such as propofol or etomidate should be used and combined with opioids and lidocaine to blunt sympathetic responses. Depolarizing or non-depolarizing neuromuscular blockade can be used to facilitate intubation, but non-depolarizing agents should be reversed if necessary before baseline evoked potential monitoring. Because volatile anesthetics decrease the amplitude and increase the latency of evoked potentials, a balanced maintenance technique with a combination of volatile anesthetic (limited to 0.5 MAC) and an opioid or dexmedetomidine infusion should be used. A total intravenous anesthetic technique with propofol and a supplemental opioid infusion can also be used.

Systemic anticoagulation with heparin is required before insertion of the graft in the arterial system, targeting an ACT of at least 250 seconds. The goal ACT should be maintained throughout the case.

MAP should be maintained close to baseline for elective TEVAR and EVAR; however, a lower MAP goal may be necessary in the setting of aneurysm rupture or acute dissection. Just before graft deployment, blood pressure should be lowered to prevent graft migration. During TEVAR, higher MAP goals (90 mm Hg) may be required to augment SCPP in high-risk patients. At the conclusion of both EVAR and TEVAR, patients should be extubated, and vasodilators should be readily available to treat emergence hypertension. A neurologic examination should be completed as soon as the patient is able to follow commands. Continuation of dexmedetomidine throughout the intraoperative and postoperative period may be helpful in both providing analgesia and making a period of strict supine positioning more tolerable.

Postoperative Care

TEVAR and EVAR patients should be closely monitored during the postoperative period with frequent neurovascular examinations. Blood pressure parameters, including systolic and MAP goals, should be clearly communicated among the interdisciplinary team. To facilitate hemostasis of groin access sites, patients are typically required to remain flat for 4 to 6 hours after closure. This minimizes the chances for vascular complications such as hematomas and pseudoaneurysms. After TEVAR, early detection of motor deficits warrants prompt intervention to improve spinal cord perfusion by using vasopressors to increase MAP and/or draining CSF via a lumbar drain. CSF drains should be transduced for continuous pressure monitoring typically with a goal at or below 10 mm Hg. Intermittent drainage by nursing staff should be limited to 10 mL every hour with further drainage directed by the critical care team. Complications, as described below, are estimated to be 16% to 30% following endovascular AAA repair, and as high as 38% following TEVAR.[50]

COMPLICATIONS

The endovascular approach to both thoracic and AAAs is associated with fewer complications. TEVAR is associated with lower mortality, SCI, and pulmonary complications within 30 days of the intervention,[51] and EVAR is associated with a lower 30-day mortality[14,52] and lower complications[53] compared with open surgery. However, there are complications unique to endovascular repair which are important to recognize. These include vascular access site-related complications, graft-related complications, and end-organ injury (**Table 2**).

Vascular Site Complications

Vascular site complications include hematoma formation, pseudoaneurysm, embolic events resulting in distal ischemia, thrombosis, and dissection. Surveillance of the vascular access sites is necessary during the early postoperative period to evaluate for hematomas and pseudoaneurysms. Hematomas can be managed with manual compression along with blood pressure control and coagulation management. Pseudoaneurysms present as pulsatile masses and may require a range of therapeutic maneuvers ranging from manual compression to ultrasound-guided thrombin injection and surgical repair. Arterial dissection and thrombosis can present with the loss of distal pulses and may necessitate emergent interventions such as thrombectomies and bypass procedures.

Table 2
Complications associated with endovascular aortic repair and thoracic endovascular aortic repair

Complications	Management
Access-Site Related	
Hematoma	Manual compression
	Surgical repair
Pseudoaneurysm	Ultrasound-guided compression
	Ultrasound-guided thrombin injection
	Surgical repair
Arterial dissection	Vascular bypass procedure
Arterial thrombosis	Thrombectomy, catheter-directed thrombolysis
Graft-Related	
Endoleak	Type I: Deploy new stent
	Type II: Conservative management
	Type III: Endovascular relining
	Type IV: Reverse anticoagulation
	Type V: Endovascular relining or Open repair
Endograft migration	Treat Type I endoleak if present
	Deploy new stent
	Convert to open repair
Endograft infection	Antibiotic therapy
	Endograft resection
End-Organ Injury	
Thromboembolic events	Management depends on organ system affected
	Medical management of AKI, CRRT
	Medical and surgical management of gut ischemia
Occlusion of arterial or endograft branches	Stenting occluded vessels
	CSF drainage, increasing MAP for SCI

Abbreviations: CSF, cerebrospinal fluid; MAP, mean arterial pressure; SCI, spinal cord injury; CRRT, continuous renal replacement therapy.

Graft-Related Complications

Graft-related complications include endoleak, migration of the endograft, problems with the endograft branches, and graft infection.[50] Endoleaks result from a failure of the graft to exclude the aneurysm from the systemic circulation (**Fig. 3**). Type I endoleaks result from blood perfusing the aneurysm sac from the proximal (Type IA) or distal (Type IB) end of the endograft. These are often diagnosed during post-deployment angiography and treated using balloon dilation of the graft or placement of a new stent.[9] Type II endoleaks result from collateral blood vessels perfusing the aneurysm and are managed conservatively. Type III endoleaks represent blood flow into the aneurysm sac either in between grafts or due to a defect in the graft. These are also managed by deploying additional stents. Type IV endoleaks occur due to extravasation of blood through normal graft material. These typically seal spontaneously after anticoagulation is reversed.[9] Type V endoleak describes expansion of the aneurysm sac in the absence of an angiographically visible leak. Endograft migration can occur due to aortic anatomy, endograft size mismatch, or a failure of the endograft seal zones. These can be prevented by oversizing the distal limbs of the endograft[54] or treating Type 1 endoleaks early. Both graft migration and graft kinking can result in thrombosis of one or more limbs of the graft. These occlusions may require endovascular or surgical therapy. Early

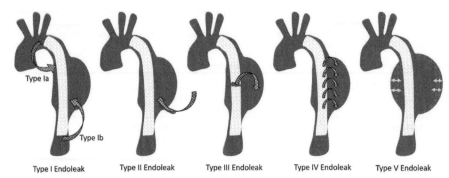

Type Ia

Type Ib

| Type I Endoleak | Type II Endoleak | Type III Endoleak | Type IV Endoleak | Type V Endoleak |

Fig. 3. Classification of endoleaks. Type I endoleaks originate from the proximal and distal seal zones of the endograft. Type II endoleaks result from collateral vessels that feed the aneurysm sac. Type III endoleaks are leaks between overlapping endografts or occur through defects in the endograft. Type IV endoleaks represent are transient leaks through the endograft fabric. Type V endoleaks are used to describe an enlarging aneurysm sac in the absence of a visualized leak. (*Adapted from* Cheruku S, Huang N, Meinhardt K, Aguirre M. Anesthetic management for endovascular repair of the thoracic aorta. Anesthesiology Clinics. 2019 Dec 1;37(4):593-607 with permission.)

graft infection after endovascular repair occurs most frequently due to endograft contamination or seeding of the endograft from a known or unknown infection present in the patient. Signs of sepsis along with radiologic evidence of fluid or air around the graft suggest this diagnosis. The treatment of endograft infection includes antibiotic therapy followed by endograft resection.[55]

End-Organ Injury

End-organ injury after endovascular aortic procedures results most frequently from embolic events, occlusion of aortic branch vessels, or occlusion of an endograft branch. Ischemic injury to the kidneys and gut can result from emboli generated by the endograft deployment device as well as manipulation of catheters and wires in the aorta. Embolic injury can be reduced by minimizing catheter manipulation in the aorta. Coverage of the renal, inferior mesenteric, superior mesenteric, celiac, and internal iliac vessels by the endograft can also result in renal, intestinal, and pelvic ischemia, respectively.[50] End-organ injury is more common in patients with previous aortic procedures and those with poor collateral circulation due to other reasons. Using branched or fenestrated endografts and stenting inadvertently occluded vessels may serve to reduce the incidence of ischemia due to occlusion of aortic branches. In TEVAR, inadvertent coverage of the takeoff of the left subclavian artery may lead to upper extremity ischemia. This complication is often prevented by performing a carotid-subclavian bypass in addition to the TEVAR.[50]

SCI is much more common after TEVAR than EVAR and likely results from coverage of the segmental arteries to the spinal cord by the endograft. Perioperative strategies to reduce the incidence of SCI include using evoked potential monitoring, prophylactic CSF drain placement in high-risk patients, optimizing oxygen delivery by maintaining cardiac output and adequate hemoglobin, maintaining SCPP, and using mild hypothermia.[43]

SUMMARY

Aortic aneurysms—both abdominal and thoracic—are a significant cause of death and disability in the United States. EVAR has since become the preferred operative treatment of most thoracic and abdominal aneurysms because of a lower rate of complications and better outcomes compared with the open approach. Patients who present for EVAR often have comorbid conditions related to their aortic pathology. These conditions should be evaluated and optimized before the procedure. Although GA is most frequently used for TEVAR, GA, neuraxial techniques, and LA with MAC can all be used for patients undergoing EVAR. The ideal anesthetic technique for EVAR is one which considers patient and procedural factors. Endovascular aortic repair is associated with potential vascular access site-related, endograft-related, and ischemic complications. Among these, SCI is a feared complication of TEVAR that requires a multidisciplinary approach to prevention and treatment. Mitigating this and other complications requires using appropriate perioperative monitors, optimizing hemodynamics, and continued close postoperative monitoring.

CLINICS CARE POINTS

- The preoperative evaluation should be comprehensive and also focus on the cardiac, pulmonary, and renal systems as patients with aneurysmal disease often have comorbidities affecting these systems.
- Patients with abnormal electrocardiograms, heart failure symptoms, or poor functional capacity should undergo transthoracic echocardiography because both left and right ventricular dysfunction is associated with an increased risk of perioperative complications.
- The benefits of general anesthesia for endovascular aortic repair (EVAR) and thoracic EVAR (TEVAR) include airway protection, controlled ventilation, breath-holding, paralysis to ensure immobility, and facilitation of the use of transesophageal echocardiography.
- Regional anesthesia and local anesthesia with sedation can be used to decrease the risk of myocardial depression, pulmonary complications in select patients when procedural considerations allow.
- Surveillance of the vascular access sites is necessary during the early postoperative period to evaluate for hematomas and pseudoaneurysms.
- After TEVAR, early detection of motor deficits warrants prompt intervention to improve spinal cord perfusion by using vasopressors to increase mean arterial pressure and/or draining cerebrospinal fluid via a lumbar drain.

DISCLOSURE

Dr S. Cheruku is supported by the Society of Critical Care Medicine VIRUS Automation Grant and the Society of Critical Care Medicine VIRUS CURE-ID Grant.

REFERENCES

1. Kuzmik GA, Sang AX, Elefteriades JA. Natural history of thoracic aortic aneurysms. J Vasc Surg 2012;56(2):565–71.
2. Upchurch GR Jr, Escobar GA, Azizzadeh A, et al. Society for Vascular Surgery clinical practice guidelines of thoracic endovascular aortic repair for descending thoracic aortic aneurysms. J Vasc Surg 2021;73(1):55S–83S.
3. Olsson C, Thelin S, Ståhle E, et al. Thoracic aortic aneurysm and dissection: increasing prevalence and improved outcomes reported in a nationwide population-based study of more than 14 000 cases from 1987 to 2002. Circulation 2006;114(24):2611–8.

4. Owens DK, Davidson KW, Krist AH, et al. Screening for abdominal aortic aneurysm: US Preventive Services Task Force recommendation statement. Jama 2019;322(22):2211–8.

5. Dubost C, Allary M, Oeconomos N. Resection of an aneurysm of the abdominal aorta: reestablishment of the continuity by a preserved human arterial graft, with result after five months. AMA Arch Surg 1952;64(3):405–8.

6. Gopaldas RR, Huh J, Dao TK, et al. Superior nationwide outcomes of endovascular versus open repair for isolated descending thoracic aortic aneurysm in 11,669 patients. J Thorac Cardiovasc Surg 2010;140(5):1001–10.

7. Conrad MF, Ergul EA, Patel VI, et al. Management of diseases of the descending thoracic aorta in the endovascular era: a Medicare population study. Ann Surg 2010;252(4):603–10.

8. Isselbacher EM. Thoracic and abdominal aortic aneurysms. Circulation 2005; 111(6):816–28.

9. Cheruku S, Huang N, Meinhardt K, et al. Anesthetic management for endovascular repair of the thoracic aorta. Anesthesiology Clin 2019;37(4):593–607.

10. Silvay G, Lurie JM, Casale M. The anaesthetic management of patients with thoracic ascending aortic aneurysms: A review. J Perioper Pract 2021;31(7–8): 281–8.

11. Elefteriades JA, Farkas EA. Thoracic aortic aneurysm: clinically pertinent controversies and uncertainties. J Am Coll Cardiol 2010;55(9):841–57.

12. Foundation ACoC, Guidelines AHATFoP, Surgery AAfT, et al. 2010 ACCF/AHA/ AATS/ACR/ASA/SCA/SCAI/SIR/STS/SVM guidelines for the diagnosis and management of patients with thoracic aortic disease. J Am Coll Cardiol 2010; 55(14):e27–129.

13. Hirsch A. American Association for Vascular Surgery/Society for Vascular Surgery; Society for Cardiovascular Angiography and Interventions; Society for Vascular Medicine and Biology; Society of Interventional Radiology; ACC/AHA Task Force on Practice Guidelines ACC/AHA 2005 guidelines for the management of patients with peripheral arterial disease (lower extremity, renal, mesenteric, and abdominal aortic): Executive summary a collaborative report from the American Association for Vascular Surgery/Society for Vascular Surgery, Society for Cardiovascular Angiography and Interventions, Society for Vascular Medicine and Biology, Society of Interventional Radiology, and the ACC/AHA Task Force on Practice Guidelines. J Am Coll Cardiol 2006;47:1239–312.

14. Kontopodis N, Galanakis N, Antoniou SA, et al. Meta-analysis and meta-regression analysis of outcomes of endovascular and open repair for ruptured abdominal aortic aneurysm. Eur J Vasc Endovasc Surg 2020;59(3):399–410.

15. Schermerhorn ML, O'Malley AJ, Jhaveri A, et al. Endovascular vs. open repair of abdominal aortic aneurysms in the Medicare population. N Engl J Med 2008; 358(5):464–74.

16. Chaikof EL, Dalman RL, Eskandari MK, et al. The Society for Vascular Surgery practice guidelines on the care of patients with an abdominal aortic aneurysm. J Vasc Surg 2018;67(1):2–77.e72.

17. Dillavou ED, Muluk SC, Makaroun MS. Improving aneurysm-related outcomes: nationwide benefits of endovascular repair. J Vasc Surg 2006;43(3):446–52.

18. Greenberg RK, Lu Q, Roselli EE, et al. Contemporary analysis of descending thoracic and thoracoabdominal aneurysm repair: a comparison of endovascular and open techniques. Circulation 2008;118(8):808–17.

19. Sadat U, Boyle JR, Walsh SR, et al. Endovascular vs open repair of acute abdominal aortic aneurysms—a systematic review and meta-analysis. J Vasc Surg 2008; 48(1):227–36.
20. Fleisher LA, Fleischmann KE, Auerbach AD, et al. 2014 ACC/AHA guideline on perioperative cardiovascular evaluation and management of patients undergoing noncardiac surgery: executive summary: a report of the American College of Cardiology/American Heart association Task Force on practice guidelines. Developed in collaboration with the American College of Surgeons, American Society of Anesthesiologists, American Society of Echocardiography, American Society of Nuclear Cardiology, Heart Rhythm Society, Society for cardiovascular Angiography and interventions, Society of cardiovascular Anesthesiologists, and Society of Vascular medicine Endorsed by the Society of Hospital medicine. J Nucl Cardiol official Publ Am Soc Nucl Cardiol 2015;22(1):162–215.
21. Omar HR, Mangar D, Camporesi EM. Preoperative cardiac evaluation of the vascular surgery patient—an anesthesia perspective. Vasc endovascular Surg 2012;46(3):201–11.
22. Ganapathi AM, Englum BR, Schechter MA, et al. Role of cardiac evaluation before thoracic endovascular aortic repair. J Vasc Surg 2014;60(5):1196–203.
23. Flu W-J, van Kuijk J-P, Hoeks SE, et al. Prognostic implications of asymptomatic left ventricular dysfunction in patients undergoing vascular surgery. J Am Soc Anesthesiol 2010;112(6):1316–24.
24. Chou J, Ma M, Gylys M, et al. Preexisting right ventricular dysfunction is associated with higher postoperative cardiac complications and longer hospital stay in high-risk patients undergoing nonemergent major vascular surgery. J Cardiothorac Vasc Anesth 2019;33(5):1279–86.
25. Ando K, Kaneko N, Doi T, et al. Prevalence and risk factors of aortic aneurysm in patients with chronic obstructive pulmonary disease. J Thorac Dis 2014;6(10): 1388.
26. Smetana GW, Lawrence VA, Cornell JE. Preoperative pulmonary risk stratification for noncardiothoracic surgery: systematic review for the American College of Physicians. Ann Intern Med 2006;144(8):581–95.
27. Piffaretti G, Mariscalco G, Bonardelli S, et al. Predictors and outcomes of acute kidney injury after thoracic aortic endograft repair. J Vasc Surg 2012;56(6): 1527–34.
28. McCullough PA, Choi JP, Feghali GA, et al. Contrast-induced acute kidney injury. J Am Coll Cardiol 2016;68(13):1465–73.
29. Scali ST, Wang SK, Feezor RJ, et al. Preoperative prediction of spinal cord ischemia after thoracic endovascular aortic repair. J Vasc Surg 2014;60(6): 1481–90, e1481.
30. Acher C, Acher C, Marks E, et al. Intraoperative neuroprotective interventions prevent spinal cord ischemia and injury in thoracic endovascular aortic repair. J Vasc Surg 2016;63(6):1458–65.
31. Kotelis D, Bianchini C, Kovacs B, et al. Early experience with automatic pressure-controlled cerebrospinal fluid drainage during thoracic endovascular aortic repair. J Endovascular Ther 2015;22(3):368–72.
32. Scali ST, Feezor RJ, Chang CK, et al. Efficacy of thoracic endovascular stent repair for chronic type B aortic dissection with aneurysmal degeneration. J Vasc Surg 2013;58(1):10–7.e11.
33. Arnaoutakis DJ, Arnaoutakis GJ, Beaulieu RJ, et al. Results of adjunctive spinal drainage and/or left subclavian artery bypass in thoracic endovascular aortic repair. Ann Vasc Surg 2014;28(1):65–73.

34. Nation DA, Wang GJ. TEVAR: Endovascular Repair of the Thoracic Aorta. Semin Intervent Radiol 2015;32(3):265–71.

35. Setacci F, Sirignano P, De Donato G, et al. Endovascular thoracic aortic repair and risk of spinal cord ischemia: the role of previous or concomitant treatment for aortic aneurysm. J Cardiovasc Surg 2010;51(2):169.

36. Geube M, Troianos C. Anesthetic Management of Thoracic Endovascular Aortic Repair. In: Cheng DCH, Martin J, David T, editors. Evidence-based Practice in perioperative cardiac anesthesia and surgery. Gewerbestrasse 11, 6330 Cham, Switzerland: Springer; 2021. p. 123–38.

37. Harky A, Ahmad MU, Santoro G, et al. Local versus general anesthesia in nonemergency endovascular abdominal aortic aneurysm repair: a systematic review and meta-analysis. J Cardiothorac Vasc Anesth 2020;34(4):1051–9.

38. Fetterman Y, Puttur Rajkumar K, Salamanca-Padilla YY. Anesthesia for Endovascular Thoracic Aortic Aneurysm Repair (TEVAR). In: Awad AS, editor. Cardiac anesthesia. Gewerbestrasse 11, 6330 Cham, Switzerland: Springer; 2021. p. 345–64.

39. Aadahl P, Lundbom J, Hatlinghus S, et al. Regional anesthesia for endovascular treatment of abdominal aortic aneurysms. J Endovascular Ther 1997;4(1):56–61.

40. Armstrong RA, Squire YG, Rogers CA, et al. Type of anesthesia for endovascular abdominal aortic aneurysm repair. J Cardiothorac Vasc Anesth 2019;33(2): 462–71.

41. Swaminathan M, Lineberger CK, McCann RL, et al. The importance of intraoperative transesophageal echocardiography in endovascular repair of thoracic aortic aneurysms. Anesth Analgesia 2003;97(6):1566–72.

42. Rocchi G, Lofiego C, Biagini E, et al. Transesophageal echocardiography–guided algorithm for stent-graft implantation in aortic dissection. J Vasc Surg 2004;40(5):880–5.

43. Awad H, Ramadan ME, El Sayed HF, et al. Spinal cord injury after thoracic endovascular aortic aneurysm repair. Can J Anesth 2017;64(12):1218–35.

44. von Aspern K, Haunschild J, Heier M, et al. Experimental near-infrared spectroscopy-guided minimally invasive segmental artery occlusion. Eur J Cardio-Thoracic Surg 2021;60(1):48–55.

45. Ali J, Cody J, Maldonado Y, et al. Near-Infrared Spectroscopy (NIRS) for Cerebral and Tissue Oximetry: Analysis of Evolving Applications. J Cardiothorac Vasc Anesth 2022;36(8 Pt A):2758–66.

46. Aucoin VJ, Eagleton MJ, Farber MA, et al. Spinal cord protection practices used during endovascular repair of complex aortic aneurysms by the US Aortic Research Consortium. J Vasc Surg 2021;73(1):323–30.

47. Arora H, Kumar PA. Prophylactic cerebrospinal fluid drainage for high-risk thoracic endovascular aortic repair: safe and effective? J Cardiothorac Vasc Anesth 2018;32(2):890–2.

48. Chaudhary O, Sharkey A, Schermerhorn M, et al. Protocolized based management of cerebrospinal fluid drains in thoracic endovascular aortic aneurysm repair procedures. Ann Vasc Surg 2021;72:409–18.

49. Scott CK, Timaran DE, Malekpour F, et al. Selective Versus Routine Spinal Drain Use for Fenestrated/Branched Endovascular Aortic Repair (F-BEVAR). Ann Vasc Surg 2021;76:168–73.

50. Daye D, Walker TG. Complications of endovascular aneurysm repair of the thoracic and abdominal aorta: evaluation and management. Cardiovasc Diagn Ther 2018;8(Suppl 1):S138.

51. Alsawas M, Zaiem F, Larrea-Mantilla L, et al. Effectiveness of surgical interventions for thoracic aortic aneurysms: a systematic review and meta-analysis. J Vasc Surg 2017;66(4):1258–68.e8.
52. Stather P, Sidloff D, Dattani N, et al. Systematic review and meta-analysis of the early and late outcomes of open and endovascular repair of abdominal aortic aneurysm. J Br Surg 2013;100(7):863–72.
53. Elkouri S, Gloviczki P, McKusick MA, et al. Perioperative complications and early outcome after endovascular and open surgical repair of abdominal aortic aneurysms. J Vasc Surg 2004;39(3):497–505.
54. Jasinski PT, Adrahtas D, Monastiriotis S, Tassiopoulos AK. Early and late endograft limb proximal migration with resulting type 1b endoleak following an EVAR for ruptured AAA. Case Reports in Vascular Medicine. 2017;2017.
55. Maleux G, Koolen M, Heye S. Complications after endovascular aneurysm repair. Semin Intervent Radiol 2009;26(1):3–9.

The Unstable Carotid Plaque

Salim Habib, MD[a,b], Muhammad Saad Hafeez, MBBS[a,b],
Theodore H. Yuo, MD, MSc[b], Kathirvel Subramaniam, MD, MPH, FASE[c,*]

KEYWORDS

- Unstable carotid plaque • Perioperative stroke • Anesthesia management
- Cardiac and noncardiac surgery

KEY POINTS

- Unstable carotid plaque is characterized by a greater burden of inflammatory atherosclerosis and translates to a higher risk of strokes.
- Plaque texture and neovascularization contribute to instability. Identification of such features can help in better patient selection for carotid revascularization.
- General anesthesia, monitored anesthesia care, and regional anesthesia have all been used with success and selection of anesthesia technique depends on center's experience, patient's comorbidities, and anticipated complexity of the procedure.

INTRODUCTION

Stroke is the fourth leading cause of death in the United States.[1] In addition to significant mortality, it also contributes to prolonged disability, imposing financial and care burdens on society.[1] Asymptomatic carotid artery disease is responsible for 11% of new strokes per year.[2] Surgical intervention is recommended for symptomatic carotid artery disease following the recommendations of the North American Symptomatic Carotid Endarterectomy Trial criteria (NASCET).[3] The Asymptomatic Carotid Atherosclerosis Study results have also been used to justify surgery in asymptomatic patients. Based on these trials, European guidelines recommend surgery in asymptomatic individuals with stenosis greater than 60%, whereas the Society for Vascular Surgery guidelines recommends the same for stenosis greater than 70%.[4,5] However, the results of these studies cannot be extrapolated to current management.[6] First, trials select surgeons with good outcomes, reducing their external validity. Second, medical management has advanced in the two decades since these

S. Habib and M.S. Hafeez combined 1st author.
[a] Department of Vascular Surgery, University of Pittsburgh Medical Center, 200 Lothrop Street, Pittsburgh, PA 15213, USA; [b] Division of Vascular Surgery, Department of Surgery, University of Pittsburgh School of Medicine, UPMC Presbyterian Hospital, 200 Lothrop Street, Pittsburgh, PA 15143, USA; [c] Department of Anesthesiology and Perioperative Medicine, University of Pittsburgh, Pittsburgh, 3471 5th Avenue Ste 402, Pittsburgh, PA 15213, USA
* Corresponding author.
E-mail address: subramaniamk@upmc.edu

Anesthesiology Clin 40 (2022) 737–749
https://doi.org/10.1016/j.anclin.2022.08.015
1932-2275/22/© 2022 Elsevier Inc. All rights reserved.
anesthesiology.theclinics.com

Abbreviations	
RR	relative risks
CD40L	Soluble CD40 ligandhs
CRP	high-sensitivity C-reactive protein
TIMP	Tissue Inhibitor of Metalloproteinase
MMPs	Matrix metalloproteinases
IFN-γ	interferon
TGF-β	Transforming growth factor beta
CMV	Cytomegalovirus
TCAR	Transcarotid Artery Revascularization
ASA	American Society of Anesthesiologists
CANTOS	Canakinumab Anti-Inflammatory Thrombosis Outcomes Study

trials. The NASCET trial showed plaque texture's role in predicting ischemic events and hence opened the discussion on risk stratification based on plaque features.[3,7] Identifying these "time-bomb" plaques has two advantages: (1) it prevents exposing patients to unnecessary surgery with a high perioperative stroke risk and (2) it recommends surgery in patients that are more likely to benefit from surgery.[8] In this review, we discuss the epidemiology, pathophysiology, and clinical presentation of the "unstable plaque", along with medical, surgical, and anesthesia aspects of its management.

EPIDEMIOLOGY

Plaque composition can predict the risk of strokes in asymptomatic individuals. The prevalence of asymptomatic stenosis varies with gender and age. Risk stratification can advise surgery for a sufficiently high-risk subgroup of this patient population.[9]

In the absence of extensive cross-sectional studies about carotid plaques, small case-control studies are the best tool to understand the epidemiology of vulnerable plaques. Secondary analysis of the Asymptomatic Carotid Surgery Trial 1 (ACST-1) shows that echolucent plaques are associated with younger age groups.[10] Conversely, intraplaque hemorrhage has been associated with older individuals.[11,12] Larson and colleagues[11] also found that patients with unstable plaque had a greater cardiovascular comorbidity burden. Individuals with vulnerable plaque had higher systolic blood pressures.[13] A higher incidence of smoking is observed in this cohort as well.[11,12]

Plaque texture correlates with lipid profiles. Individuals with vulnerable plaques have lower HDL levels, higher total cholesterol levels, and higher triglyceride levels.[11,13] Inflammatory markers such as white blood cells and fibrinogen are elevated, reflecting more severe atherosclerotic disease.[13] In addition to these, other biomarkers such as serum amyloid -A, cytokines, and hemostatic factors can assist in the classification of plaques.[14] Adherence to statins to treat dyslipidemia can help to reduce carotid intimal medial thickness, thus "stabilizing" the plaque.[15] These differences in medical compliance translate to a greater risk of stroke eventually.[10]

PATHOPHYSIOLOGY

Understanding the pathophysiological process of atheroma formation is key to understanding the differences between stable and unstable plaques. Arterial walls have been shown to adapt to the frictional forces, or shear stress, caused by blood flow at the endothelial surface. Disorganized blood flow and shear stress trigger atheroma formation which begins with increased permeability of endothelial cells to low-density lipoprotein (LDL).[16,17] The LDL particles accumulate in the subendothelial matrix and undergo several modifications, most importantly oxidation, which renders them proin-flammatory.[18] Monocytes are recruited to the lesion, convert into macrophages and begin actively eliminating the LDL particles, giving rise to droplet-filled cells known as foam cells.[18] The secretion of proinflammatory cytokines by these foam cells maintains a chronic local inflammatory response at the lesion.[18] The progressive death of some macrophages leads to the formation of a necrotic core which is a key factor in the in-flammatory process that renders plaques vulnerable to disruption.[19] In parallel, once macrophages become unable to keep up with the excessive amount of lipids, vascular smooth muscle cells (VSMCs) get activated and migrate into the subendothelium.[20] VSMCs convert into fibroblast-like cells and produce an extracellular matrix (ECM) which is constituted mainly of collagen and proteoglycans. This ECM gives the atheroma its fibrous cap and stabilizes the lesion in place.[21] It is considered that the bal-ance between inflammatory processes and ECM deposition is what determines the sta-bility of a plaque.[20] As such, stable plaques are characterized by chronic inflammatory reactions, thick fibrous caps, and small necrotic cores. Unstable and ruptured plaques are on the contrary characterized by active inflammatory reactions that lead to fibrous cap thinning and necrotic core growth.[22] Many inflammatory (eg, sCD40 L, hs-CRP, TIMP, MMPs, IFN-γ) and anti-inflammatory biomarkers (eg, TGF-β) have been described in the literature; the balance between their activities is also believed to affect the stability of the fibrous caps and therefore the vulnerability of plaques.[7,23]

Intraplaque neovascularization is another culprit for plaque instability. Symptomatic lesions show larger neovessels with more irregularities.[24–26] Rupture of such vessels leads to intraplaque hemorrhage with subsequent fibrous cap tear and exposure of flowing blood to the necrotic core.[24–26] The extensive neogenesis in unstable plaques has been associated with greater concentrations of vascular endothelial growth factor (VEGF).[20,27] The latter plays a dual role of being an angiogenic factor but also an in-flammatory cytokine.[20,27]

Once a stream of blood, rich in platelets and coagulation factors, meets tissue-presenting cells and the thrombogenic lipid core of a ruptured plaque, a thrombus gets formed.[28,29]

CLINICAL PRESENTATION

Carotid artery disease can be asymptomatic, or it may present with neurologic man-ifestations due to embolic episodes or distal hypoperfusion. Plaque ulceration leads to embolic fragments that cause distal occlusion in the distribution of the internal carotid artery. It can manifest abruptly as retinal infarction, presenting as blindness or amau-rosis fugax, or cerebral infarction (stroke or transient ischemic attack). Alternatively, chronic microembolization can produce subtle cerebral atrophy and vascular demen-tia.[30] Gradual reductions in cerebrovascular reserve carry a greater risk of future stroke events.[31] During physical examination, carotid auscultation can detect a bruit when plaque produces turbulent flow. The presence of a carotid bruit is associated with an increased risk of cerebrovascular disease, however, its utility in asymptomatic individuals is limited by poor predictive value.[32]

Although the pattern of presentation is not different when an unstable plaque is pre-sent, there is a greater incidence of stroke.[33] The natural history of asymptomatic ca-rotid artery disease, grouped by plaque morphology, was first published by Moore and colleagues.[34] Their finding that plaque texture modifies stroke risk has been echoed in the decades since.

Plaque echolucency is associated with an elevated risk of ipsilateral stroke.[35] In post hoc analysis of the ACST-1, soft echolucent plaque was associated with a 2.5

times higher risk of ipsilateral stroke in individuals managed medically.[10] In their 2016 meta-analysis, Jashari and colleagues[33] summarized that an echolucent plaque predicted future cardiovascular events in asymptomatic patients (RR = 2.72, P<.05) and recurrent symptoms in symptomatic patients (RR = 2.97, P<.05). A secondary analysis of the Asymptomatic Carotid Stenosis and Risk of Stroke (ACSRS) trial corroborates that not all plaques are created equal. Plaques with a high degree of echolucency accounted for 94% of the ischemic events. Predominantly echogenic centers and calcified caps were associated with a low event rate.[36]

Plaque characteristics that can be detected by noninvasive modalities such as ultrasound are essential for clinical management. Intraplaque hemorrhage can predict future cerebrovascular events.[12] The volume of the juxta-luminal hypoechoic area is predictive of ischemic events in asymptomatic individuals.[37] A cutoff point of 8 mm^2 has been suggested to have a good diagnostic value.[38] Proximity of the necrotic plaque core to the lumen is associated with symptomatic presentation.[39,40] Higher carotid intima-medial thickness is also associated with higher stroke risk.[41]

Microemboli from a carotid plaque is associated with a 7 to 10 times greater risk of stroke in asymptomatic patients.[42,43] These can be detected using transcranial Doppler studies, which can also identify other morphologic features. A model that checks for ulcers and microemboli can identify more high-risk asymptomatic patients.[42] This is in contrast to the current trends in the United States, where 90% of interventions are performed for asymptomatic patients without prior risk scoring.[43]

Progression of carotid plaque is associated with a two times higher risk of stroke. Although it may not be cost-effective to introduce screening protocols, knowledge of predictors of regression such as statin use can be used to guide management in such a subgroup.[44]

LABORATORY TESTING

There is growing interest in biomarkers associated with carotid artery disease. Early research was motivated by a now-debunked belief that traditional cardiovascular risk factors are absent in up to half of patients with atherosclerotic disease. Current interest is based on better understanding the natural history of carotid plaque and risk stratification.[45] Moreover, tracking levels of these biomarkers can indirectly indicate the efficacy of medical therapies.[14] For example, statin administration has been associated with a reduction in intima-medial thickness and improvements in lipid profiles.[15]

The differences in the balance of lipoproteins are reflective of systemic atherosclerosis and predict progression, stroke risk, and even the type of stroke. LDL levels correlate directly with stroke risk, whereas high-density lipoprotein (HDL) levels vary inversely with the incidence of stroke.[46] Apolipoprotein ratios similarly correlate with stroke risk. ApoB and apoE levels are associated with an earlier and greater likelihood of strokes respectively.[46,47] ApoA and apoJ are associated with a lower likelihood and less severe stroke respectively.[46]

C-reactive protein (CRP) is the most extensively studied of inflammatory cytokines. In their 2011 systematic review, Avgerinos and colleagues[14] summarized that CRP has been linked with ischemic stroke across the majority of studies on the subject. High levels of fibrinogen have been suggested to improve the predictive ability of CRP assays in predicting stroke risk.[48] Prospective data from the CANTOS trial shows that management of inflammation with biologics can reduce cardiovascular events. Reductions in CRP levels were used in this analysis to follow the improvements in inflammation.[49] With regard to clinical utility, other candidate biomarkers that have been studied include interleukin-6, matrix metalloproteinases, infectious agents, D-dimer, osteoprotegerin, various cell adhesion molecules, CD40 ligand, adiponectin, and leptin.[14,46] However, individually none of these biomarkers have shown high enough sensitivity in identifying the vulnerable plaque.[46]

IMAGING

Noninvasive imaging is the standard to diagnose carotid artery disease.[5] The role of angiography in diagnosis is limited due to the prohibitive procedural stroke incidence, despite its superior accuracy in measuring the degree of stenosis.[6,50] Ultrasound is preferred to visualize the plaque as it is cost-effective, easily available at the bedside, noninvasive, and does not expose the patient to high doses of radiation.[51] Ultrasound examination can delineate the degree of stenosis, carotid intima-medial thickness, plaque morphology, and plaque volume.[52] Novel variations of ultrasound can shorten the time required for volume assessment.[53] Contrast-enhanced ultrasound based on microbubbles with sulfur hexafluoride stabilized by phospholipids can additionally identify plaque neovascularization.[54] Doppler monitoring can detect microemboli emitted from a plaque.[43] The detailed information obtained from a single ultrasound examination of the plaque can guide prescription patterns as well as motivate patients to make appropriate lifestyle changes.[55] The main limitation of ultrasound techniques is their operator-dependent nature that reduces its accuracy, interobserver agreement, and incorporation into regular practice.

MANAGEMENT

For a long time, the treatment of carotid stenosis was based on the patients' symptomatic status or degree of carotid stenosis. However, with the evolving understanding of unstable plaques, especially through new vascular imaging techniques, it has become clear that the stability of a plaque is what determines the risks of cerebrovascular accidents rather than the degree of arterial stenosis.[56] The review below summarizes the most up-to-date management of carotid stenosis.

Regardless of plaque characteristics or the presence of symptoms, all patients with signs of carotid stenosis require lifestyle changes and intensive medical therapy (IMT) to decrease the risks of cerebrovascular events.[57] Management of modifiable risk factors including smoking, drinking, hypertension, hyperlipidemia, and diabetes mellitus is strongly recommended.[58] All patients should be started on aspirin as their anti-inflammatory and antithrombotic effects have been established to benefit atherosclerosis management.[20,27,59] High-intensity statins are also recommended as they slow atherosclerosis and prevent plaque destabilization.[20,57] Furthermore, the combination of antihypertensives with statins has been reported to have additive benefits for secondary prevention of strokes.[60] Although all patients are recommended IMT, the decision to proceed to surgery can be delicate.

Following the 1990s randomized clinical trials, the European Carotid Surgery Trial[61] (ECST) and the NASCET,[62,63] most guidelines recommend carotid endarterectomy (CEA) for symptomatic stenosis of 50% to 99% and asymptomatic stenosis of 70% to 99%.[57,64] For symptomatic patients with stenosis less than 50% and asymptomatic patients with stenosis below 60%, these trials do not recommend CEA as it does not decrease the risks of strokes and is associated with high postoperative morbidity. With the growing evidence that the risk of stroke is not equivalent for all patients with similar grades of stenosis, these aforementioned guidelines are being continuously challenged, especially for asymptomatic disease.[20,65] The selection of patients for revascularization based on plaque characteristics continues to generate research interest.

There is emerging evidence that plaque morphology, besides the presence of symptoms or the degree of stenosis, should play a major role in the selection of patients for revascularization.[66] The European Society of Vascular Surgery (ESVS) provides a list of clinical and imaging features that have been associated with an increased risk of late stroke among patients with asymptomatic carotid stenosis (ACS) of 50% to 99%.[5] These imaging features include cerebral findings such as silent infarctions and impaired cerebral vascular reserve, and carotid plaque characteristics such as plaque echolucency, intra-plaque hemorrhage, stenosis progression, and large juxta-luminal black area on computerized plaque analysis.[5] Furthermore, the assessment of patients' risk of stroke based on biological markers has also recently gained interest.[14,46] Potential markers include inflammatory markers (CRP, fibrinogen, MMPs), infectious markers (CMV, helicobacter), hemostatic markers (D-dimers, PAI), and vascular calcification markers (osteopontin, osteoprotegerin).[14,46] Randomized clinical trials are still needed to incorporate such markers into current clinical practice.r

For patients selected for revascularization, the choice of surgical approach should be made. CEA is the oldest approach and has been the standard of surgical care. The interest in adopting minimally invasive approaches in all surgical fields has led to the development of carotid angioplasty and stenting (CAS). However, as per the major society guidelines,[57,64] in the absence of anatomic and physiologic high risks for surgical procedures or anesthesia exposure, CEA remains the preferred option over CAS. CEA is recommended for tortuous vessels, highly stenotic vessels, and vessels with anatomies preventing safe deployment of the embolic protection device or stent during CAS.[67] History of previous CEA, radiation to the neck, radical neck dissection, and contralateral laryngeal palsy would favor the choice of CAS.[67] When CAS is chosen, the transcarotid approach is considered safer than transfemoral approach.[64]

The benefit of surgical interventions as compared with IMT is recently being requestioned. A comparison between the results reported in the Asymptomatic Carotid Atherosclerosis Study[68] (ACAS) and the subsequent Asymptomatic Carotid Surgery Trial (ACST)[69] reveals a decline in annual stroke risks which can be associated with the improvement in available medical therapies and the increased use of lipid-lowering agents. Although both trials favor CEA over medical treatment, the IMT they studied are nowadays considered rudimentary as they rely solely on aspirin and comorbidity management. Newer trials comparing IMT alone versus surgical intervention (CEA or CAS) in addition to IMT are needed.

PERIOPERATIVE IMPLICATIONS

For elective cardiac and noncardiac surgery, presence of symptoms or high-risk criteria (age, renal disease, and transient ischemic attacks/stroke) should direct carotid duplex imaging preoperatively. Routine scanning of the carotid artery in patients without symptoms or high-risk features is not indicated.[70] Literature on preoperative management of the cardiac surgical patient is extensive but scant on noncardiac surgery.[71-73] Although carotid revascularization is indicated for high-grade symptomatic stenosis (>70%) before elective cardiac surgery, the decision-making for asymptomatic patients, lesser degrees of stenosis, and urgent cardiac surgery should depend on several other factors; priority to highly symptomatic vascular territory, local expertise, and the plaque characteristics.[74] The plaque characteristics should be considered for decision making and highly unstable plaques can be considered for intervention before or concomitant with cardiac surgery. The incidence of postoperative stroke detected clinically varies between 0.1% and 1% after noncardiac surgery but silent stroke (detectable lesions in MRI without clinical manifestations) can occur in 8% to

10% of patients undergoing noncardiac surgery.[75] The contribution of unstable carotid lesions to perioperative stroke in noncardiac surgery is not known but general principles of management apply. Elective surgery in a patient with symptomatic carotid stenosis (>70%) can be postponed for carotid intervention if the risk of carotid intervention is acceptable (less than 6%).[75]

Anesthesia management of patients with unstable atheromatous plaques will involve all principles of perioperative stroke prevention. Maintenance of adequate oxygen delivery to the brain is the goal and the principles of management will include adequate ventilation, treatment of anemia below hemoglobin 8 g/dL and maintaining mean arterial pressure above 70 mm Hg.[76,77] Carotid artery manipulation with access of internal jugular puncture should be avoided and central venous access contralateral to the side with unstable carotid plaque is safer strategy. Earlier detection of intraoperative of neurologic insult from unstable carotid plaques can be facilitated by multimodal neuromonitoring.[78] Intraoperative neuromonitoring may include cerebral oximetry, electroencephalogram, somatosensory evoked potentials, and transcranial Doppler either alone or in combination depending on the patient and surgical factors. Regional anesthesia may be preferred for suitable surgical procedures so that onset of any neurologic deficits can be diagnosed earlier in conscious patients.[79] In addition to goal-directed intraoperative management under general anesthesia (GA), patients should be reversed and checked for neurologic status in patients with unstable carotid plaques undergoing surgery. Earlier imaging in patients with suspected neurologic dysfunction can direct mechanical thrombectomy or embolectomy, and these interventions can improve the outcomes after stroke if done within 6 hours or even within 24 hours in some patients.[80]

Trans Carotid Artery Revascularization Procedure

Literature on anesthesia management of CEA is already extensively discussed elsewhere and is not within the scope of this review.[81,82] However, the authors will discuss the TCAR procedure more often used for patients with carotid artery stenosis nowadays. Compared with carotid artery stenting through the femoral artery, TCAR reverses blood flow during the procedure of carotid stenting so that unstable plaques manipulated during the procedure are diverted away from the brain.[83] TCAR was associated with a lower incidence of death and stroke compared with transfemoral carotid artery stenting.[83] ROADSTER clinical trial (a single arm, multicenter study) evaluated the safety and efficacy of TCAR for carotid artery stenting. Between 2012 and 2014, 208 patients were enrolled, and the success rate was 99%. Composite outcomes of stroke, myocardial infarction (MI), and death occurred in 3.5% and stroke alone in 1.4% of patients.[84] ROADSTER-2 clinical trials examined high-risk patients (n = 692) and the success rate was 96.5%. Stroke, MI, and death as composite outcomes occurred in 3.2% of patients with stroke alone in 1.9% of patients.[85]

Preoperative evaluation and preparation are completed similar to any vascular surgery patient with significant comorbidities. Type of anesthesia depends on the patient's ability to lie still and supine on the operating table and presence of comorbidities such as obesity, sleep apnea, and difficult airway. Superficial cervical plexus block and local infiltration are used as adjuvants to monitored anesthesia care (MAC) and GA. Burton and colleagues[86] evaluated the association of anesthesia type with perioperative adverse events during TCAR using the American College of Surgeons National Surgical Quality Improvement (ACS NSQIP) registry (n = 632). MAC was used in 73% of patients and was associated with lower 30-day mortality, shorter case duration, decreased length of stay, and pulmonary complications. This study examined patients operated on between 2012 and 2016. Mukherjee and colleagues[87] examined a large national database from the society for vascular surgery to compare the effect of GA and MAC on clinical outcomes after TCAR (number of patients = 2609). In contrast to Burton and colleagues's[87] report, GA was administered in 82% of patients. Composite primary outcome of stroke, MI, and mortality was detected in 2.3% of GA versus 2.6% in local anesthesia patients. When proper selection criteria are employed, both MAC and GA seem to be safe for this procedure.

Apart from standard ASA monitoring, invasive arterial blood pressure and wide bore IV access are established before starting the procedure. Heparin is used to maintain activated clotting time above 250 s. Blood pressure is maintained 15% to 20% above baseline or above 140 to 160 mm Hg systolic to maintain perfusion through the circle of Willis during reversal of flow from the common carotid artery to the femoral vein. Patients with advanced lung disease and patients with the contralateral carotid disease may develop intolerance to flow reversal and can be managed by adjusting the reversal flow rate and faster completion of the procedure.[88] Flow through the circle of Willis can be monitored with cerebral oximetry during flow reversal and electroencephalography/somatosensory evoked potentials (EEG/SSEP) during GA. After stent deployment, systolic blood pressure can be lowered and maintained above 100 mm Hg. During manipulations, patients can suffer severe bradycardia or asystole and anticholinergic medications can be administered prophylactically or should be ready on the bedside. Patients should be monitored postoperatively for neurologic function and bleeding.

In summary, patients with unstable carotid plaques can pose significant perioperative stroke risk. Defining the plaque characteristics with carotid duplex imaging preoperatively can direct risk assessment, appropriate preoperative interventions such as stenting or surgical endarterectomy, intraoperative management, and earlier treatment of perioperative stroke.

CLINICS CARE POINTS

- Patient selection for operations to treat carotid artery disease should incorporate an assessment of plaque morphology guided by imaging studies.

- All patients with carotid artery disease should be recommended lifestyle changes, such as weight loss, smoking cessation, and intensive medical therapy.

- Current guidelines are based on early trials, which recommend surgical revascularization over best medical therapy. However, the introduction of modern medications is being investigated by ongoing trials, which may lead to a revision of these recommendations.

- Biological markers are actively being studied as tools to improve patient selection for operative management, but randomized data is necessary before testing for these markers becomes the standard of care.

DISCLOSURE

No relevant disclosures for this article from the authors.

REFERENCES

1. Virani SS, Alonso A, Benjamin EJ, et al. Heart Disease and Stroke Statistics—2020 Update: A Report From the American Heart Association. Circulation 2020; 141(9):e139–596.

2. Naylor AR. Why is the management of asymptomatic carotid disease so controversial? Surgeon 2015;13(1):34–43 (In en).
3. Ferguson GG, Eliasziw M, Barr HW, et al. The North American Symptomatic Carotid Endarterectomy Trial : surgical results in 1415 patients. Stroke 1999;30(9): 1751–8 (In eng).
4. AbuRahma AF, Avgerinos E, Chang RW, et al. SOCIETY FOR VASCULAR SURGERY CLINICAL PRACTICE GUIDELINES FOR MANAGEMENT OF EXTRACRANIAL CEREBROVASCULAR DISEASE. J Vasc Surg 2021;0(0) (In English).
5. Naylor AR, Ricco JB, de Borst GJ, et al. Editor's Choice - Management of Atherosclerotic Carotid and Vertebral Artery Disease: 2017 Clinical Practice Guidelines of the European Society for Vascular Surgery (ESVS). Eur J Vasc Endovasc Surg 2018;55(1):3–81 (In eng).
6. Walker MD, Marler JR, Goldstein M, et al. Endarterectomy for Asymptomatic Carotid Artery Stenosis. JAMA 1995;273(18):1421–8.
7. Skagen K, Skjelland M, Zamani M, et al. Unstable carotid artery plaque: new insights and controversies in diagnostics and treatment. Croat Med J 2016;57(4): 311–20 (In eng).
8. Abbott AL, Brunser AM, Giannoukas A, et al. Misconceptions regarding the adequacy of best medical intervention alone for asymptomatic carotid stenosis. J Vasc Surg 2020;71(1):257–69 (In eng).
9. de Weerd M, Greving JP, Hedblad B, et al. Prevalence of asymptomatic carotid artery stenosis in the general population: an individual participant data meta-analysis. Stroke 2010;41(6):1294–7 (In eng).
10. Huibers A, de Borst GJ, Bulbulia R, et al. Plaque Echolucency and the Risk of Ischaemic Stroke in Patients with Asymptomatic Carotid Stenosis Within the First Asymptomatic Carotid Surgery Trial (ACST-1). Eur J Vasc Endovasc Surg 2016; 51(5):616–21 (In eng).
11. Larson AS, Brinjikji W, Savastano LE, et al. Carotid Intraplaque Hemorrhage Is Associated with Cardiovascular Risk Factors. Cerebrovasc Dis (Basel, Switzerland) 2020;49(4):355–60 (In eng).
12. Singh N, Moody AR, Gladstone DJ, et al. Moderate carotid artery stenosis: MR imaging-depicted intraplaque hemorrhage predicts risk of cerebrovascular ischemic events in asymptomatic men. Radiology 2009;252(2):502–8 (In eng).
13. Mathiesen EB, Bønaa KH, Joakimsen O. Echolucent plaques are associated with high risk of ischemic cerebrovascular events in carotid stenosis: the tromsø study. Circulation 2001;103(17):2171–5 (In eng).
14. Avgerinos ED, Kadoglou NP, Moulakakis KG, et al. Current role of biomarkers in carotid disease: a systematic review. Int J Stroke 2011;6(4):337–45 (In eng).
15. Riccioni G, Vitulano N, Mancini B, et al. One-year treatment with rosuvastatin reduces intima-media thickness in 45 hypercholesterolemic subjects with asymptomatic carotid artery disease. Pharmacology 2010;85(2):63–7 (In eng).
16. Silver AE, Vita JA. Shear-stress-mediated arterial remodeling in atherosclerosis: too much of a good thing? Circulation 2006;113(24):2787–9.
17. Resnick N, Yahav H, Shay-Salit A, et al. Fluid shear stress and the vascular endothelium: for better and for worse. Prog Biophys Mol Biol 2003;81(3):177–99.
18. Bobryshev YV, Ivanova EA, Chistiakov DA, et al. Macrophages and Their Role in Atherosclerosis: Pathophysiology and Transcriptome Analysis. Biomed Res Int 2016;2016:9582430.
19. Seimon T, Tabas I. Mechanisms and consequences of macrophage apoptosis in atherosclerosis. J Lipid Res 2009;50(Suppl):S382–7.

20. Migdalski A, Jawien A. New insight into biology, molecular diagnostics and treatment options of unstable carotid atherosclerotic plaque: a narrative review. Ann Transl Med 2021;9(14):1207.
21. Hansson GK. Inflammation, atherosclerosis, and coronary artery disease. N Engl J Med 2005;352(16):1685–95.
22. Spagnoli LG, Bonanno E, Sangiorgi G, et al. Role of inflammation in atherosclerosis. J Nucl Med 2007;48(11):1800–15 (In eng).
23. Silvestre-Roig C, de Winther MP, Weber C, et al. Atherosclerotic plaque destabilization: mechanisms, models, and therapeutic strategies. Circ Res 2014;114(1): 214–26 (In eng).
24. McCarthy MJ, Loftus IM, Thompson MM, et al. Angiogenesis and the atherosclerotic carotid plaque: an association between symptomatology and plaque morphology. J Vasc Surg 1999;30(2):261–8 (In eng).
25. Mofidi R, Crotty TB, McCarthy P, et al. Association between plaque instability, angiogenesis and symptomatic carotid occlusive disease. Br J Surg 2001; 88(7):945–50 (In eng).
26. Giannoni MF, Vicenzini E. Focus on the "unstable" carotid plaque: detection of intraplaque angiogenesis with contrast ultrasound. Present state and future perspectives. Curr Vasc Pharmacol 2009;7(2):180–4 (In eng).
27. Wijeratne T, Menon R, Sales C, et al. Carotid artery stenosis and inflammatory biomarkers: the role of inflammation-induced immunological responses affecting the vascular systems. Ann Transl Med 2020;8(19):1276 (In eng).
28. Halvorsen B, Otterdal K, Dahl TB, et al. Atherosclerotic plaque stability–what determines the fate of a plaque? Prog Cardiovasc Dis 2008;51(3):183–94 (In eng).
29. Owens AP 3rd, Mackman N. Role of tissue factor in atherothrombosis. Curr Atheroscler Rep 2012;14(5):394–401 (In eng).
30. Moore WS. Moore's Vascular and Endovascular Surgery, Ninth Edition - Chapter 19 Extracranial Cerebrovascular Disease: The Carotid Artery. Ninth ed.
31. Gupta A, Chazen JL, Hartman M, et al. Cerebrovascular reserve and stroke risk in patients with carotid stenosis or occlusion: a systematic review and meta-analysis. Stroke 2012;43(11):2884–91 (In eng).
32. Pickett CA, Jackson JL, Hemann BA, et al. Carotid bruits and cerebrovascular disease risk: a meta-analysis. Stroke 2010;41(10):2295–302 (In eng).
33. Jashari F, Ibrahimi P, Bajraktari G, et al. Carotid plaque echogenicity predicts cerebrovascular symptoms: a systematic review and meta-analysis. Eur J Neurol 2016;23(7):1241–7 (In eng).
34. Moore WS, Boren C, Malone JM, et al. Natural history of nonstenotic, asymptomatic ulcerative lesions of the carotid artery. Arch Surg 1978;113(11):1352–9 (In eng).
35. Topakian R, King A, Kwon SU, et al. Ultrasonic plaque echolucency and emboli signals predict stroke in asymptomatic carotid stenosis. Neurology 2011;77(8): 751–8 (In eng).
36. Nicolaides AN, Kakkos SK, Griffin M, et al. Effect of image normalization on carotid plaque classification and the risk of ipsilateral hemispheric ischemic events: results from the asymptomatic carotid stenosis and risk of stroke study. Vascular 2005;13(4):211–21 (In eng).
37. Kakkos SK, Griffin MB, Nicolaides AN, et al. The size of juxtaluminal hypoechoic area in ultrasound images of asymptomatic carotid plaques predicts the occurrence of stroke. J Vasc Surg 2013;57(3):609–18.e1 [discussion: 617–8]. [in English].

38. Griffin MB, Kyriacou E, Pattichis C, et al. Juxtaluminal hypoechoic area in ultrasonic images of carotid plaques and hemispheric symptoms. J Vasc Surg 2010;52(1):69–76 (In eng).
39. Bassiouny HS, Sakaguchi Y, Mikucki SA, et al. Juxtalumenal location of plaque necrosis and neoformation in symptomatic carotid stenosis. J Vasc Surg 1997; 26(4):585–94 (In eng).
40. Lal BK, Hobson RW, Hameed M, et al. Noninvasive identification of the unstable carotid plaque. Ann Vasc Surg 2006;20(2):167–74 (In eng).
41. Kitamura A, Iso H, Imano H, et al. Carotid Intima-Media Thickness and Plaque Characteristics as a Risk Factor for Stroke in Japanese Elderly Men. Stroke 2004;35(12):2788–94.
42. Madani A, Beletsky V, Tamayo A, et al. High-risk asymptomatic carotid stenosis: ulceration on 3D ultrasound vs TCD microemboli. Neurology 2011;77(8):744–50 (In eng).
43. Spence JD. Transcranial Doppler monitoring for microemboli: a marker of a high-risk carotid plaque. Semin Vasc Surg 2017;30(1):62–6 (In eng).
44. Kakkos SK, Nicolaides AN, Charalambous I, et al. Predictors and clinical significance of progression or regression of asymptomatic carotid stenosis. J Vasc Surg 2014;59(4):956–67.e1 (In en).
45. Khot UN, Khot MB, Bajzer CT, et al. Prevalence of conventional risk factors in patients with coronary heart disease. JAMA 2003;290(7):898–904 (In eng).
46. Puig N, Jiménez-Xarrié E, Camps-Renom P, et al. Search for Reliable Circulating Biomarkers to Predict Carotid Plaque Vulnerability. Int J Mol Sci 2020;21(21): 8236. https://www.mdpi.com/1422-0067/21/21/8236.
47. Khan TA, Shah T, Prieto D, et al. Apolipoprotein E genotype, cardiovascular biomarkers and risk of stroke: Systematic review and meta-analysis of 14 015 stroke cases and pooled analysis of primary biomarker data from up to 60 883 individuals. Int J Epidemiol 2013;42(2):475–92.
48. Tanne D, Benderly M, Goldbourt U, et al. C-reactive protein as a predictor of incident ischemic stroke among patients with preexisting cardiovascular disease. Stroke 2006;37(7):1720–4 (In eng).
49. Ridker PM, MacFadyen JG, Everett BM, et al. Relationship of C-reactive protein reduction to cardiovascular event reduction following treatment with canakinumab: a secondary analysis from the CANTOS randomised controlled trial. Lancet 2018;391(10118):319–28 (In eng).
50. Netuka D, Belšán T, Broulíková K, et al. Detection of carotid artery stenosis using histological specimens: a comparison of CT angiography, magnetic resonance angiography, digital subtraction angiography and Doppler ultrasonography. Acta Neurochir (Wien) 2016;158(8):1505–14 (In eng).
51. Golemati S, Patelaki E, Gastounioti A, et al. Motion synchronisation patterns of the carotid atheromatous plaque from B-mode ultrasound. Sci Rep 2020;10(1):11221 (In eng).
52. Lee W. General principles of carotid Doppler ultrasonography. Ultrasonography 2014;33(1):11–7 (In eng).
53. Khan AA, Koudelka C, Goldstein C, et al. Semiautomatic quantification of carotid plaque volume with three-dimensional ultrasound imaging. J Vasc Surg 2017; 65(5):1407–17 (In eng).
54. Faggioli GL, Pini R, Mauro R, et al. Identification of Carotid 'Vulnerable Plaque' by Contrast-enhanced Ultrasonography: Correlation with Plaque Histology, Symptoms and Cerebral Computed Tomography. Eur J Vasc Endovasc Surg 2011; 41(2):238–48 (In en).

55. Korcarz CE, DeCara JM, Hirsch AT, et al. Ultrasound Detection of Increased Carotid Intima-Media Thickness and Carotid Plaque in an Office Practice Setting: Does It Affect Physician Behavior or Patient Motivation? J Am Soc Echocardiogr 2008;21(10):1156–62.

56. Brinjikji W, Huston J 3rd, Rabinstein AA, et al. Contemporary carotid imaging: from degree of stenosis to plaque vulnerability. J Neurosurg 2016;124(1):27–42 (In eng).

57. Kleindorfer DO, Towfighi A, Chaturvedi S, et al. 2021 Guideline for the Prevention of Stroke in Patients With Stroke and Transient Ischemic Attack: A Guideline From the American Heart Association/American Stroke Association. Stroke 2021;52(7): e364–467.

58. Woo SY, Joh JH, Han SA, et al. Prevalence and risk factors for atherosclerotic carotid stenosis and plaque: A population-based screening study. Medicine (Baltimore) 2017;96(4):e5999.

59. Taylor DW, Barnett HJ, Haynes RB, et al. Low-dose and high-dose acetylsalicylic acid for patients undergoing carotid endarterectomy: a randomised controlled trial. ASA and Carotid Endarterectomy (ACE) Trial Collaborators. Lancet 1999; 353(9171):2179–84 (In eng).

60. Hackam DG, Spence JD. Combining multiple approaches for the secondary prevention of vascular events after stroke: a quantitative modeling study. Stroke 2007;38(6):1881–5.

61. Randomised trial of endarterectomy for recently symptomatic carotid stenosis: final results of the MRC European Carotid Surgery Trial (ECST). Lancet 1998; 351(9113):1379–87 (In eng).

62. MRC European Carotid Surgery Trial: interim results for symptomatic patients with severe (70-99%) or with mild (0-29%) carotid stenosis. European Carotid Surgery Trialists' Collaborative Group. Lancet 1991;337(8752):1235–43 (In eng).

63. Barnett HJM, Taylor DW, Eliasziw M, et al. Benefit of Carotid Endarterectomy in Patients with Symptomatic Moderate or Severe Stenosis. N Engl J Med 1998; 339(20):1415–25.

64. AbuRahma AF, Avgerinos ED, Chang RW, et al. The Society for Vascular Surgery implementation document for management of extracranial cerebrovascular disease. J Vasc Surg 2022;75(1s):26s–98s (In eng).

65. Paraskevas KI, Veith FJ, Ricco J-B. Best medical treatment alone may not be adequate for all patients with asymptomatic carotid artery stenosis. J Vasc Surg 2018;68(2):572–5.

66. Hennerici MG. The unstable plaque. Cerebrovasc Dis 2004;17(Suppl 3):17–22 (In eng).

67. Brott TG, Brown RD Jr, Meyer FB, et al. Carotid revascularization for prevention of stroke: carotid endarterectomy and carotid artery stenting. Mayo Clin Proc 2004; 79(9):1197–208 (In eng).

68. Endarterectomy for asymptomatic carotid artery stenosis. Executive Committee for the Asymptomatic Carotid Atherosclerosis Study. Jama 1995;273(18): 1421–8 (In eng).

69. Halliday A, Harrison M, Hayter E, et al. 10-year stroke prevention after successful carotid endarterectomy for asymptomatic stenosis (ACST-1): a multicentre randomised trial. Lancet 2010;376(9746):1074–84 (In eng).

70. Mufti HN, Alshaltoni RS, AlGahtani A, et al. Role of Carotid Artery Ultrasound Duplex Prior to Cardiac Surgery in Adults in Predicting Neurocognitive Complications. Cureus 2020;12(10):e11211 (In eng).

71. Li Y, Jenny D, Castaldo J. Cardiac surgery, carotid stenosis, and stroke prevention. Hosp Pract (1995) 2010;38(2):29–39 (In eng).

72. Morgante A, Di Bartolo M. Impact of a carotid stenosis on cardiac surgery: marker more than risk factor. G Chir 2019;40(5):381–8 (In eng).
73. Pinto Sousa P, Teixeira G, Gonçalves J, et al. Carotid Stenosis in Cardiac Surgery Patients. Rev Port Cir Cardiotorac Vasc 2017;24(3–4):126 (In eng).
74. Das P, Clavijo LC, Nanjundappa A, et al. Revascularization of carotid stenosis before cardiac surgery. Expert Rev Cardiovasc Ther 2008;6(10):1393–6 (In eng).
75. Benesch C, Glance LG, Derdeyn CP, et al. Perioperative Neurological Evaluation and Management to Lower the Risk of Acute Stroke in Patients Undergoing Noncardiac, Nonneurological Surgery: A Scientific Statement From the American Heart Association/American Stroke Association. Circulation 2021;143(19): e923–46 (In eng).
76. Wesselink EM, Kappen TH, Torn HM, et al. Intraoperative hypotension and the risk of postoperative adverse outcomes: a systematic review. Br J Anaesth 2018;121(4):706–21 (In eng).
77. Carson JL, Guyatt G, Heddle NM, et al. Clinical Practice Guidelines From the AABB: Red Blood Cell Transfusion Thresholds and Storage. Jama 2016; 316(19):2025–35 (In eng).
78. Shmigel'skiĭ AV, Usachev D, Lukshin VA, et al. [Multimodal neuromonitoring in the early diagnosis of brain ischemia during carotid arterial reconstruction]. Anesteziol Reanimatol 2008;(2):16–22 (In rus).
79. Rocha-Neves J, Pereira-Macedo J, Ferreira A, et al. Impact of intraoperative neurologic deficits in carotid endarterectomy under regional anesthesia. Scand Cardiovasc J 2021;55(3):180–6 (In eng).
80. Powers WJ, Rabinstein AA, Ackerson T, et al. Guidelines for the Early Management of Patients With Acute Ischemic Stroke: 2019 Update to the 2018 Guidelines for the Early Management of Acute Ischemic Stroke: A Guideline for Healthcare Professionals From the American Heart Association/American Stroke Association. Stroke 2019;50(12):e344–418 (In eng).
81. Lehot JJ, Durand PG. [Anesthesia for carotid endarterectomy]. Rev Esp Anestesiol Reanim 2001;48(10):499–507 (In spa).
82. Yepes Temiño MJ, Lillo Cuevas M. [Anesthesia for carotid endarterectomy: a review]. Rev Esp Anestesiol Reanim 2011;58(1):34–41 (In spa).
83. Schermerhorn ML, Liang P, Eldrup-Jorgensen J, et al. Association of Transcarotid Artery Revascularization vs Transfemoral Carotid Artery Stenting With Stroke or Death Among Patients With Carotid Artery Stenosis. Jama 2019;322(23): 2313–22 (In eng).
84. Kwolek CJ, Jaff MR, Leal JI, et al. Results of the ROADSTER multicenter trial of transcarotid stenting with dynamic flow reversal. J Vasc Surg 2015;62(5): 1227–34 (In eng).
85. Kashyap VS, Schneider PA, Foteh M, et al. Early Outcomes in the ROADSTER 2 Study of Transcarotid Artery Revascularization in Patients With Significant Carotid Artery Disease. Stroke 2020;51(9):2620–9 (In eng).
86. Burton BN, Finneran Iv JJ, Harris KK, et al. Association of Primary Anesthesia Type with Postoperative Adverse Events After Transcarotid Artery Revascularization. J Cardiothorac Vasc Anesth 2020;34(1):136–42 (In eng).
87. Mukherjee D, Collins DT, Liu C, et al. The study of transcarotid artery revascularization under local versus general anesthesia with results from the Society for Vascular Surgery Vascular Quality Initiative. Vascular 2020;28(6):784–93 (In eng).
88. Teter K, Rockman C, Lamparello P, et al. Risk Factors for and Intraoperative Management of Intolerance to Flow Reversal in TCAR. Ann Vasc Surg 2022;79:41–5 (In eng).

Regional Anesthesia for Vascular Surgery and Pain Management

Vicente Garcia Tomas, MD[a],*, Nicole Hollis, MD[b],
Jean-Pierre P. Ouanes, DO[c]

KEYWORDS

- Regional anesthesia • Carotid endarterectomy • Cervical plexus block
- Brachial plexus block • Lumbar plexus • Femoral nerve block • Sciatic nerve block

KEY POINTS

- Regional anesthesia for carotid endarterectomy (CEA) has several reported outcome benefits over general anesthesia.
- Superficial cervical plexus block, whether using the superficial or intermediate technique, provides clinically effective surgical anesthesia for CEA while avoiding the potential complications of the deep block.
- End-stage renal disease is increasing worldwide: hemodialysis through an arteriovenous fistula is the preferred method of renal replacement therapy as it carries lower risks of sepsis and mortality.
- Regional anesthesia for lower extremity vascular procedures may reduce graft failure rate and may reduce phantom limb pains in lower extremity amputation.

INTRODUCTION

Cardiovascular death remains a major cause of late mortality following vascular surgical procedures.[1] Vascular surgery is associated with greater cardiac morbidity and overall mortality than other forms of noncardiac surgery.[2] The patient population undergoing vascular surgical procedures present as a challenge because often these patients have other systemic comorbidities, including coronary artery disease, hypertension, diabetes mellitus, congestive heart failure, and renal impairment. Regional anesthesia (RA) serves as an adjunct as well as an alternative to general anesthesia (GA) in patients undergoing vascular procedures.

[a] Department of Anesthesiology, Regional Anesthesia and Acute Pain Medicine, Northwestern University Feinberg School of Medicine Chicago, 251 E. Huron St F5-704, Chicago, IL 60611, USA; [b] Department of Anesthesiology, West Virginia University, 1 Medical Center Drive PO Box 8255, Morgantown, WV 26508, USA; [c] Cornell Medicine, Hospital for Special Surgery, Florida, 300 Palm Beach Lakes Boulevard, West Palm Beach, FL 33401, USA
* Corresponding author.
E-mail address: vicente.garciatomas@nm.org

Anesthesiology Clin 40 (2022) 751–773
https://doi.org/10.1016/j.anclin.2022.08.016   anesthesiology.theclinics.com
1932-2275/22/© 2022 Elsevier Inc. All rights reserved.

An additional challenge for use of RA techniques in vascular patients is related to the common use of anticoagulants in this patient population. The American Society of Regional Anesthesia (ASRA) published guideline recommendations for the management of RA in patients receiving antithrombotic or thrombolytic therapy, which are updated periodically.[3] ASRA recommends following these guidelines when performing neuraxial procedures as well as deep plexus or peripheral nerve blocks. A summary of the guidelines for some of the most commonly used anticoagulants is presented in **Table 1**.

In this article, the authors review RA techniques for carotid endarterectomy (CEA), arteriovenous fistula (AVF) creation, and lower extremity bypass surgery and amputation.

General Concepts for Block Performance

Patient preparation

Before performing RA techniques, a thorough review of the patient's history, focusing on the use of anticoagulant medications, existing neuropathies, concomitant respiratory disease, and potential airway issues that could be worsened by specific blocks should be obtained. Risks, benefits, and alternatives to RA should be discussed with patients. Intravenous access should be established, and standard ASA monitors applied before performing any block. If sedation is planned to be administered to decrease patient anxiety, supplemental oxygen should be immediately available. Several RA techniques are amenable to catheter placement and or long-acting local anesthetics with additives to prolong the analgesia in the postoperative period.

Carotid Endarterectomy

The choice of primary anesthesia for CEA has been a topic of debate for five decades. The debate is over the advantages and disadvantages of the type of anesthesia pertaining to monitoring and neurologic complications. The argument of RA versus GA is based on monitoring the adequacy of cerebral perfusion during carotid cross-clamping and its relationship to perioperative neurologic events. GA offers the benefits of controlled airway and patient positioning but lacks highly sensitive and specific neurological monitoring. RA offers the benefit of using the awake patient as a direct monitor for cerebral perfusion. If a patient demonstrates neurologic impairment during carotid artery clamping, the surgeon places a shunt to restore cerebral perfusion. The risks of shunt placement include microembolization and vascular trauma. Under GA, shunt placement maybe done prophylactically, not at all, or if indicated by indirect monitoring demonstrating decreased cerebral perfusion.[4]

The techniques of local and cervical blocks for carotid surgery were originally described in the early 1960s.[5] The body of literature on outcome-related benefits of RA has grown over the decades. RA has been reported to the decreased risk of stroke[6,7] and myocardial infarction (MI).[8,9] RA is shown to provide better intraoperative and postoperative hemodynamic stability with less vasoactive utilization.[10–12] Other immediate postoperative benefits include decreased postoperative cognitive dysfunction and opioid use compared with GA.[13–15] Some studies have shown that RA reduces the rate of shunt placement,[11,16] operating time,[11,16] and hospital length of stay.[8] In 2007, a systematic review found statistically significant reductions in stroke, death, and MI. However, the investigators concluded that the number of patients included in the individual trial was too low to allow any conclusions on the differences in outcome between the anesthetic techniques.[17] In 2008, a large multicenter randomized controlled trial (general anesthesia vs local anesthesia [GALA]) was conducted to investigate the choice of anesthesia in CEA.[12] The results

Table 1
Regional anesthesia in the patient receiving antithrombotic or thrombolytic therapy

Anticoagulant		Discontinuation Before Puncture	Discontinuation Before Catheter Removal	Administration After Block/ Catheter Removal
Unfractionated heparin, intravenous		4–6 h and verify normal coagulation status		1 h
Unfractionated heparin, subcutaneous				
Thromboprophylaxis	Low dose: 5000 U BID or TID	4–6 h or assess coagulation status	4–6 h	Immediately
	Higher dose: 7500–10,000 U BID or daily dose of ≤ 20,000 U	12 h and assessment of coagulation status	Safety not established	
Therapeutic	individual dose > 10,000 U or >20,000 U total daily dose	24 h and assessment of coagulation status		
Low-molecular-weight heparin				
Prophylactic dose		12 h	12 h (single daily dosing only: indwelling catheters should be removed before twice-daily dosing regimen)	12 h/4 h
Therapeutic dose	Enoxaparin 1 mg/Kg BID, or 1.5 mg/Kg daily	24 h	Indwelling catheter not recommended	24 h/4 h
Anti-factor Xa agents (rivaroxaban, apixaban)		72 h	Indwelling catheter not recommended	6 h
Warfarin		6 d, and normalization of INR	In patients with low-dose warfarin and indwelling catheters, monitor INR daily. Remove catheter when INR<1.5	
Nonsteroidal anti-inflammatory drugs		No restrictions		

(continued on next page)

Table 1
(*continued*)

Anticoagulant	Discontinuation Before Puncture	Discontinuation Before Catheter Removal	Administration After Block/ Catheter Removal
Ticlopidine	10 d	Indwelling catheters may be maintained for 1–2 d if no loading dose	Immediately if no loading dose. 6 h if loading dose
Clopidogrel	5–7 d		
Prasugrel	7–10 d	Indwelling catheter not recommended	Immediately if no loading dose. 6 h if loading dose
Ticagrelor	5–7 d	Indwelling catheter not recommended	Immediately if no loading dose. 6 h if loading dose
GP IIb/IIIa inhibitors	Avoid neuraxial techniques until platelet function has recovered	Contraindicated within 4 wk of surgery	
Cilostazol	2 d	Remove catheter before reinstitution of cilostazol	6 h after catheter removal
Dipyridamole	24 h	Remove catheter before reinstitution of dipyridamole	6 h after catheter removal
Cangrelor	3 h	Remove catheter before reinstitution of cangrelor	8 h after catheter removal
Herbal medications	No restrictions		

showed no significant difference in the rates of stroke, MI, or mortality. A subgroup analysis from the GALA trial has since suggested that RA and local anesthesia (LA) are associated with better postoperative neurocognitive outcomes, supported by neurobiochemical assays.[18] Following that study, some publications with large sample sizes found significant differences in outcomes between GA and RA[19] prompting an updated systematic review and meta-analysis in 2020.[20] More recently, a 2021 Cochrane review found the incidence of stroke and death was lower with RA, but the investigators believed it was not convincingly different between the two groups because the evidence was low quality. They concluded that the current evidence supports the choice of either approach as high-quality evidence limited.[21]

Regional blockade for CEA was historically accomplished with deep cervical plexus block (CPB), with or without a superficial CPB. However, several randomized, controlled trials have shown that a superficial CPB alone is as effective as when it is combined with a deep CPB with respect to operative conditions and patient satisfaction.[22–25] A systematic review in 2007 showed that when a combined block is performed, the odds ratio of serious complications is 2 and of conversion to GA is 5 compared with superficial CPB alone.[26] These data provide a compelling argument for omitting the deep CPB.

Intermediate CPB[26–30] or ultrasound (US)-guided (USG) intermediate CPB combined with USG infiltration of local anesthetic to the perivascular area of the carotid artery[31–34] has been described to reduce the amount of intraoperative local anesthetic supplementation by surgeon. One study quantified noted with that this technique reduced the rate of surgical supplementation to less than 20%.[32]

RA can be accomplished with cervical epidural anesthesia; however, the risks outweigh the benefits. This technique is associated with increased incidence of hypotension, bradycardia, and bilateral phrenic nerve palsy, without improvement in analgesia or operating conditions.[35]

RA for CEA is a relatively straight forward technique that is highly successful as the sole anesthetic for CEA. Incomplete surgical block may be attributable to failure to provide anesthesia to the carotid sheath and pain near midline which is presumably mediated by contralateral fibers.[34,36–39] Some surgical supplementation of LA should be expected.

ANATOMY
Nerves

The cervical plexus is made up of spinal nerves from C1 to C4. There are two distinct portions of the plexus: deep and superficial. The deep plexus is contained within the deep prevertebral fascia or perivertebral fascia that envelopes the prevertebral muscles of the neck. The superficial plexus (sensory only) initially travels posterior and pierces the prevertebral fascia and travels in the space superficial to preverbal fascia and deep to the superficial fascia (the investing fascia of the sternocleidomastoid muscle [SCM]). The nerves pierce through the superficial fascia and terminate as the cutaneous branches: lesser occipital, great auricular, transverse cervical, and supraclavicular nerves (**Fig. 1**).[39–41]

The deep plexus nerves stay below the prevertebral fascia and travel anteromedially and form a loop (ansa cervicalis) which innervates various neck muscles within the prevertebral fascia. The anterior rami of C3 and C4 join C5 to give rise to the phrenic nerve. The deep cervical plexus nerves anastomose or travel with the spinal accessory nerve, hypoglossal nerve, facial nerve, vagus nerve, glossopharyngeal nerve, and sympathetic trunk.[39]

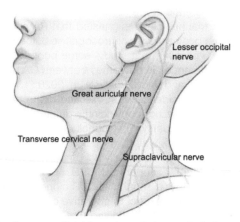

Fig. 1. Schematic of the four superficial branches of the cervical plexus as it emerges from the posterior boarder of the sternocleidomastoid muscle. (*Adapted from* Shane Tubbs R, Loukas M, Martinez-Pereira M, Cejas C, Bui CJ, Reina MA, et al. Surgical Anatomy of the Cervical Plexus and Its Branches. Elsevier Health Sciences; 2021.)

Cervical Fascia

The structural classification of cervical fasciae has been the subject of controversy despite more modern techniques for preserving and studying fascial.[38] The complexity and debate among the fascia layers in the neck are beyond the scope of this article. For simplicity, we will use the following nomenclature (**Fig. 2**).

Superficial fascia: The investing fascia of the SCM.

Deep fascia: The prevertebral fascia also known as perivertebral fascia because technically the term "prevertebral fascia" should be used for the anterior portion of the fascia. This fascia contains the deep muscles of the neck.

Carotid sheath: Fibrous sheath that contain the carotid artery, jugular vein, vagus nerve, sympathetic plexus, and lymph nodes.[34,42–45]

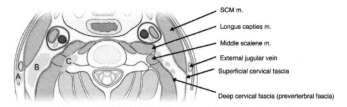

Fig. 2. Target sites for local anesthetic deposition of the CPB. (A) Superficial approach to the superficial CPB injection is at the posterior boarder of the SCM in the subcutaneous tissue. (B) Intermediate approach to the superficial CPB injection is deep to the superficial fascia of the SCM and superficial to the prevertebral fascia. (C) Deep CPB injection is deep to the prevertebral fascia and adjacent to the transverse process of the cervical vertebra. The superficial and deep cervical fascial layers are outlined in blue and green. Blue: deep layer of cervical fascia (prevertebral fascia); Green: superficial cervical fascia: investing layer of SCM fascia. (*Modified from* Shane Tubbs R, Loukas M, Martinez-Pereira M, Cejas C, Bui CJ, Reina MA, et al. Surgical Anatomy of the Cervical Plexus and Its Branches. Elsevier Health Sciences; 2021.)

Cervical plexus blockade
The superficial CPB is conventionally described as a subcutaneous injection technique performed at the midportion of the posterior border of the SCM muscle targeting superficial branches of the cervical plexus.[10,14] The same result also be accomplished by blocking the nerves deep to the SCM. The intermediate CPB targets the superficial cervical plexus nerves deep to the superficial fascia just below the SCM. The deep CPB is essentially a paravertebral block deep to the prevertebral fascia and adjacent to the cervical spinal nerve root. The paravertebral location of the deep block provides blockade of both the superficial and deep nerves together as they exit the transverse process.

Patient preparation and equipment. Sterile technique: Prepare the block site with a sterile prep solution like chlorhexidine/isopropyl alcohol or betadine solution.

Needle: Short bevel block needle (various gauges/lengths acceptable 50 to 100 mm ± echogenic block needle), for example, a 22-G 50-mm echogenic block needle.

Local anesthetics: Various concentrations and volumes have been described (bupivacaine, ropivacaine, lidocaine, mepivacaine), for example, 0.375% bupivacaine 5-15 mL.

US with a high-frequency linear probe, for example, set depth to 3 cm.

The patient is positioned in the supine or semirecumbent position, with the head turned away from the site of surgery.

Deep Cervical Plexus Block

Landmark technique
The block can be performed as a single injection at the level of C4 or as multiple injections at C2, C3, and C4.[21,26,44] Draw a line connecting the mastoid process to the transverse process of C6, the latter being the most prominent transverse cervical process palpated just inferior to the cricoid cartilage and posterior to the clavicular head of the SCM. Along this line, palpate or use ultrasonography to mark the transverse process of C2 located 1.5 to 2 cm caudad to the mastoid process, C3 located 3 to 4 cm, C4 located 4.5 to 6 cm. LA is injected superficially along the entire marked line as the skin wheal. For each level, insert the needle perpendicular to the skin, with slight caudad and posterior orientation. Advance the needle slowly until contact is made with the transverse process, approximately 1 to 3 cm deep. Withdraw the needle 1 to 2 mm and inject 4 to 5 mL of local anesthetic in fractionated aliquots, with intermittently aspirating for blood (vertebral artery typically is within 1 cm of the target). A single injection technique may alternatively be performed at the level of C4. A total of 15 mL of local anesthetic as a single injection or spread over three levels is typically used.

Ultrasound-guided technique
There have been multiple descriptions of the USG deep CPB. Either injecting LA into the space between the prevertebral fascia and the cervical transverse process under US guidance[46,47] or injected local anesthetics after the needle touched the target cervical transverse process under USG.[48,49]

Place the US in the transverse orientation at the midpoint of the posterior border of the SCM at approximately the level of the cricoid cartilage, visualizing the tapering edge of the SCM. Identify the relevant sonoanatomy (**Fig. 3**) and then move the probe medially to center the nerve roots on the screen. A slight cephalad or caudad tilt of the US probe may improve the visualization of the nerve roots. Trace the nerve roots distally by moving the probe caudal and then proximally by moving the probe cephalad. While scanning proximally, identify the nerve roots where they exit the

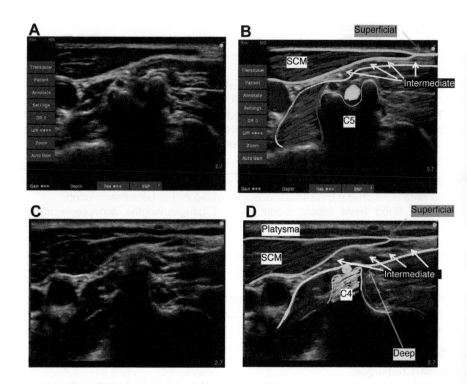

Fig. 3. Ultrasound image and corresponding highlighted at C5 and C4. (*A*) Ultrasound image at C5. (*B*) Ultrasound image at C5, green tracing representing prevertebral fascia; blue tracing representing superficial cervical fascia; and blue arrow injection point for superficial CPB. White arrows indicate location for injection of intermediate approach to the superficial CPB. Green arrow indicates injection point for deep cervical plexus block. (*C*) Ultrasound image at C4. (*D*) Ultrasound image at (*C*), green tracing representing prevertebral fascia and blue tracing representing superficial cervical fascia. Blue arrow indicates injection point for superficial CPB superficial to the superficial cervical fascia. White arrows indicate location for injection of the intermediate approach to the superficial CPB. Note that this injection is between the superficial and deep cervical fascia. Green arrow indicates injection point for deep cervical plexus block. Note that this injection is near the posterior tubercle of the C4 transverse process and deep to the prevertebral fascia.

transversus process of the cervical spine. There are unique characteristic C7, C6, and C5 anterior and posterior tubercles of the transverse process that help identify the correct cervical vertebra. Scanning cephalad and caudad identifies transverse processes and roots of C7–C4 to establish correct vertebral level (**Fig. 4**).

After sterile prep and skin wheal, a block needle is advanced in plane under US visualization until the needle tip is in close proximity to the lateral aspect of the transverse process and close to the nerve root. After negative aspiration inject local anesthetic and visualize the spread during injection. A 5 mL of local may be injected and repeated at C3 and C2 or a larger volume of local injected at this single level (~ 15 mL) in divided doses (see **Fig. 3**).

Superficial Cervical Plexus Block

The superficial CPB is performed superficial to the deep fascia. The block can be performed in the intermediate location sometimes called *intermediate cervical plexus*

Anterior   Posterior

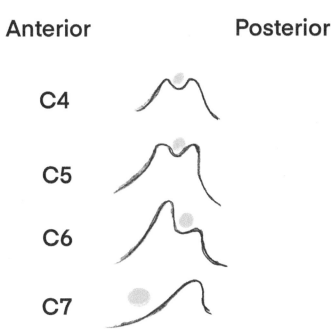

C4

C5

C6

C7

Fig. 4. Cervical vertebra C4–C7. Note the unique characteristics of the anterior (AT) and posterior tubercles (PT) of the cervical vertebrae's transverse processes (TP). C7 has a shallow AT. C6's TP has a prominent AT known as Chassaignac's tubercle. C5 and C4 have similar height AT and PT. This information can be helpful in orientation of which vertebra one is visualizing and helpful in counting up to C4.

block (between the deep and superficial fascia) or in the superficial location (superficial to the superficial fascia) in the subcutaneous tissue.

Landmark technique (superficial)
The superficial CPB is performed as a subcutaneous field block, with the needle inserted at the posterior boarder of the SCM.

After sterile prep and skin wheal, a block needle, the needle is inserted and guided just deep to the posterior border of the SCM (0.5 cm) and 5 mL of local anesthetic delivered. The needle is then redirected and local is injected in the subcutaneous tissue superiorly with an additional 5 mL of local injected. The needle is then redirected inferiorly, and an additional 5 mL of local anesthetic is delivered.[50,51]

Landmark technique (intermediate)
The intermediate cervical plexus is performed by injecting local anesthetic just deep to the superficial cervical fascia. In identical fashion to the superficial CPB, the needle is inserted posterior to the SCM and advanced until a loss of resistance or fascial click is felt, approximately 1 to 2 cm deep. A 15 to 25 mL of local anesthetic injected with intermittent aspiration in this space.[36]

Ultrasound guided (superficial)
Place the US in the transverse orientation at the midpoint of the posterior border of the SCM at approximately the level of the cricoid cartilage, visualizing the tapering edge of the SCM. The superficial cervical plexus may be visualized at this level.

Superficial cervical plexus block: After sterile prep and skin wheal, a block needle is advanced in plane under US visualization until the needle is at the posterior aspect of the lateral boarder of the SCM just deep to the skin and platysma muscle but not deep to the superficial investing fascia of the SCM. A 3 to 20 mL of local anesthetic is injected with intermittent aspiration (see **Fig. 3**).

Ultrasound guided (intermediate)

Intermediate cervical plexus block: Same US technique as the superficial CPB. If the plexus is not visible, target the intermuscular plane deep to the tapering edge of the SCM and superficial to the anterior and middle scalene muscles. Once the target is identified, clean the skin with antiseptic and create a skin wheal. Advance the block needle under US guidance with some LA hydrodissection to open the target space. A 10 to 15 mL of LA is injected in this location (see **Fig. 3**).

PERIVASCULAR INJECTION

Position the US probe transversely just above the clavicle to identify the common carotid artery in cross-section. Move the US probe cephalad and trace the carotid artery to the bifurcation. After sterile skin prep and skin wheal, advance the block needle in plane from the lateral border of the SCM until abutting the bifurcation point. After negative aspiration, LA is injected in this plane to achieve a half-moon shape spread.[31,33]

Postprocedure Care

The onset time of the described blocks is approximately 10 to 20 minutes, depending on type, concentration, and volume of local anesthetic used. To test for adequate anesthesia, assess for loss of sensation to pinprick in the C2, C3, and C4 dermatome. Monitor the patient for signs of intrathecal, epidural, or intravascular injection as well as symptomatic phrenic nerve blockade. A discussion should be had with the surgical team about the expectation of requiring local supplementation, particularly to the carotid sheath.

Avoiding Complications

The overall complication rate for all types of CPB is low. The composite of serious complications (including spinal anesthesia, respiratory distress, intravascular injection, and local anesthetic systemic toxicity) occurred in approximately 1% of patients receiving deep cervical blockade in a 2007 meta-analysis.[26] Virtually no serious block-related complications were reported in patients receiving a superficial CPB.

Complications specific to cervical plexus blockade are discussed below based on block site.

DEEP

Deep CPBs can produce major complications such as intravascular injection, epidural or subarachnoid injection, and phrenic nerve palsy due to its deep endpoint.[22,52] USG deep CPB technique is reported as a simple procedure that is relatively safe.[47,49] Opperer and colleagues[53] studied the characteristics and side effects of CPBs by depth of injection and found diaphragmatic dysfunction was most pronounced in patients receiving deep CPB. Data regarding cranial nerve block associated with single deep CPBs are rare.[25,54,55] It is possible that LA from deep CPBs can spread to the glossopharyngeal, vagus, hypoglossal, and accessory nerves, because extensive neural anastomoses exist between the lower cranial nerves and the upper cervical nerves.[42,55] In patients with preexisting contralateral vagus (or recurrent laryngeal) or hypoglossal nerve injury, it can lead to total airway obstruction unilateral deep CPB.[55,56]

Carotid sheath: Anesthesiologists have become proficient at blocking the incisional pain of the carotid sheath and carotid artery.[44,57] However, the direct infiltration of local anesthetic to the perivascular area of the carotid artery can produce some adverse effects due to cranial nerve palsy[31–35,56–59] in addition to the impairment of baroreceptor reflex.[34]

Overall surgical anesthesia is not compromised when the deep CPB is omitted. The superficial CBP technique minimizes the risk of the deep block with same clinical efficacy as the deep for CEA.

Arteriovenous Fistula

AVF is the method of vascular access of choice for hemodialysis due to its lower complication and mortality rates compared with arteriovenous grafts (AVGs) and central venous dialysis catheters.[60–63] AVFs are reported to have a high primary failure and low to moderate patency rates.[64] Several factors contribute to the successful creation and maturation of an AVF, including preoperative arterial and venous diameter and postoperative flow through the fistula.[65] Poor flow predisposes to thrombosis and fistula failure. RA has been shown to affect these factors, in addition to avoiding GA-associated complications in patients with chronic kidney disease, who often have associated co-morbidities.[66,67] Compared with GA, RA is associated with a shorter postoperative length of hospital stay and fewer admissions after this type of procedures.[68,69] The sympathectomy-like effect associated with RA reduces vasospasm and increases venous and arterial diameter as well as blood flow in the intraoperative and early postoperative periods. This effect may allow for AVF creation in patients originally planned for AVG placement.[70] Increased fistula blood flow may lead to faster fistula maturation and increased 3-month access utilization, while possibly reducing the need for temporary tunneled dialysis catheters for slower or non-maturing fistulas and their associated complications.[69] However, this conclusion has been challenged by a retrospective analysis associating GA with lower rates of early AVF failure.[71] Beyond this initial period, a retrospective review by Levin and colleagues[69] was unable to demonstrate differences in 1-year access occlusion or reintervention based on the anesthesia type. Conversely, a randomized control trial comparing AVF creation under RA or LA demonstrated higher primary patency as well as functional patency at 12 months in the RA group.[72] These findings are consistent with those of a recent meta-analysis.[73]

The surgical field for AVF creation may include a combination of the following nerve territories: musculocutaneous, medial antebrachial cutaneous, medial brachial cutaneous, radial, axillary, and intercostobrachial. A successful blockade of these areas may be accomplished through brachial plexus block at the supraclavicular, infraclavicular, or axillary levels, with exception of the intercostobrachial nerve, which requires a separate block. Multiple injection techniques may result in faster onset of adequate blockade and greater success.[74–76] However, these benefits have been challenged by previous studies.[77–79]

Nerve block equipment

- Sterile technique
- 5 or 10 cm 21G short bevel block needle
- 20 to 30 mL of local anesthetic
- US guidance with high-frequency linear probe

Supraclavicular Nerve Block

Patient preparation
The patient in supine or semi-recumbent position and the head turned to the contra-lateral side.

Technique
The US probe is placed in the supraclavicular fossa, providing a cross-sectional view of the subclavian artery and brachial plexus (**Fig. 5**). At this level, the brachial plexus is composed of trunks and their subsequent divisions, which appear as hypoechoic structures, located superior and lateral to the artery. The first rib appears as a hyper-echoic structure with its corresponding acoustic shadow inferior to the plexus and artery. After sterile preparation, the needle is advanced in a lateral-to-medial fashion into the corner pocket[80] between the subclavian artery and first rib, below the plexus, where the initial injection of local anesthetic is deposited. If adequate spread of local anesthetic is not visualized, the needle may be redirected to ensure the entire plexus is exposed to the local anesthetic solution. The needle can be repositioned with careful hydrodissection between the trunks of the plexus with local anesthetic.

Avoiding complications
The supraclavicular nerve block consistently results in varying degrees of transient phrenic palsy.[81] Although this is well tolerated in healthy patients, caution must be exercised when considering this block in patients with significant respiratory morbidity.

Infraclavicular Nerve Block

Patient preparation
Patient supine or semi-recumbent, head turned away, arm abducted 90°, and externally rotated to allow for cephalad displacement of clavicle.

Technique
The transducer is placed perpendicular to the clavicle in the deltopectoral groove, just medial to the coracoid process. At this level, the brachial plexus is composed of the medial, lateral, and posterior cords, named after their position relative to the axillary artery (**Fig. 6**). The axillary artery, vein, and the three cords are visualized in cross-section deep to the pectoralis minor muscle. The needle is introduced in a cephalad-to-caudad direction and advanced in plane to the point between the axillary artery and the posterior cord of the brachial plexus. Injection of local anesthetic at this point leads to a separation of the posterior cord from the axillary artery and spread of the solution toward the medial cord. If spread is considered to be suboptimal around all three cords, additional local anesthetic can be deposited around the lateral cord by

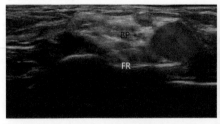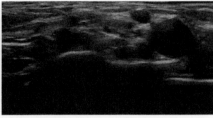

Fig. 5. Supraclavicular nerve block. The brachial plexus (BP) lies anterior and lateral to the subclavian artery (A), overlying the first rib (FR).

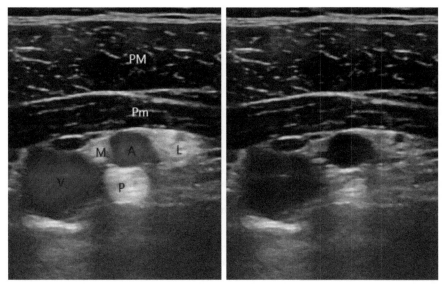

Fig. 6. Infraclavicular nerve block. The brachial plexus medial (M), lateral (L), and posterior (P) cords are located in the vicinity of the axillary artery (A) and axillary vein (V), beneath the pectoralis major (PM) and pectoralis minor (Pm) muscles. The exact position of the cords is highly variable between patients.

partially withdrawing the needle and around the medial cord by advancing the needle over the axillary artery.

Avoiding complications
Compared with supraclavicular nerve block, the risk of phrenic palsy is negligible.

Axillary Brachial Plexus Block

Patient preparation
Patient supine, head turned away, arm abducted 90°, and externally rotated.

Technique
The probe is placed at the axillary level perpendicular to the arm, and its position is adjusted to obtain a cross-sectional view of the axillary artery. The axilla is a highly vascularized space with several veins typically located in the vicinity of the artery. The radial, median, and ulnar nerves are visualized as hyperechoic structures around the artery (**Fig. 7**). Although there is significant individual variation in the position of the nerves, the radial nerve lies most often posterior to the artery. The musculocutaneous nerve is also visualized in the plane between the coracobrachialis and biceps muscles or within either one of them. The block needle is advanced in plane from the anterior aspect of the probe toward the area posterior to the axillary artery where local anesthetic is injected to surround the radial nerve. Subsequently, the needle is withdrawn and redirected toward the median and ulnar nerves, where additional injections are performed to surround the nerves with local anesthetic. Last, the needle is redirected toward the musculocutaneous nerve where the final injection is performed.

Avoiding complications
Frequent aspiration and slow injection are important measures to decrease the risk of intravascular injection. Lack of spread visualization when injecting local anesthetic

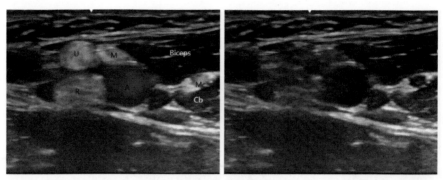

Fig. 7. Axillary brachial plexus nerve block. The radial (R), median (M), and ulnar (U) nerves are located around the axillary artery (A). The musculocutaneous nerve (Mc) appears in the plane between the biceps muscle and coracobrachialis muscle (Cb).

may signify an intravascular placement of the needle. In this situation, injection should be halted, and the needle position adjusted before resuming the injection. Owing to the superficial location and easy compressibility of the structures in the axillary neurovascular bundle, this approach is sometimes favored in patients with mild derangements in their coagulation profile.

Intercostobrachial Nerve Block

Patient preparation
Patient supine, head turned away, arm abducted 90°, and externally rotated.

Technique
This block can be performed as a subcutaneous field ring at the axillary level. The block needle is introduced at the proximal side of the axilla, advancing the needle toward the inferior axillary area while injecting local anesthetic to form a subcutaneous ring.

LOWER EXTREMITY VASCULAR SURGERY: ARTERIAL BYPASS AND AMPUTATION

GA, neuraxial anesthesia, and RA are the potential methods used during lower extremity bypass surgery.[82] RA has been an anesthetic method used as an adjunct as well as an alternative to GA for lower extremity vascular procedures.[83] The proposed benefits of regional anesthetic techniques are improved hemodynamic stability, reducing respiratory morbidity, decreased catecholamine surge, and sympathectomy: all resulting in improved lower extremity blood flow and excellent quality postoperative analgesia. However, RA may not be suitable as a primary anesthetic technique in patients unable to lie flat due to cardiac, respiratory, or musculoskeletal problems for prolonged procedures.[84] The type of anesthesia used is usually determined at the discretion of the anesthesiologist and surgeon.

In patients undergoing lower extremity surgical revascularization, RA offers an alternative or adjunct to GA. The type of anesthesia influences the hemodynamic changes and surgical stress responses during surgery. A combined femoral and sciatic nerve block is an option for lower extremity vascular surgical procedures.[85]

In patients undergoing lower extremity amputation, RA techniques offer a decrease in perioperative pain. An additional benefit of RA may be a decrease in phantom limb pain, phantom sensations, and stump pain in the perioperative period; however, it is unclear of how long these benefits may last. It is thought that RA techniques prevent the establishment of central sensitization which may play a role in reducing the incidence of chronic pain.[86]

The cutaneous innervation of the lower extremity is provided by the lumbar and lumbosacral plexi. The upper leg is primarily innervated by the lumbar plexus, and below the knee is primarily innervated by the lumbosacral plexus. The lumbar plexus includes primary contributions from the femoral nerve, the obturator nerve, and the lateral femoral cutaneous nerve. The femoral nerve provides sensory to the anteromedial thigh and medial aspect of the leg below the knee and foot. The femoral nerve provides motor fibers to the quadriceps muscles. The obturator nerve provides sensory to the medial thigh and knee joint. The obturator nerve also supplies motor branches to the adductor muscles of the hip. The lateral femoral cutaneous nerve provides sensory to the anterolateral thigh.[87] The sciatic nerve originates from the lumbosacral plexus. The sciatic nerve exits the pelvis through the greater sciatic foramen deep to the piriformis muscle and progresses down the posterior compartment of the thigh deep to the long head of the biceps femoris muscle. The sciatic nerve provides sensory distribution to the posterior thigh, posterior knee, and most of the lower leg, ankle, and foot. The sciatic nerve also supplies motor branches to the muscles of the posterior compartment of the thigh. The primary nerves of interest for lower extremity bypass surgery and above the knee and below the knee amputations are the femoral and sciatic nerves. USG approaches to the femoral and sciatic nerve blocks are described below.

Femoral Nerve Blockade

Equipment

- Sterile technique
- 100-mm short-bevel nerve block needle or Tuohy needle for catheter placement
- 20 mL of local anesthetic: Depends on surgical indication
- US guidance with a high-frequency linear probe

Patient preparation

The patient is positioned supine with legs extended. The US machine is positioned opposite the side to be blocked.

Technique

A femoral nerve block is performed under US guidance. The high-frequency linear US transducer is placed over the inguinal crease to identify the femoral artery and nerve. At the level of the femoral artery before splitting, identify the femoral nerve 1 to 2 cm lateral to the artery. The femoral nerve should be on top of the iliacus muscle and underneath fascia lata and fascia iliaca (**Fig. 8**). A block needle is inserted under the US transducer in a latera-to-medial direction. The needle tip passes through fascia lata and fascia iliaca until the tip of the needle is lateral to the femoral nerve. Administration of local anesthetic, 5 mL at a time, is performed after confirming negative aspiration. Local anesthetic should be surrounding the femoral nerve under fascia iliaca. A catheter can be threaded to provide continuous analgesia.[88,89]

Postprocedural care

A successful femoral nerve block will result in weakness of the quadriceps femoris muscle and a decrease in sensation over the anterior and medial thigh. There is a risk of falling secondary to quadriceps weakness, and patients should be monitored accordingly. Other potential complications with a femoral nerve block include nerve injury, local anesthetic toxicity, bleeding, and infection.

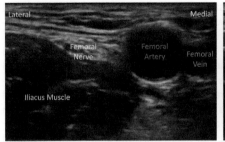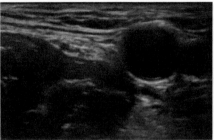

Fig. 8. Femoral nerve ultrasound. Femoral nerve is seen lateral to the femoral artery and femoral vein.

Sciatic nerve blockade. The sciatic nerve can be blocked at a variety of locations along the lower extremity. The anterior, transgluteal, and subgluteal approaches are described here.

Equipment
- Sterile technique
- 100-mm short-bevel block needle or Tuohy needle for catheter placement
- 20 mL of local anesthetic
- US guidance with a low-frequency curvilinear probe

Patient preparation The anterior approach to the sciatic nerve is performed at the bedside with the patient in the supine position, and the table flat with the patient's hip abducted to assist with transducer and needle placement. The US machine should be positioned on the opposite side of the bed facing the operator.

The transgluteal approach to the sciatic nerve is performed at the bedside with the patient in the lateral position with the hip and knee flexed and the table flat. The US machine should be positioned on the opposite side of the bed facing the operator.

The subgluteal approach to the sciatic nerve is performed at the bedside with the patient in the lateral decubitus position. The US machine should be positioned on the opposite side of the bed facing the operator.

Technique Anterior approach to the sciatic nerve: The curvilinear US transducer is placed over the inguinal crease to identify the femoral artery and the sciatic nerve (**Fig. 9**). The sciatic nerve is visualized between the adductor magnus and hamstring

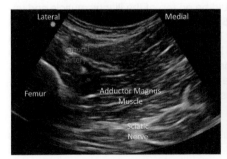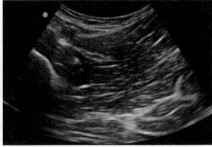

Fig. 9. Sciatic nerve (anterior approach) ultrasound. The femoral artery and nerve are imaged superficial to the sciatic nerve which is visualized between the adductor magnus and hamstring muscles.

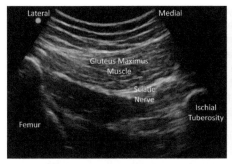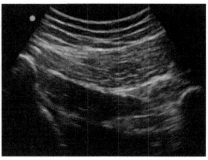

Fig. 10. Sciatic nerve (transgluteal approach) ultrasound. The sciatic nerve is a triangular shape deep to the gluteus maximus muscle between the femur and the ischial tuberosity.

muscles. A block needle is inserted under the US probe in-plane in a medial-to-lateral direction toward the sciatic nerve. If nerve stimulation is also being used, the contact of the needle tip with the sciatic nerve will trigger a motor response. Administration of 1 to 2 mL of local anesthetic is injected to confirm the adequate distribution. Administration of 10 to 15 mL of local anesthetic, 5 mL at a time, is performed after confirming negative aspiration.

Transgluteal approach to the sciatic nerve: The curvilinear US transducer is placed at the level of the ischial tuberosity and the greater trochanter of the femur (**Fig. 10**). The sciatic nerve is located deep to the gluteus maximus muscle. A block needle is inserted under the US probe in-plane in a lateral-to-medial direction toward the sciatic nerve. If nerve stimulation is also being used, the contact of the needle tip with the sciatic nerve will trigger a motor response. Administration of 1 to 2 mL of local anesthetic is injected to confirm the adequate distribution. Administration of 10 to 15 mL of local anesthetic, 5 mL at a time, is performed after confirming negative aspiration.

Subgluteal approach to the sciatic nerve: The curvilinear US transducer is placed transversely over the posterior thigh at the gluteal crease (**Fig. 11**). The femur is

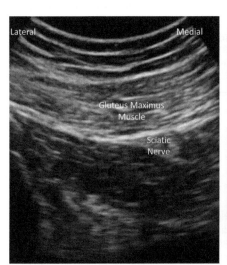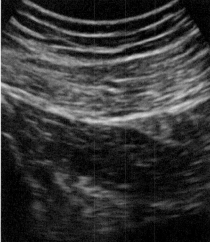

Fig. 11. Sciatic nerve (subgluteal approach) ultrasound. The sciatic nerve is positioned deep to the gluteus maximus muscle.

located, and the probe is slide proximally to the level of the greater trochanter. The probe is then slide medially from the greater trochanter to visualize the sciatic nerve deep to the gluteus maximus. A block needle is inserted under the US probe in-plane in a lateral-to-medial direction toward the sciatic nerve. If nerve stimulation is also being used, the contact of the needle tip with the sciatic nerve will trigger a motor response. Administration of 1 to 2 mL of local anesthetic is injected to confirm the adequate distribution. Administration of 10 to 15 mL of local anesthetic, 5 mL at a time, is performed after confirming negative aspiration.[9]

Postprocedural care A successful sciatic nerve block will result in weakness of the muscles in the posterior compartment of the thigh and decreased sensation of the posterior thigh, the posterior aspect of the knee, and most of the lower leg, ankle, and foot. Potential complications with a sciatic nerve block include nerve injury, local anesthetic toxicity, bleeding, and infection.

SUMMARY

RA is an acceptable option as the primary anesthetic for a variety of vascular surgery procedures. Regional techniques eliminate the risks associated with performing GA in a patient population that frequently suffers from significant comorbidities. Furthermore, RA confers the additional benefit of improved pain control perioperatively reducing the risk of adverse effects related to systemic analgesics and opioids in particular. Beyond these benefits, robust evidence of improved outcomes associated with RA is lacking, for which reason GA remains an acceptable choice for these procedures.

CLINICS CARE POINTS

- When performing a supraclavicular nerve block, we recommend following an intertruncal approach, where local anesthetic is used to hydrodissect the three trunks of the brachial plexus and deposited in the adipose tissue them. This approach facilitates adequate spread of local anesthetic around the plexus while reducing the risk of intraneural injection.

- Owing to high variability in the position of the brachial plexus cords around the axillary artery, we recommend performing dynamic scanning of the brachial plexus at this level (cords) before an infraclavicular nerve block. This practice facilitates adequate identification of the exact position of the cords, thereby increasing block success reducing the risk of nerve injury.

DISCLOSURE

The authors have nothing to disclose.

REFERENCES

1. Simons JP, Baril DT, Goodney PP, et al, Vascular Study Group of New England. The effect of postoperative myocardial ischemia on long-term survival after vascular surgery. J Vasc Surg 2013;58(6):1600–8.
2. Bode RH, Lewis KP, Zarich SW, et al. Cardiac outcome after peripheral vascular surgery. Comparison of general and regional anesthesia. Anesthesiology 1996; 84:3–13.

3. Horlocker TT, Vandermeulen E, Kopp SL, et al. Regional Anesthesia in the Patient Receiving Antithrombotic or Thrombolytic Therapy: American Society of Regional Anesthesia and Pain Medicine Evidence-Based Guidelines (Fourth Edition). Reg Anesth Pain Med 2018;43(3):263–309, published correction appears in Reg Anesth Pain Med. 2018 Jul;43(5):566. Vandermeuelen, Erik [corrected to Vandermeulen, Erik].

4. Shah DM, Darling RC 3rd, Chang BB, et al. Carotid endarterectomy in awake patients: its safety, acceptability, and outcome. J Vasc Surg 1994;19(6):1015–9 [discussion: 1020].

5. Spencer FC, Eiseman B. Technique of carotid endarterectomy. Surg Gynecol Obstet 1962;115:115–7.

6. Corson JD, Chang BB, Shah DM, et al. The influence of anesthetic choice on carotid endarterectomy outcome. Arch Surg 1987;122(7):807–12.

7. Lutz HJ, Michael R, Gahl B, et al. Local versus general anaesthesia for carotid endarterectomy–improving the gold standard? Eur J Vasc Endovasc Surg 2008;36:145–9.

8. Leichtle SW, Mouawad NJ, Welch K, et al. Outcomes of carotid endarterectomy under general and regional anesthesia from the American College of Surgeons' National Surgical Quality Improvement Program. J Vasc Surg 2012;56:81–8.

9. Becquemin JP, Paris E, Valverde A, et al. Carotid surgery. Is regional anesthesia always appropriate? J Cardiovasc Surg (Torino) 1991;32(5):592–8.

10. Sternbach Y, Illig KA, Zhang R, et al. Hemodynamic benefits of regional anesthesia for carotid endarterectomy. J Vasc Surg 2002;35:333–9.

11. Watts K, Lin PH, Bush RL. The impact of anesthetic modality on the outcome of carotid endarterectomy. Am J Surg 2004;188:741–7.

12. Lewis SC, Warlow CP, Bodenham AR, et al. General anaesthesia versus local anaesthesia for carotid surgery (GALA): a multicentre, randomised controlled trial. Lancet 2008;372:2132–42.

13. Mracek J, Holeckova I, Chytra I, et al. The impact of general versus local anesthesia on early subclinical cognitive function following carotid endarterectomy evaluated using P3 event-related potentials. Acta Neurochir 2012;154:433–8.

14. Messner M, Albrecht S, Lang W, et al. The superficial cervical plexus block for postoperative pain therapy in carotid artery surgery. A prospective randomised controlled trial. Eur J Vasc Endovasc Surg 2007;33:50–4.

15. Markovic D, Vlajkovic G, Sindjelic R, et al. Cervical plexus block versus general anesthesia in carotid surgery: single center experience. Arch Med Sci 2012;8(6):1035–40.

16. Dakour Aridi H, Paracha N, Nejim B, et al. Anesthetic type and hospital outcomes after carotid endarterectomy from the Vascular Quality Initiative database. J Vasc Surg 2018;67:1419–28.

17. Guay J. Regional or general anesthesia for carotid endarterectomy? Evidence from published prospective and retrospective studies. J Cardiothorac Vasc Anesth 2007;21(1):127–32.

18. Weber CF, Friedl H, Hueppe M, et al. Impact of general versus local anesthesia on early postoperative cognitive dysfunction following carotid endarterectomy: GALA Study Subgroup Analysis. World J Surg 2009;33(7):1526–32.

19. Liu J, Martinez-Wilson H, Neuman MD, et al. Outcome of carotid endarterectomy after regional anesthesia versus general anesthesia - a retrospective study using two independent databases. Transl Perioper Pain Med 2014;1:14–21.

20. Harky A, Chan JSK, Kot TKM, et al. General Anesthesia Versus Local Anesthesia in Carotid Endarterectomy: A Systematic Review and Meta-Analysis. J Cardiothorac Vasc Anesth 2020;34(1):219–34.

21. Rerkasem A, Orrapin S, Howard DP, et al. Local versus general anaesthesia for carotid endarterectomy. Cochrane Database Syst Rev 2021;10:CD000126.

22. Pandit JJ, Bree S, Dillon P, et al. A comparison of superficial versus combined (superficial and deep) cervical plexus block for carotid endarterectomy: a prospective, randomized study. Anesth Analg 2000;91:781–6.

23. Martusevicius R, Swiatek F, Joergensen LG, et al. Ultrasound-guided locoregional anaesthesia for carotid endarterectomy: a prospective observational study. Eur J Vasc Endovasc Surg 2012;44:27–30.

24. Stoneham MD, Doyle AR, Knighton JD, et al. Prospective, randomized comparison of deep or superficial cervical plexus block for carotid endarterectomy surgery. Anesthesiology 1998;89:907–12.

25. de Sousa AA, Filho MA, Faglione W, et al. Superficial vs combined cervical plexus block for carotid endarterectomy: a prospective, randomized study. Surg Neurol 2005;63:22–5.

26. Ivanec Z, Mazul-Sunkol B, Lovricevic I, et al. Superficial versus combined (deep and superficial) cervical plexus block for carotid endarterectomy. Acta Clin Croat 2008;47(2):81–6.

27. Pandit JJ, Satya-Krishna R, Gration P. Superficial or deep cervical plexus block for carotid endarterectomy: a systematic review of complications. Br J Anaesth 2007;99:159–69.

28. Koköfer A, Nawratil J, Felder TK, et al. Ropivacaine 0.375% vs. 0.75% with prilocaine for intermediate cervical plexus block for carotid endarterectomy: a randomised trial. Eur J Anaesthesiol 2015;32:781–9.

29. Calderon AL, Zetlaoui P, Benatir F, et al. Ultrasound-guided intermediate cervical plexus block for carotid endarterectomy using a new anterior approach: a two-centre prospective observational study. Anaesthesia 2015;70:445–51.

30. Leblanc I, Chterev V, Rekik M, et al. Safety and efficiency of ultrasound-guided intermediate cervical plexus block for carotid surgery. Anaesth Crit Care Pain Med 2016;35(2):109–14. https://doi.org/10.1016/j.accpm.2015.08.004.

31. Alilet A, Petit P, Devaux B, et al. Ultrasound-guided intermediate cervical block versus superficial cervical block for carotid artery endarterectomy: the randomized-controlled CERVECHO trial. Anaesth Crit Care Pain Med 2017; 36:91–5.

32. Mądro P, Dąbrowska A, Jarecki J, et al. Anaesthesia for carotid endarterectomy. Ultrasound-guided superficial/intermediate cervical plexus block combined with carotid sheath infiltration. Anaesthesiol Intensive Ther 2016;48:234–238.94.

33. Rössel T, Kersting S, Heller AR, et al. Combination of high-resolution ultrasound-guided perivascular regional anesthesia of the internal carotid artery and intermediate cervical plexus block for carotid surgery. Ultrasound Med Biol 2013; 39:981–6.

34. Seidel R, Zukowski K, Wree A, et al. Ultrasound-guided intermediate cervical plexus block and perivascular local anesthetic infiltration for carotid endarterectomy: a randomized controlled trial. Anaesthesist 2016;65:917–24.

35. Hakl M, Michalek P, Sevcik P, et al. Regional anaesthesia for carotid endarterectomy: an audit over 10 years. Br J Anaesth 2007;99(3):415–20.

36. Ramachandran SK, Picton P, Shanks A, et al. Comparison of intermediate vs subcutaneous cervical plexus block for carotid endarterectomy. Br J Anaesth 2011; 107:157–63.

37. Umbrain VJ, van Gorp VL, Schmedding E, et al. Ropivacaine 3.75 mg/ml, 5 mg/ml, or 7.5 mg/ml for cervical plexus block during carotid endarterectomy. Reg Anesth Pain Med 2004;29:312–6.
38. Capek S, Tubbs RS, Spinner RJ. Do cutaneous nerves cross the midline? Clin Anat 2015;28:96–100.
39. Kim J-S, Ko JS, Bang S, et al. Cervical plexus block. Korean J Anesthesiol 2018; 71(4):274–88.
40. Moore K, Dalley AF, Agur AM. Clinically oriented anatomy. 7th edition. Balimore: Lippincott Williams & Wilkins; 2014. p. 988.
41. Havet E, Duparc F, Tobenas-Dujardin AC, et al. Morphometric study of the shoulder and subclavicular innervation by the intermediate and lateral branches of supraclavicular nerves. Surg Radiol Anat 2007;29:605–10.
42. Guidera AK, Dawes PJ, Stringer MD. Cervical fascia: a terminological pain in the neck. ANZ J Surg 2012;82:786–91.
43. Shoja MM, Oyesiku NM, Shokouhi G, et al. Aomprehensive review with potential significance during skull base and neck operations, Part II: glossopharyngeal, vagus, accessory, and hypoglossal nerves and cervical spinal nerves 1-4. Clin Anat 2014;27:131–44.
44. Einav S, Landesberg G, Prus D, et al. A case of nerves. Reg Anesth 1996;21: 168–70.
45. Winnie AP, Ramamurthy S, Durrani Z, et al. Interscalene cervical plexus block: a single-injection technic. Anesth Analg 1975;54:370–5.
46. Perisanidis C, Saranteas T, Kostopanagiotou G. Ultrasound-guided combined intermediate and deep cervical plexus nerve block for regional anaesthesia in oral and maxillofacial surgery. Dentomaxillofac Radiol 2013;42:29945724.
47. Saranteas T, Kostopanagiotou GG, Anagnostopoulou S, et al. A simple method for blocking the deep cervical nerve plexus using an ultrasound-guided technique. Anaesth Intensive Care 2011;39:971–2.
48. Wan Q, Yang H, Li X, et al. Ultrasound-guided versus fluoroscopy-guided deep cervical plexus block for the treatment of cervicogenic headache. Biomed Res Int 2017;2017:4654803.
49. Sandeman DJ, Griffiths MJ, Lennox AF. Ultrasound guided deep cervical plexus block. Anaesth Intensive Care 2006;34:240–4.
50. Brown DL. Atlas of regional anesthesia. Philadelphia: Saunders; 2010.
51. Gray AT. Atlas of ultrasound-guided regional anesthesia. Philadelphia: Saunders; 2013.
52. Carling A, Simmonds M. Complications from regional anaesthesia for carotid endarterectomy. Br J Anaesth 2000;84:797–800.
53. Opperer M, Kaufmann R, Meissnitzer M, et al. Depth of cervical plexus block and phrenic nerve blockade: a randomized trial. Reg Anesth Pain Med 2022;47(4): 205–11. https://doi.org/10.1136/rapm-2021-102851.
54. Pintaric TS, Hocevar M, Jereb S, et al. A prospective, randomized comparison between combined (deep and superficial) and superficial cervical plexus block with levobupivacaine for minimally invasive parathyroidectomy. Anesth Analg 2007;105:1160–3.
55. Harris RJ, Benveniste G. Recurrent laryngeal nerve blockade in patients undergoing carotid endarterectomy under cervical plexus block. Anaesth Intensive Care 2000;28:431–3.
56. Weiss A, Isselhorst C, Gahlen J, et al. Acute respiratory failure after deep cervical plexus block for carotid endarterectomy as a result of bilateral recurrent laryngeal nerve paralysis. Acta Anaesthesiol Scand 2005;49:715–9.

57. Casutt M, Breitenmoser I, Werner L, et al. Ultrasound-guided carotid sheath block for carotid endarterectomy: a case series of the spread of injectate. Heart Lung Vessel 2015;7:168–76.

58. Masters RD, Castresana EJ, Castresana MR. Superficial and deep cervical plexus block: technical considerations. AANA J 1995;63:235–43.

59. Kwok AO, Silbert BS, Allen KJ, et al. Bilateral vocal cord palsy during carotid endarterectomy under cervical plexus block. Anesth Analg 2006;102:376–7.

60. Lok CE. Fistula first initiative: advantages and pitfalls. Clin J Am Soc Nephrol 2007;2(5):1043–53.

61. Ravani P, Gillespie BW, Quinn RR, et al. Temporal risk profile for infectious and noninfectious complications of hemodialysis access. J Am Soc Nephrol 2013; 24(10):1668–77.

62. Bray BD, Boyd J, Daly C, et al. Vascular access type and risk of mortality in a national prospective cohort of haemodialysis patients. QJM 2012;105(11): 1097–103.

63. Arhuidese IJ, Orandi BJ, Nejim B, et al. Utilization, patency, and complications associated with vascular access for hemodialysis in the United States. J Vasc Surg 2018;68(4):1166–74.

64. Al-Jaishi AA, Oliver MJ, Thomas SM, et al. Patency rates of the arteriovenous fistula for hemodialysis: a systematic review and meta-analysis. Am J Kidney Dis 2014;63(3):464–78.

65. Farber A, Imrey PB, Huber TS, et al. Multiple preoperative and intraoperative factors predict early fistula thrombosis in the Hemodialysis Fistula Maturation Study. J Vasc Surg 2016;63(1):163–70.e6.

66. Mathew A, Devereaux PJ, O'Hare A, et al. Chronic kidney disease and postoperative mortality: a systematic review and meta-analysis. Kidney Int 2008;73(9): 1069–81.

67. Howell SJ, Sear YM, Yeates D, et al. Risk factors for cardiovascular death after elective surgery under general anaesthesia. Br J Anaesth 1998;80(1):14–9.

68. Cole NM, Vlassakov K, Brovman EY, et al. Regional anesthesia for arteriovenous fistula surgery may reduce hospital length of stay and reoperation rates. Vasc Endovascular Surg 2018;52(6):418–26.

69. Levin SR, Farber A, Malas MB, et al. Association of anesthesia type with outcomes after outpatient brachiocephalic arteriovenous fistula creation. Ann Vasc Surg 2020;68:67–75.

70. Jorgensen MS, Farres H, James BLW, et al. The role of regional versus general anesthesia on arteriovenous fistula and graft outcomes: a single-institution experience and literature review. Ann Vasc Surg 2020;62:287–94.

71. Beaulieu RJ, Locham S, Nejim B, et al. General anesthesia is associated with reduced early failure among patients undergoing hemodialysis access. J Vasc Surg 2019;69(3):890–7.e5.

72. Aitken E, Kearns R, Gaianu L, et al. Long-term functional patency and cost-effectiveness of arteriovenous fistula creation under regional anesthesia: a randomized controlled trial. J Am Soc Nephrol 2020;31(8):1871–82.

73. Cerneviciute R, Sahebally SM, Ahmed K, et al. Regional versus local anaesthesia for haemodialysis arteriovenous fistula formation: a systematic review and meta-analysis. Eur J Vasc Endovasc Surg 2017;53(5):734–42.

74. Arab SA, Alharbi MK, Nada EM, et al. Ultrasound-guided supraclavicular brachial plexus block: single versus triple injection technique for upper limb arteriovenous access surgery. Anesth Analg 2014;118(5):1120–5.

75. Choi JJ, Kwak HJ, Jung WS, et al. Sonographic guidance for supraclavicular brachial plexus blocks: single vs. double injection cluster approach. Pain Physician 2017;20(6):529–35.

76. Choudhary N, Kumar A, Kohli A, et al. Single-point versus double-point injection technique of ultrasound-guided supraclavicular block: A randomized controlled study. J Anaesthesiol Clin Pharmacol 2019;35(3):373–8.

77. Roy M, Nadeau MJ, Côté D, et al. Comparison of a single- or double-injection technique for ultrasound-guided supraclavicular block: a prospective, randomized, blinded controlled study. Reg Anesth Pain Med 2012;37(1):55–9.

78. Tran DQ, Muñoz L, Zaouter C, et al. A prospective, randomized comparison between single- and double-injection, ultrasound-guided supraclavicular brachial plexus block. Reg Anesth Pain Med 2009;34(5):420–4.

79. Tran DQ, Bertini P, Zaouter C, et al. A prospective, randomized comparison between single- and double-injection ultrasound-guided infraclavicular brachial plexus block. Reg Anesth Pain Med 2010;35(1):16–21.

80. Soares LG, Brull R, Lai J, et al. Eight ball, corner pocket: the optimal needle position for ultrasound-guided supraclavicular block. Reg Anesth Pain Med 2007;32(1):94–5.

81. Tedore TR, Lin HX, Pryor KO, et al. Dose-response relationship between local anesthetic volume and hemidiaphragmatic paresis following ultrasound-guided supraclavicular brachial plexus blockade. Reg Anesth Pain Med 2020;45(12):979–84.

82. Singh N, Sidawy AN, Dezee K, et al. The effects of the type of anesthesia on outcomes of lower extremity infrainguinal bypass. J Vasc Surg 2006;44(5):964–70.

83. Sgroi MD, McFarland G, Mell MW. Utilization of regional versus general anesthesia and its impact on lower extremity bypass outcomes. J Vasc Surg 2019;69(6):1874–9.

84. Fraser K, Raju I. Anaesthesia for lower limb revascularization surgery. BJA Education 2015;15(5):225–30.

85. Yazigi A, Madi-Gebara S, Haddad F, et al. Intraoperative myocardial ischemia in peripheral vascular surgery: general anesthesia vs combined sciatic and femoral nerve blocks. J Clin Anesth 2005;17(7):499–503.

86. Sahin SH, Colak A, Arar C, et al. A retrospective trial comparing the effects of different anesthetic techniques on phantom pain after lower limb amputation. Curr Ther Res Clin Exp 2011;72(3):127–37.

87. Awad IT, Duggan EM. Posterior lumbar plexus block: anatomy, approaches, and techniques. Reg Anesth Pain Med 2005;30(2):143–9.

88. Hadzic A, editor. Hadzic's textbook of regional anesthesia and acute pain management. 2nd ed. New York, USA: McGraw-Hill Education; 2017.

89. Vloka JD, Hadzic A, Drobnik L, et al. Anatomical landmarks for femoral nerve block: a comparison of four needle insertion sites. Anesth Analgesia 1999;89(6):1467.

Critical Care of the Vascular Surgery Patient

Milad Sharifpour, MD, MS[a],*, Edward A. Bittner, MD, PhD, MSEd, FCCM[b]

KEYWORDS

- Critical care • Vascular surgery • Postoperative complications • Aortic surgery
- TEVAR

KEY POINTS

- Patients undergoing major vascular procedures often have multiple comorbidities and are at high risk for postoperative complications.
- Major postoperative complications after vascular surgery often affect multiple organ systems.
- Critical care of the vascular surgery patient reduces postoperative complications and improves the outcome.

INTRODUCTION

Patients that have undergone major vascular surgery require admission to the ICU for postoperative care and management of potential complications. The management of vascular disease is complex and includes both medical and surgical interventions. Diseases can be classified as nonocclusive, whereby there is restricted blood flow, or occlusive, whereby the vessels are completely obstructed. Aneurysmal disease occurs when vessel walls weaken. The surgical treatment of these lesions includes replacing the diseased segment with a vascular graft or excluding it with an endovascular stent. Occlusive vascular disease can occur because of atherosclerotic emboli or thrombosis and can be treated by embolectomy, bypass, or endovascular procedures. Recent advances in surgical technology have shifted treatment options from open surgical to endovascular approach. Despite advances in patient selection, surgical technique, and anesthetic management, patients who undergo major vascular surgery, whether open or endovascular, remain at increased risk for postoperative complications.[1] The high prevalence of systemic atherosclerosis and comorbidities (diabetes mellitus, COPD, coronary artery disease, obstructive sleep apnea (OSA),

[a] Department of Anesthesiology, Cedars Sinai Medical Center, 8700 Beverly Boulevard #8211, Los Angeles, CA 90048, USA; [b] Critical Care-Anesthesiology Fellowship, Department of Anesthesia, Critical Care and Pain Medicine, Harvard Medical School, Massachusetts General Hospital, Boston MA 02114, USA
* Corresponding author.
E-mail address: Milad.sharifpour@cshs.org

Anesthesiology Clin 40 (2022) 775–790
https://doi.org/10.1016/j.anclin.2022.08.017
1932-2275/22/© 2022 Elsevier Inc. All rights reserved.

chronic kidney disease, and so forth), prolonged surgery, large intraoperative blood loss and the associated hemodynamic shifts, systemic inflammatory response to surgery, and the ischemia-reperfusion associated with cross-clamping and unclamping the aorta leads to increased postoperative morbidity and mortality.[2] Patients who require emergency vascular surgery are at the highest risk for perioperative morbidity and mortality as they are often physiologically and hemodynamically not optimized.

Postoperative critical care for patients that have undergone major vascular surgery is focused on enhancing myocardial oxygen supply, optimizing circulatory volume status, early extubation and mobilization, achieving hemostasis, and pain control. Early identification and management of postoperative complications is the key to improving patient outcomes. These complications are summarized in **Table 1**.

Open Aortic Surgery

Cardiac Complications: Postoperative cardiac complications are common in patients who undergo major vascular surgery due to the high prevalence of atherosclerotic disease and include myocardial ischemia, congestive heart failure, and arrhythmias.[3] Postoperatively, myocardial function can change for many reasons (from systemic inflammatory response to new coronary ischemia). In clinical situations of low cardiac output, a transthoracic echocardiogram (TTE) can guide therapy. Acute management of low cardiac output involves treating the underlying cause (often ischemic), and support care (fluids, inotropes, mechanical circulatory support devices). Postoperative EKG monitoring with two precordial leads (V_3 and V_5) has greater than 95% sensitivity for detecting postoperative myocardial infarction (POMI).[4]

Myocardial Ischemia

Myocardial ischemia can manifest in several ways including acute hemodynamic instability (from decreased cardiac output), postoperative ECG changes, or an elevation in troponin. Ischemia can be the result of coronary thrombosis, or decreased flow across a stable fixed lesion. Troponin can also rise in response to significant myocardial strain, especially in the presence of renal impairment. Echocardiography is necessary for evaluating cardiac function and detecting new wall motion abnormalities. The presence of regional wall motion abnormalities should prompt input from a cardiologist regarding the need for coronary angiography and revascularization. Maintaining adequate organ perfusion using a combination of inotropes, vasopressors, and intravenous (IV) fluids when warranted reduces the risk of ischemic complications.

Perioperative myocardial infarction defined by elevated troponin levels, occurs in 3% to 12% of the patients who undergo major vascular surgery, and is associated with a three-fold increased risk of cardiac arrest and death.[5,6] The pathophysiology of POMI is complex and poorly understood. Tachycardia plays a role in the development of cardiac ischemia while flow-mediated hypoperfusion, exacerbated by hypotension and thrombosis, secondary to hypercoagulability and inflammation are also contributing factors. Reducing myocardial oxygen demand is key to reducing the incidence of postoperative myocardial complications. Optimization of hemodynamics, maintenance of normothermia and treatment of shivering, and adequate control of pain are crucial. Patients should be maintained on their usual cardiac medications perioperatively; withdrawal of ß-blockers in patients on long-term therapy is associated with increased mortality, while discontinuation of statins postoperatively is a predictor of adverse postoperative cardiac events.[7,8] Antiplatelet therapy requires individualized consideration, particularly in the presence of coronary artery stents.

Hypertension and tachycardia increase myocardial oxygen demand and the risk of myocardial ischemia and therefore should be treated with antihypertensive agents,

Table 1
Postoperative complications after open aortic surgery and strategies to prevent them

Complication	Management Strategy
Neurologic	
Spinal Cord Ischemia	Monitoring for early signs of SCI
Epidural Hematoma	Maintain appropriate CSF pressure
Stroke	Ensure adequate SCPP
Pain	Frequent neurologic checks to assess lower extremity strength, bowel/bladder continence
	Monitoring for early signs/symptoms of CVA
	Multimodal pain management strategy
Cardiovascular	
Postoperative MI	Monitoring for symptoms/signs of myocardial ischemia, myocardial biomarker checks
Arrythmias	
Heart failure/cardiogenic shock	Early resumption or initiation of aspirin, beta-blocker, and statins
Limb ischemia	
	Avoid hypertension/hypotension
	Careful management of intravascular volume
	Monitoring peripheral pulses hourly by palpation or Doppler signals
	Monitoring for compartment syndrome
	Daily inspection of surgical incisions
Pulmonary	
Atelectasis	Postextubation incentive spirometry and noninvasive positive pressure ventilation
Pleural effusions	
Pulmonary edema	Diuresis when appropriate
Pneumonia	Expedite ventilator weaning process
Respiratory failure	Early extubation when possible
ARDS	Ventilator-associated pneumonia prevention bundle
	Lung protective ventilation strategy
Renal	
AKI	Maintain euvolemia and adequate renal perfusion pressure
	Avoid nephrotoxins
Hematologic	
Hemorrhage	Monitor for bleeding complications and retroperitoneal hematoma
HIT	
	Conservative blood transfusion strategy unless evidence of organ ischemia or hypotension
	Thromboembolic prophylaxis
Gastrointestinal	
Ileus	Early resumption of oral feeding or early institution of enteral feeding
Mesenteric ischemia	
Stress ulceration	Monitoring for early signs of mesenteric ischemia
Abdominal compartment syndrome	Stress gastritis prophylaxis when indicated
	Early resumption of enteral feeding
	Monitoring for abdominal compartment syndrome

which commonly include short-acting calcium channel blocker (nicardipine, clevidipine) or ß-blocker (esmolol) infusions. Hypertension also exacerbates the risk of bleeding and should be treated promptly. A target systolic blood pressure within 20% of the patient's baseline value is often recommended.

Fluid management requires attention to detail both during the initial resuscitation and on the second and third postoperative days, when the mobilization of interstitial fluids (third space fluids) tends to occur. Patients commonly require additional fluid resuscitation in the immediate postoperative period to maintain adequate end-organ perfusion. However, by the second or third postoperative day, interstitial fluid shifts back into the intravascular space and leads to volume overload and necessitates diuresis. Hypervolemia should be treated with loop diuretics, or renal replacement therapy if indicated, as volume overload is associated with adverse cardiac (arrhythmias), respiratory (pulmonary edema), renal (AKI), and gastrointestinal (bowel edema, delayed bowel function) outcomes. Volume status can be assessed by close monitoring of clinical examination, urine output, laboratory values and noninvasive cardiac monitoring including transthoracic echocardiography.

Pulmonary complications: Postoperative pulmonary complications (PPC) are reported in up to 30% of the patients undergoing open thoracoabdominal aortic repair and are associated with increased ICU length of stay and mortality.[9,10] PPCs include atelectasis, pleural effusions, pulmonary edema, pneumonia, the need for supplemental oxygen, noninvasive positive pressure ventilation, reintubation, or failure to wean from mechanical ventilator and the need for tracheostomy, and ARDS.[11] Preoperative risk factors include tobacco use, COPD, and OSA. Intraoperative risk factors include surgical division of the diaphragm, phrenic nerve injury, prolonged one-lung ventilation, ischemia-reperfusion associated with aortic cross-clamping and unclamping, and the systemic release of inflammatory mediators, infusion of large volumes of IV fluids transfusion of blood products and the associated fluid shifts.

Many patients, who undergo vascular surgery, are extubated in the operating room. Those that remain intubated likely had complex operations with large volume fluid resuscitation or transfusion or may have had trouble with intraoperative ventilation requirements. Postoperatively, intubated patients should receive lung protective mechanical ventilation with tidal volumes of 6 to 8 mL/Kg of predicted body weight and moderate amounts of PEEP, which may attenuate the risk of PPCs.[12,13] Thoracic epidural analgesia for intra- and postoperative pain control reduces intraoperative opioid consumption, while providing superior postoperative pain control, and further reduces the risk of PPCs.[14] It is essential to achieve reversal of neuromuscular blockade before extubation. Head of the bed should be elevated to 30° to reduce airway edema and the risk of ventilator-associated pneumonia, and the patients should undergo diuresis, when ready, to minimize pulmonary and airway edema before extubation. Administration of dexamethasone, 8 to 10 mg every 8 hours for 24 hours, may be beneficial for reducing airway edema associated with fluid infusions and prolonged double-lumen tube use. Early extubation facilitates patient mobilization and reduces the risk of ventilator-associated pneumonia. Application of continuous positive airway pressure or use of high flow nasal cannula after extubation has been associated with fewer pulmonary complications. The benefit is believed to result from maintaining functional residual capacity, which prevents atelectasis formation, shunting, and hypoxemia, and improves the work of breathing.[15] For patients who require prolonged ventilator support, early tracheostomy can be beneficial for early mobilization and expedited transfer out of the ICU.

Neurologic Complications

Spinal cord ischemia: Spinal cord ischemia (SCI) resulting in paraparesis, or paraplegia is a devastating complication of surgery on the thoracoabdominal aorta. The reported incidence of SCI following open thoracoabdominal aortic surgery is 2% to 8%, compared with 4% to 7% after endovascular repair.[16–18] The extent (highest risk in patients with Crawford class II aneurysm) and location of the aneurysm, prior abdominal aortic surgery, hypotension, duration of aortic cross-clamp, and emergent surgery increase the risk of SCI.[18,19] SCI may be identified immediately after emerging from general anesthesia, or days to weeks later. It commonly presents as anterior spinal artery syndrome, with the loss of motor function, pain, and temperature sensation, while vibration and proprioception may remain intact.

Frequent neurologic examinations facilitate prompt diagnosis and treatment and reduce the risk of permanent deficit. Treatment includes increasing spinal cord perfusion pressure (SCPP) by raising mean arterial pressure (MAP) to 90 mm Hg, using phenylephrine or norepinephrine infusions, and cerebral spinal fluid (CSF) drainage with the use of a lumbar drain.[20] CSF drainage improves SCPP by decreasing CSF pressure. It has been shown to reduce the risk of SCI and can improve or reverse a postoperative neurologic deficit.[21-24] CSF pressure is maintained below 10 mm Hg to optimize spinal cord perfusion, as SCPP is determined by the difference between MAP and CSF pressure (or central venous pressure, whichever is higher).

SCPP = MAP – CSF Pressure (or CVP)

CSF drainage should not exceed 20 mL/h as excessive drainage may increase the risk of subdural hematoma and subarachnoid hemorrhage.[20,25] CSF drainage is typically started intraoperatively and is maintained for 72 hours.[2,20-22] While multiple therapeutic adjuncts including barbiturates, steroids, naloxone, or free radical scavengers have been proposed for the management of SCI after vascular surgery, strong data supporting their benefit is lacking.

Epidural hematoma: Placement of a lumbar drain using an 14G Touhy needle may result in bleeding and the formation of an epidural hematoma with resulting cord compression and paraplegia. The incidence of epidural hematoma is 2 to 20 cases per 100,000 lumbar drain insertions.[26-28] A high index of clinical suspicion, combined with diagnostic neurologic examination and a prompt MRI study are essential. It is important to note that many lumbar drains are MRI compatible, whereas spring-wound epidural catheters are not. Rapid surgical decompression (within 8 hours of the onset of symptoms) is key to achieving resolving neurologic deficits.

Stroke: Patients undergoing major vascular surgical procedures are at increased risk of stroke due to patient characteristics and conditions related to systemic atherosclerosis such as high blood pressure, coronary artery disease, diabetes, and procedural factors such as atherosclerotic plaque embolization or profound intraoperative hypotension. The incidence of stroke in patients undergoing noncarotid, major vascular surgery is 0.2% to 0.6%, compared with 3% in patients undergoing carotid endarterectomy.[29] Majority of perioperative strokes are ischemic and caused by embolic events and hypoperfusion.[30,31] Perioperative stroke is associated with increased length of ICU stay and mortality.[29] Diagnostic work up includes noncontrast head CT to rule out acute intracranial hemorrhage, followed by an MRI/MRA of head and neck to evaluate for arterial obstruction. Treatment is focused on endovascular embolectomy when indicated, antiplatelet and statin therapy, and preventing secondary injury by maintaining adequate CPP, and avoiding hyperglycemia and hyperthermia. A consultation with a neurocritical care specialist should be promptly obtained.

Pain: Inadequate treatment of pain related to surgery may be associated with increased complications and prolonged recovery time. Postoperative pain is recognized as one of the many factors contributing to the surgical stress response, and pain control is known to reduce myocardial oxygen demand. Modern pain management uses multimodal therapies; options available for postoperative analgesia depend on the type of surgery and the use of anticoagulants and antiplatelet agents that may preclude the use of regional techniques. Epidural analgesia provides superior analgesia when compared with the use of intravenous opiates, especially during movement, and may reduce the duration of mechanical ventilation, overall rates of myocardial infarction, acute respiratory failure, gastrointestinal and renal complications.[14]

Renal Complications: Acute kidney injury (AKI) is a common complication after vascular surgery and occurs in 20% to 49% of the patients undergoing aortic surgery, depending on the criteria used to define AKI, and is associated with worse outcomes.[1] Preoperative risk factors for postoperative AKI include the history of chronic kidney disease, anemia, and emergent surgery.[1] Intraoperative risk factors include hypotension, hypovolemia, embolic debris, juxta- or suprarenal aortic cross-clamping, and the duration of cross-clamping. Intraoperative partial left heart bypass and distal perfusion of renal arteries with cold crystalloid reduces renal ischemic time and attenuates the risk of postoperative AKI.

Maintenance of adequate intravascular volume and cardiac output in the postoperative period optimizes kidney perfusion. Nephrotoxins such as nonsteroidal anti-inflammatory medications, aminoglycoside antibiotics, and intravenous contrast dye should be avoided.[1] Of note, perioperative infusion of dopamine, furosemide, mannitol, and N-acetylcysteine have not been shown to reduce the risk of perioperative AKI. If AKI develops, meticulous management of fluids, electrolytes, and acid–base status is imperative. Renal replacement therapy should be instituted promptly when clinically indicated.

Gastrointestinal Complications

Mesenteric ischemia is a potentially fatal complication of aortic surgery.[32–34] It affects 2% of the patients undergoing elective aortic surgery, with mortality up to 65%.[33] Mesenteric hypoperfusion may be caused by embolic, thrombotic, or mechanical obstruction of arterial blood flow. The resulting bowel ischemia triggers a systemic inflammatory response leading to distant organ damage and often worsens any previously ongoing coagulopathy.[33] Delayed diagnosis is associated with transmural ischemia and increased mortality. Abdominal pain out of proportion to physical examination, persistent lactic acidosis, ongoing fluid requirement, and refractory shock are signs of mesenteric ischemia and require immediate surgical attention.[33] Workup includes serial abdominal examinations, gastric decompression, early surgical consultation, and an abdomen and pelvis CT angiogram. Diagnosis can be confirmed by flexible sigmoidoscopy or colonoscopy but should not delay surgical intervention. Patients with transmural bowel necrosis require exploratory laparotomy with the resection of the involved segment and diverting ostomy, whereas patients with reversible mucosal ischemia are treated with bowel rest and broad-spectrum antibiotics.

Ileus: Prolonged postoperative ileus occurs in 10% of the patients who have undergone open aortic surgery.[35] Mobilization of abdominal viscera, bowel edema from intraoperative fluid administration, and perioperative use of opioids are risk factors for ileus. Utilization of thoracic epidural analgesia may facilitate faster return of bowel function by reducing perioperative opioid use and unopposed parasympathetic innervation of the bowels.[36,37] Prokinetic agents can be beneficial in the absence of bowel obstruction.

Abdominal compartment syndrome (ACS): Patients who receive large volumes of intravenous fluids, blood, and blood products intraoperatively, and those with mesenteric ischemia, are at increased risk for developing abdominal compartment syndrome.[38] ACS is more common in patients who have undergone an emergency repair (due to a significant retroperitoneal hematoma and edema).[38] ACS can impair the function of nearly every organ system, resulting in impaired cardiac function, decreased venous return, impaired ventilation with hypoxemia and hypercarbia, renal impairment, diminished gut perfusion, and elevated intracranial pressure. Diagnosis of ACS includes an intra-abdominal pressure of more than 20 mm Hg associated with evidence of new organ failure. Management consists of supportive care such as using neuromuscular blockers and early surgical decompression.[39]

Pancreatitis: Acute pancreatitis after open abdominal aortic repair is a rare but serious complication that occurs in 1% to 2% of patients.[40] It can result from direct trauma and manipulation during surgical dissection or ischemia. Treatment is supportive.

Hematologic Complications

Postoperative Hemorrhage: Postoperative hemorrhage occurs in up to 5% of patients after aortic surgery and may require surgical reexploration, further increasing morbidity and mortality.[41]

Large intraoperative blood loss, extensive surgical dissection, systemic heparinization, mesenteric ischemia, and hypothermia all combine to increase the risk of postoperative hemorrhage.[42,43] The differential diagnosis for hemodynamic instability in the postoperative period should include hemorrhage until proven otherwise. Bleeding from aortotomy suture lines is a potentially devastating complication of aortic surgery. Fluid administration and blood transfusion should be provided in conjunction with vasopressor support as appropriate. Hypertension exacerbates the risk of bleeding and should be promptly treated. Hypothermia, acidosis, and hypocalcemia should also be aggressively treated, and coagulation abnormalities should be corrected promptly, guided by thromboelastography when available.[44] The attending surgeon should be notified immediately. If the patient is hemodynamically "stable," a CT angiogram to investigate the source of bleeding should be obtained.

In the absence of ongoing bleeding and hemodynamic instability (vasopressor requirement) and ischemic signs/symptoms or concerns for SCI, a hemoglobin transfusion threshold of 7 g/dL is reasonable.[45,46] Patients with hemodynamic instability, hypovolemia, or signs/symptoms of ischemia may benefit from a higher hemoglobin target. Thrombocytopenia is common in the early postoperative period secondary to platelet consumption in the setting of persistent bleeding or sequestration by aortic graft material. Less commonly, heparin-induced thrombocytopenia (HIT) may result in the development of heparin-dependent, platelet-activating antibodies. While rare, HIT should always be considered in thrombocytopenic patients with a history of heparin exposure.

Thromboembolism: Patients undergoing vascular surgery are at increased risk for lower extremity deep venous thrombosis (DVT) (up to 10%) and prophylactic measures should be instituted as soon as deemed safe.[47,48] Advanced age, morbid obesity, limb ischemia, venous injury, lengthy surgery, and prolonged immobilization are predisposing factors to DVT formation. Patients who have undergone vascular surgery are often hypercoagulable, increasing their risk of DVT or arterial graft occlusion, and should receive antithrombotic measures postoperatively. Early ambulation and perioperative use of thoracic epidural analgesia are associated with reduced incidence of perioperative lower extremity DVT.[14]

Lower extremity ischemia: Ischemia due to embolic or thrombotic complications can occur in 2% to 5% of the patients undergoing aortic surgery.[49] Frequent evaluation of lower extremity pulses or Doppler signals facilitates early detection and intervention.

Endocrinologic Complications: Postoperative hyperglycemia is common among patients undergoing vascular surgery and is associated with increased risk of wound infection, graft failure, increased length of ICU stay, and mortality.[50,51] Blood glucose should be maintained below 180 mg/dL and blood glucose > 180 mg/dL should be treated with intravenous insulin infusion.[52]

Infection

Infection of the graft, stent, or surgical site can result in major morbidity or mortality. For this reason, correct timing, and dosing of perioperative antibiotics are important. Postoperatively adherence to wound management, ICU "care bundles," hand hygiene, general aseptic technique, and glucose control are important for preventing infection.

Endovascular Aneurysm Repair and Hybrid Operations

EVAR has emerged as a less invasive and potentially safer alternative to open surgical repair. EVAR avoids thoracotomy or laparotomy, aortic cross-clamping, and is generally associated with reduced blood loss, less postoperative pain, and a shorter recovery. EVAR was initially limited to patients considered to be at high risk for conventional open surgical repair. However, increased clinical experience, together with improvements in endograft design and delivery techniques have expanded its application. Today, EVAR is used for elective and emergent repair of thoracic and abdominal aneurysms, pseudoaneurysms, aortic dissections, and traumatic aortic injuries if there are suitable "landing zones" for the stents that do not compromise other major vessels, and the size of the femoral and common iliac arteries needs to be assessed to ensure access. The procedure involves the delivery and deployment of one or more self-expanding aortic grafts within the aorta under fluoroscopic guidance, through percutaneous access via the femoral artery or, less frequently, the brachial artery. Fenestrated and branched stent grafts are used to maintain perfusion of the visceral arteries that originate from the covered aortic segment. Hybrid procedures, which combine open surgery and endovascular stenting, use the creation of an extra-anatomical bypass to the branch arteries of the aorta and expand the indications for endovascular stenting. For example, in patients undergoing thoracic endovascular aortic repair (TEVAR), an open left carotid-subclavian bypass is performed to prevent upper extremity ischemia in patients when the repair requires covering the ostium of the left subclavian artery.

Much of the postoperative critical care provided for an open aortic repair applies to an endovascular repair as well. Complications associated with EVAR are summarized in **Table 2** and include:

Vascular access injury: Frequent injuries include iliofemoral lacerations and rupture, pseudoaneurysm formation, and retroperitoneal hematoma. The sheath size can be large and, in some patients, can constitute a sizable part of the femoral artery, increasing the risk of injury. Consequently, large hematomas can develop, leading to anemia and hemodynamic instability. Occasionally these hematomas can be masking false aneurysms created by the puncture. Ultrasound and further vascular intervention may be required.

Device-related problems: Malposition, migration, or embolization of the graft can occur. Malposition is the most common of these problems and can result in organ ischemia (commonly renal). Device-related problems require urgent intervention in the interventional suite.

Hemorrhage: There can be unrecognized blood loss "under the drapes" from the femoral access site, resulting in hypovolemia. Endoleak, defined as persistent blood

Table 2
Postoperative complications after TEVAR/EVAR and mitigation strategies

Early Complications	
Vascular access site injury	Assessment of thigh hematoma formation,
Stroke	assessment of distal pulses
SCI	Frequent neurologic checks for S/Sx of stroke
AKI	Maintaining MAP > 80 mm Hg and adequate CPP.
Post implantation syndrome	CSF drainage as indicated
	Maintaining euvolemia and avoiding nephrotoxins
	Supportive care

Late Complications
Device-related problems: malposition, migration
Endoleak
Stent graft infection
Aorto-esophageal fistula

flow outside the lumen of the endoprosthesis and within the aneurysm sac following endovascular graft stenting, can occur in up to 30% of cases and result in drops in hemoglobin (or if serious may result in sudden hemodynamic instability). Hypothermia resulting from the patient spending prolonged time in a cold interventional suite may worsen coagulopathy and hemorrhage.

Acute kidney injury: The incidence of AKI after elective EVAR is 0.7% to 2.0%.[53,54] This can result from hypovolemia, bleeding, contrast-induced nephropathy, or malposition of a stent occluding renal artery. Hydration during and after the procedure may help reduce the risk.

Spinal cord ischemia: Placement of thoracic aortic stents can be associated with SCI. The longer the length of the segment of aorta stented, the greater the risk of cord ischemia.

Infection: The endovascular graft is foreign material and can become infected following an episode of bacteremia. The groin puncture site (or any hybrid operation wounds around this area) can also become infected. Infected pseudoaneurysms can be particularly difficult to manage, involving surgery and continued antibiotics.

Postimplantation syndrome: A clinical syndrome that is thought to result from endothelial activation by the endograft. It manifests as a mild leukocytosis, fever, and elevation of C-reactive protein. Postimplantation syndrome is commonly associated with large segment coverage and the use of multiple stent devices. Post implantation syndrome is associated with prolonged length of stay.[55]

Carotid Endarterectomy

Most patients do not require admission to ICU after undergoing carotid endarterectomy. However, patients undergoing CEA suffer from widespread atherosclerosis and are at increased risk for neurologic and cardiac complications. Potential postoperative complications after CEA include hypo- or hypertension, myocardial infarction, stroke, postoperative bleeding, cervical hematoma, and nerve injury and are summarized in **Table 3**.

Hypotension: Removal of the carotid plaque, and the associated stenosis, during surgery results in transmission of increased arterial pulsation to the carotid baroceptor, which can result in reflex bradycardia and hypotension. Postoperative vasopressor support may be necessary. If such support is required, it typically lasts no

Table 3
Postoperative complications after carotid endarterectomy and strategies to prevent them

Complication	Management Strategy
Neurologic	
Stroke	Monitoring for early signs of CVA
Cerebral Hyperperfusion syndrome	Maintain appropriate cerebral perfusion pressure
Cranial nerve injury	Frequent neurologic examinations
Cardiovascular	
Postoperative MI	Monitoring for symptoms/signs of myocardial
Arrythmias	ischemia, check myocardial biomarkers
Heart failure	Early resumption or initiation of aspirin, beta-
Postoperative hypotension	blocker, and statins
Postoperative hypertension	Avoid hypertension/hypotension
	Early resumption of beta-blockers
	Judicious fluid management
	Vasopressor infusions
	Early resumption of home antihypertensive agents
Pulmonary	
Airway compromise (neck hematoma)	Correction of coagulopathies, early surgical
Vocal cord dysfunction/aspiration	decompression
	Monitoring for hoarseness and signs/symptoms of
	aspiration

longer than 6 to 24 hours. It is important to remember that CEA is typically performed with little blood loss and does not result in significant fluid shifts. Therefore, treating postoperative hypotension with fluids is often inappropriate and can result in congestive heart failure. Persistent hypotension should prompt further diagnostic workup, including invasive hemodynamic monitoring and echocardiography to assess cardiac function.

Hypertension: Carotid sinus damage during surgical dissection or its infiltration by local anesthetics can impair the normal baroreceptor sensitivity of the carotid sinus, resulting in postoperative hypertension. Patients with poorly controlled preoperative hypertension are at increased risk for postoperative hypertension. Severe hypertension increases the risk of bleeding, wound hematoma, and cardiac and neurologic complications, such as cerebral hyperperfusion syndrome. Perioperative hypertension should be promptly treated with infusion of short-acting antihypertensive agents (eg, nicardipine, clevidipine) until baroreceptor function is restored.

Cervical hematoma: Postoperative neck hematoma occurs in 3.4% of the patients undergoing CEA and may lead to airway compromise.[56] Immediate intubation and decompression of the neck in the operating room or postanesthesia care unit may be necessary to prevent airway compromise. Intubation will often be more difficult than the previous intubation in the OR due to the distortion of the airway anatomy and edema. Coagulopathy and uncontrolled hypertension increase the risk of hematoma formation and should be corrected immediately. A large cervical hematoma may also compress the internal carotid artery and adjacent cranial nerves.

Myocardial Infarction: Postoperative MI occurs in up to 2% of the patients undergoing CEA and is associated with increased short- and long-term mortality.[57–59] Management is focused on optimizing myocardial oxygen supply and demand, antiplatelet and statin therapy, and percutaneous coronary intervention to restore blood flow if indicated.

Stroke: Postoperative stroke occurs in 3% to 5% of the patients undergoing carotid endarterectomy and is the second most common cause of death after CEA.[60–62] Majority of strokes are ischemic in nature and are due to embolic or thrombotic events. Postoperative stroke can also be secondary to global hypoperfusion or hemorrhage. Strict blood pressure control is of utmost importance as hypotension may lead to global hypoperfusion and ischemia, and uncontrolled hypertension increases the risk of hemorrhage and cerebral hyperperfusion syndrome (CHS). Hypotension should primarily be treated with vasopressor infusions (phenylephrine, norepinephrine, vasopressin), and fluids only when warranted, and hypertension should be treated with infusions of short-acting calcium channel blockers (nicardipine, clevidipine). Any changes in the neurologic examination should be immediately investigated by CT/CT angiography of the brain or MRI/MRA of the brain. A neurology or neurocritical care consultation should be obtained to further direct patient care (thrombectomy or intra-arterial thrombolytic therapy). Patients should receive antiplatelet and statin therapy.

Cerebral hyperperfusion syndrome: CHS occurs in 0% to 3% of the patients after CEA. It is characterized by ipsilateral headache, hypertension, seizure, and altered mental status.[63,64] CHS is caused by impaired cerebral autoregulation of the surgically reperfused cerebral hemisphere, which is exposed postoperatively to higher cerebral perfusion resulting from improved arterial inflow. High-grade carotid stenosis, severe bilateral carotid disease, and postoperative hypertension are major risk factors for the development of cerebral hyperperfusion. If not treated promptly, it progresses to intracerebral hemorrhage, cerebral edema, and death.[65] Postoperative hypertension increases the risk of CHS, and strict blood pressure control is of utmost importance. A noncontrast head CT should be obtained to rule out hemorrhage and evaluate for cerebral edema. Critical care treatment is focused on the control of blood pressure. Antihypertensives that do not cause vasodilation (labetalol, clonidine) are favored.

Cranial nerve injury: Cranial nerve injury is common after CEA, occurring in up to 39% of the patients, with only a small proportion being permanent. Most cranial nerve injuries are secondary to retraction trauma; less frequently, they are the result of nerve transection.[66,67] The recurrent laryngeal nerve, hypoglossal nerve, and marginal mandibular nerve are most affected. Injury to vagus nerve and branches (recurrent and superior laryngeal nerves) can result in paralysis of the ipsilateral vocal cord, resulting in hoarseness and the loss of effective cough. Fortunately, the injury is temporary in most cases. If a nerve injury is clinically suspected, phonation and swallowing should be evaluated before the institution of oral intake to prevent aspiration. When vocal cord dysfunction is suspected, fiberoptic examination by an otolaryngologist should be completed to assess the need for further treatment.

Lower Limb Revascularization Procedures

Lower extremity ischemia is a common result of generalized atherosclerosis and is characterized by claudication, a lower extremity muscular pain that is induced by increased physical exertion and is relieved by rest. Critical limb ischemia, which results from the progression of chronic atherosclerotic disease, presents with pain at rest and may present with nonhealing ulceration or gangrene of the lower extremity. A sudden decrease in limb perfusion from embolism or plaque rupture with thrombosis presents more acutely, with severe pain and a pale extremity with absent pulses. Surgical bypasses (aortofemoral, femoropopliteal, and femorodistal bypass grafting) and endovascular procedures are performed to reestablish blood flow. The optimal bypass grafting technique is based on the location and the morphology of the obstructive lesions. However, there is an increasing tendency toward endovascular procedures. Patients who undergo lower extremity bypass are managed in a monitored setting for 24 to 48 hours. Complications associated with lower extremity revascularization procedures are similar to those associated with other major vascular procedures. Mortality after peripheral bypass surgery ranges between 2% and 8% and is primarily related to myocardial ischemia.[68]

Graft failure: Graft patency is monitored by routine evaluation of distal pulses and perfusion every hour for six to 8 hours, then every four to 6 hours. Loss of a palpable pulse or a Doppler signal, a cool pale extremity, or severe pain are signs of graft failure and warrant immediate attention. Graft failure can occur due to technical complications, or because of hypoperfusion from hypotension, due to an adverse cardiac event, bleeding, or sepsis, or from a hypercoagulable state. In case of suspected graft failure, imaging should be performed emergently, and reintervention should be considered.

Compartment syndrome: Reperfusion of an ischemic extremity after revascularization can result in compartment syndrome. Frequent monitoring of the reperfused extremity is essential for the early detection of compartment syndrome. Affected limb should be treated with fasciotomy. Creatine phosphokinase (CPK) levels should be followed for evidence of rhabdomyolysis, and patients should be kept euvolemic to minimize the risk of postoperative renal failure.

Bleeding: Both elective and emergency procedures need monitoring for potential bleeding, hematoma, or pseudoaneurysm development.

SUMMARY

Postoperative management of the patient undergoing major vascular surgery presents unique and complex challenges for the critical care provider. Patients undergoing vascular surgery commonly have multiple comorbidities and the surgical procedure impacts every major organ system. Postoperative complications after major vascular surgery are common and associated with increased morbidity and mortality. The spectrum of complications depends on the disease itself, its urgency, and the surgical procedure. Critical care management of these patients requires an understanding of the underlying disease process, surgical procedure, and a high index of suspicion for procedure-specific complications. A multidisciplinary approach is most likely to optimize the quality of postoperative care which is essential for successful recovery.

CLINICS CARE POINTS

- Persistent lactic acidosis, hypotension, and fluid requirement in patients who have undergone open thoracoabdominal aortic repair should prompt an evaluation for bowel ischemia. Surgical consultation and a CT scan maybe required for further evaluation.

- Changes in lower extremity motor strength (weakness, paraplegia), pain, or temperature sensation in patients who have undergone open or endovascular repair of thoracoabdominal aorta indicates spinal cord ischemia. MAP should be raised to 90 mm Hg and CSF drainage should be instituted immediately.

- Many patients who have undergone noncarotid major vascular surgery may require volume resuscitation in the immediate postoperative period. Volume resuscitation should be guided by clinical signs/symptoms (mentation, urine output, skin temperature), vital signs (normotension), and laboratory values such as lactic acid or based deficit. Transthoracic echocardiography, when available, should be utilized to guide fluid resuscitation.

DISCLOSURE

The authors have nothing to disclose.

REFERENCES

1. Hobson C, Lysak N, Huber M, et al. Epidemiology, outcomes, and management of acute kidney injury in the vascular surgery patient. J Vasc Surg 2018;68(3): 916–28.
2. Crimi E, Hill CC. Postoperative ICU management of vascular surgery patients. Anesthesiol Clin 2014;32(3):735–57.
3. Kertai MD, Klein J, van Urk H, et al. Cardiac complications after elective major vascular surgery. Acta Anaesthesiol Scand 2003;47(6):643–54.
4. Landesberg G, Mosseri M, Wolf Y, et al. Perioperative myocardial ischemia and infarction: identification by continuous 12-lead electrocardiogram with online ST-segment monitoring. Anesthesiology 2002;96(2):264–70.
5. Juo YY, Mantha A, Ebrahimi R, et al. Incidence of myocardial infarction after high-risk vascular operations in adults. JAMA Surg 2017;152(11):e173360.
6. McFalls EO, Ward HB, Moritz TE, et al. Coronary-artery revascularization before elective major vascular surgery. N Engl J Med 2004;351(27):2795–804.
7. Task Force for Preoperative Cardiac Risk Assessment and Perioperative Cardiac Management in Non-cardiac Surgery, European Society of Cardiology (ESC), Poldermans D, et al. Guidelines for pre-operative cardiac risk assessment and perioperative cardiac management in non-cardiac surgery. Eur Heart J 2009; 30(22):2769–812.
8. Kertai MD, Boersma E, Westerhout CM, et al. A combination of statins and beta-blockers is independently associated with a reduction in the incidence of periop-erative mortality and nonfatal myocardial infarction in patients undergoing abdominal aortic aneurysm surgery. Eur J Vasc Endovasc Surg 2004;28(4): 343–52.
9. Etz CD, Di Luozzo G, Bello R, et al. Pulmonary complications after descending thoracic and thoracoabdominal aortic aneurysm repair: predictors, prevention, and treatment. Ann Thorac Surg 2007;83(2):S870–92.
10. Svensson LG, Hess KR, Coselli JS, et al. A prospective study of respiratory failure after high-risk surgery on the thoracoabdominal aorta. J Vasc Surg 1991;14(3): 271–82.
11. Miskovic A, Lumb AB. Postoperative pulmonary complications. Br J Anaesth 2017;118(3):317–34.
12. Serpa Neto A, Cardoso SO, Manetta JA, et al. Association between use of lung-protective ventilation with lower tidal volumes and clinical outcomes among pa-tients without acute respiratory distress syndrome: a meta-analysis. JAMA 2012;308(16):1651–9.
13. Acute Respiratory Distress Syndrome Network, Brower RG, Matthay MA, et al. Ventilation with lower tidal volumes as compared with traditional tidal volumes for acute lung injury and the acute respiratory distress syndrome. N Engl J Med 2000;342(18):1301–8.
14. Freise H, Van Aken HK. Risks and benefits of thoracic epidural anaesthesia. Br J Anaesth 2011;107(6):859–68.
15. Kindgen-Milles D, Müller E, Buhl R, et al. Nasal-continuous positive airway pres-sure reduces pulmonary morbidity and length of hospital stay following thora-coabdominal aortic surgery. Chest 2005;128(2):821–8.

16. Coselli JS, Bozinovski J, LeMaire SA. Open surgical repair of 2286 thoracoabdominal aortic aneurysms. Ann Thorac Surg 2007;83(2):S862–92.
17. Estrera AL, Miller CC 3rd, Chen EP, et al. Descending thoracic aortic aneurysm repair: 12-year experience using distal aortic perfusion and cerebrospinal fluid drainage. Ann Thorac Surg 2005;80(4):1290–6.
18. Svensson LG, Crawford ES, Hess KR, et al. Experience with 1509 patients undergoing thoracoabdominal aortic operations. J Vasc Surg 1993;17(2):357–70.
19. Cambria RP, Clouse WD, Davison JK, et al. Thoracoabdominal aneurysm repair: results with 337 operations performed over a 15-year interval. Ann Surg 2002; 236(4):471–9.
20. Chatterjee S, Preventza O, Orozco-Sevilla V, et al. Critical care management after open thoracoabdominal aortic aneurysm repair. J Cardiovasc Surg (Torino) 2021; 62(3):220–9.
21. Cinà CS, Abouzahr L, Arena GO, et al. Cerebrospinal fluid drainage to prevent paraplegia during thoracic and thoracoabdominal aortic aneurysm surgery: a systematic review and meta-analysis. J Vasc Surg 2004;40(1):36–44.
22. Coselli JS, LeMaire SA, Köksoy C, et al. Cerebrospinal fluid drainage reduces paraplegia after thoracoabdominal aortic aneurysm repair: results of a randomized clinical trial. J Vasc Surg 2002;35(4):631–9.
23. Hill AB, Kalman PG, Johnston KW, et al. Reversal of delayed-onset paraplegia after thoracic aortic surgery with cerebrospinal fluid drainage. J Vasc Surg 1994; 20(2):315–7.
24. Tsusaki B, Grigore A, Cooley DA, et al. Reversal of delayed paraplegia with cerebrospinal fluid drainage after thoracoabdominal aneurysm repair. Anesth Analg 2002;94(6):1674.
25. Wynn MM, Mell MW, Tefera G, et al. Complications of spinal fluid drainage in thoracoabdominal aortic aneurysm repair: a report of 486 patients treated from 1987 to 2008. J Vasc Surg 2009;49(1):29–35.
26. Rosero EB, Joshi GP. Nationwide incidence of serious complications of epidural analgesia in the United States. Acta Anaesthesiol Scand 2016;60(6):810–20.
27. Li SL, Wang DX, Ma D. Epidural hematoma after neuraxial blockade: a retrospective report from China. Anesth Analg 2010;111(5):1322–4.
28. Moen V, Dahlgren N, Irestedt L. Severe neurological complications after central neuraxial blockades in Sweden 1990-1999. Anesthesiology 2004;101(4):950–9.
29. Sharifpour M, Moore LE, Shanks AM, et al. Incidence, predictors, and outcomes of perioperative stroke in noncarotid major vascular surgery. Anesth Analg 2013; 116(2):424–34.
30. Harris EJ Jr, Moneta GL, Yeager RA, et al. Neurologic deficits following noncarotid vascular surgery. Am J Surg 1992;163(5):537–40.
31. Axelrod DA, Stanley JC, Upchurch GR Jr, et al. Risk for stroke after elective noncarotid vascular surgery. J Vasc Surg 2004;39(1):67–72.
32. Steele SR. Ischemic colitis complicating major vascular surgery. Surg Clin North Am 2007;87(5):1099–ix.
33. Achouh PE, Madsen K, Miller CC 3rd, et al. Gastrointestinal complications after descending thoracic and thoracoabdominal aortic repairs: a 14-year experience. J Vasc Surg 2006;44(3):442–6.
34. Williamson JS, Ambler GK, Twine CP, et al. Elective repair of abdominal aortic aneurysm and the risk of colonic ischaemia: systematic review and meta-analysis. Eur J Vasc Endovasc Surg 2018;56(1):31–9.
35. Valentine RJ, Hagino RT, Jackson MR, et al. Gastrointestinal complications after aortic surgery. J Vasc Surg 1998;28(3):404–12.

36. Jørgensen H, Wetterslev J, Møiniche S, et al. Epidural local anaesthetics versus opioid-based analgesic regimens on postoperative gastrointestinal paralysis, PONV and pain after abdominal surgery. Cochrane Database Syst Rev 2000;4: CD001893.

37. de Leon-Casasola OA, Karabella D, Lema MJ. Bowel function recovery after radical hysterectomies: thoracic epidural bupivacaine-morphine versus intravenous patient-controlled analgesia with morphine: a pilot study. J Clin Anesth 1996;8(2):87–92.

38. Malbrain ML, Cheatham ML, Kirkpatrick A, et al. Results from the international conference of experts on intra-abdominal hypertension and abdominal compartment syndrome. i. definitions. Intensive Care Med 2006;32(11):1722–32.

39. Cheatham ML, Malbrain ML, Kirkpatrick A, et al. Results from the international conference of experts on intra-abdominal hypertension and abdominal compartment syndrome. II. recommendations. Intensive Care Med 2007;33(6):951–62.

40. Hashimoto L, Walsh RM. Acute pancreatitis after aortic surgery. Am Surg 1999; 65(5):423–6.

41. Cinà CS, Clase CM. Coagulation disorders and blood product use in patients undergoing thoracoabdominal aortic aneurysm repair. Transfus Med Rev 2005; 19(2):143–54.

42. Gertler JP, Cambria RP, Brewster DC, et al. Coagulation changes during thoracoabdominal aneurysm repair. J Vasc Surg 1996;24(6):936–45.

43. Hardy JF, de Moerloose P, Samama CM. Members of the Groupe d'Intérêt en Hémostase Périopératoire. Massive transfusion and coagulopathy: pathophysiology and implications for clinical management. Can J Anaesth 2006;53(6 Suppl): S40–58.

44. Rahe-Meyer N, Solomon C, Winterhalter M, et al. Thromboelastometry-guided administration of fibrinogen concentrate for the treatment of excessive intraoperative bleeding in thoracoabdominal aortic aneurysm surgery. J Thorac Cardiovasc Surg 2009;138(3):694–702.

45. Hébert PC, Wells G, Blajchman MA, et al. A multicenter, randomized, controlled clinical trial of transfusion requirements in critical care. Transfusion Requirements in Critical Care Investigators, Canadian Critical Care Trials Group. N Engl J Med 1999;340(6):409–17, published correction appears in N Engl J Med 1999 Apr 1;340(13):1056.

46. Bursi F, Barbieri A, Politi L, et al. Perioperative red blood cell transfusion and outcome in stable patients after elective major vascular surgery. Eur J Vasc Endovasc Surg 2009;37(3):311–8.

47. Khan NK, Oksala NK, Suominen V, et al. Risk of symptomatic venous thromboembolism after abdominal aortic aneurysm repair in long-term follow-up of 1021 consecutive patients. J Vasc Surg Venous Lymphat Disord 2021;9(1):54–61.

48. de Maistre E, Terriat B, Lesne-Padieu AS, et al. High incidence of venous thrombosis after surgery for abdominal aortic aneurysm. J Vasc Surg 2009;49(3): 596–601.

49. Behrendt CA, Dayama A, Debus ES, et al. Lower Extremity Ischemia after Abdominal Aortic Aneurysm Repair. Ann Vasc Surg 2017;45:206–12.

50. Tarbunou YA, Smith JB, Kruse RL, et al. Outcomes associated with hyperglycemia after abdominal aortic aneurysm repair. J Vasc Surg 2019;69(3):763–73.e3.

51. Long CA, Fang ZB, Hu FY, et al. Poor glycemic control is a strong predictor of postoperative morbidity and mortality in patients undergoing vascular surgery. J Vasc Surg 2019;69(4):1219–26.

52. American Diabetes Association. Standards of medical care in diabetes–2010. Diabetes Care 2010;33(Suppl 1):S11–61 [published correction appears in Diabetes Care. 2010;33(3):692].

53. Lederle FA, Freischlag JA, Kyriakides TC, et al. Outcomes following endovascular vs open repair of abdominal aortic aneurysm: a randomized trial. JAMA 2009; 302(14):1535–42.

54. Becquemin JP, Pillet JC, Lescalie F, et al. A randomized controlled trial of endovascular aneurysm repair versus open surgery for abdominal aortic aneurysms in low- to moderate-risk patients. J Vasc Surg 2011;53(5):1167–73.e1.

55. Arnaoutoglou E, Kouvelos G, Milionis H, et al. Post-implantation syndrome following endovascular abdominal aortic aneurysm repair: preliminary data. Interact Cardiovasc Thorac Surg 2011;12(4):609–14.

56. Doig D, Turner EL, Dobson J, et al. Incidence, impact, and predictors of cranial nerve palsy and haematoma following carotid endarterectomy in the international carotid stenting study. Eur J Vasc Endovasc Surg 2014;48(5):498–504.

57. International Carotid Stenting Study investigators, Ederle J, Dobson J, et al. Carotid artery stenting compared with endarterectomy in patients with symptomatic carotid stenosis (International Carotid Stenting Study): an interim analysis of a randomised controlled trial. Lancet 2010;375(9719):985–97 [published correction appears in Lancet. 2010;376(9735):90. Nasser, H-C [corrected to Nahser, H-C].

58. Müller MD, Lyrer P, Brown MM, et al. Carotid artery stenting versus endarterectomy for treatment of carotid artery stenosis. Cochrane Database Syst Rev 2020;2(2):CD000515.

59. Liu Z, Shi Z, Wang Y, et al. Carotid artery stenting versus carotid endarterectomy: systematic review and meta-analysis. World J Surg 2009;33(3):586–96.

60. Wu TY, Anderson NE, Barber PA. Neurological complications of carotid revascularisation. J Neurol Neurosurg Psychiatry 2012;83(5):543–50.

61. Hill MD, Brooks W, Mackey A, et al. Stroke after carotid stenting and endarterectomy in the Carotid Revascularization Endarterectomy versus Stenting Trial (CREST). Circulation 2012;126(25):3054–61.

62. Sfyroeras GS, Bessias N, Moulakakis KG, et al. New cerebral ischemic lesions after carotid endarterectomy. Ann Vasc Surg 2013;27(7):883–7.

63. Reigel MM, Hollier LH, Sundt TM Jr, et al. Cerebral hyperperfusion syndrome: a cause of neurologic dysfunction after carotid endarterectomy. J Vasc Surg 1987;5(4):628–34.

64. Naylor AR, Ruckley CV. The post-carotid endarterectomy hyperperfusion syndrome. Eur J Vasc Endovasc Surg 1995;9(4):365–7.

65. van Mook WN, Rennenberg RJ, Schurink GW, et al. Cerebral hyperperfusion syndrome. Lancet Neurol 2005;4(12):877–88.

66. Kakisis JD, Antonopoulos CN, Mantas G, et al. Cranial Nerve Injury After Carotid Endarterectomy: Incidence, Risk Factors, and Time Trends. Eur J Vasc Endovasc Surg 2017;53(3):320–35.

67. Grieff AN, Dombrovskiy V, Beckerman W, et al. Anesthesia Type is Associated with Decreased Cranial Nerve Injury in Carotid Endarterectomy. Ann Vasc Surg 2021;70:318–25.

68. Collins TC, Nelson D, Ahluwalia JS. Mortality following operations for lower extremity peripheral arterial disease. Vasc Health Risk Manag 2010;6:287–96. Published 2010 May 6.

Chronic Pain Considerations in Patients with Cardiovascular Disease

Corinne M. Layne-Stuart, DO*, Anna L. Carpenter, MD

KEYWORDS

- Chronic pain • Vascular disease • Postamputation pain • Phantom limb pain
- Ischemic pain • Central poststroke pain • Hemiplegic shoulder pain
- Thoracic out syndrome

KEY POINTS

- Cardiovascular disease encompasses a wide range of disorders and affects a large portion of the United States population; many of these patients will also endure chronic pain as a direct or indirect result of their disease process.
- Treating chronic pain associated with cardiovascular disease can be intricate and necessitates a multifaceted, multidisciplinary approach to optimize patient outcomes.
- Improvements and developments in advanced technological treatment options for various vascular/ischemic pain states have dramatically expanded patient care choices and ability to achieve better and more sustained pain relief.
- Medical comorbidities and psychological factors are highly important components of the patient assessment and optimal treatment plan as a multitude of patient outcomes will be affected by these aspects of their disease and care processes.

INTRODUCTION

Cardiovascular disease (CVD) is prevalent in the United States (US) and includes a multitude of arterial, venous, and lymphatic disorders. CVD affects 48% of adults in the United States, 121.5 million people, according to the 2019 update of heart disease and stroke statistics from the American Heart Association.[1]

Unfortunately, many patients who suffer from cardiovascular disease must also endure resultant chronic pain. The challenges facing these patients and the providers

Disclosure statement: Neither of the authors has any commercial or financial conflicts of interest to disclose.
Funding: This research did not receive any specific grant from funding agencies in the public, commercial, or not-for-profit sectors.
Department of Anesthesiology, Division of Chronic Pain Medicine, Center for Integrative Pain Management, West Virginia University, 1075 Van Voorhis Road, Morgantown, WV 26505, USA
* Corresponding author.
E-mail address: cmlaynestuart@hsc.wvu.edu

Anesthesiology Clin 40 (2022) 791–802
https://doi.org/10.1016/j.anclin.2022.08.018
1932-2275/22/© 2022 Elsevier Inc. All rights reserved.

anesthesiology.theclinics.com

who treat them are many, including coexisting disease, limited treatment options, and continued progression of underlying pathology.

Pain associated with cardiovascular disease often involves multiple mechanisms including inflammatory, nociceptive and neuropathic. Inflammatory pain is defined as the perception and affective response to noxious stimuli as a result of inflammatory response associated with tissue damage. This pain is characterized by: heat, redness, hypersensitivity, swelling, and loss of function. Nociceptive pain results from actual or threatened damage to nonneural tissue (induced following thermal, chemical, and/or mechanical insult) resulting in the stimulation of peripheral nociceptors.[2] Neuropathic pain is pain caused by a lesion or disease of the somatosensory nervous system.[2] Neuropathic pain symptoms vary, but can include descriptions of sharp, shooting, stabbing, tingling, numb sensations. The sympathetic nervous system may also be involved in the conversion of pain from acute to chronic. This is thought to occur by 2 different mechanisms. The first mechanism occurs when physiological changes, which arise as the result of a peripheral nerve injury, lead to chemical coupling between afferent and sympathetic neurons. The sympathetic nervous system may also become involved when sympathetic nerve terminals, located in peripheral tissue, work as mediator elements in the setting of tissue damage without nerve injury.[3] Delineation and identification of primary causative mechanisms can be challenging, but is necessary to tailor treatment to the individual patient and optimize outcomes.[4]

Throughout this article, we will discuss multiple pain-inducing vascular disease states as well as pain-inducing sequelae of cardiovascular disease processes.

PERIPHERAL ARTERY DISEASE

Peripheral artery disease (PAD) is the narrowing or blockage of arteries, primarily due to atherosclerosis.[5] This generally causes pain due to insufficient blood supply and ischemia.[5] Critical limb ischemia (CLI) is the phenomenon of severe PAD in the lower extremities which leads to chronic pain at rest, ulcers or gangrene in one or both lower extremities.[6] Critical limb ischemia is treated by revascularization if possible.[5] There is, however, a subset of patients who have failed revascularization or are not candidates for this type of therapy. In this situation, first-line therapy includes analgesics along with vasodilators and anticoagulants.[5] Second-line treatment includes spinal cord stimulation and sympathetic blocks.[5] Third-line treatment includes sympathectomy.[5]

The evidence for spinal cord simulation (SCS) for the treatment of pain secondary to critical limb ischemia is generally supportive. The mechanism of pain relief of SCS in this population is not well understood. Multiple theories exist, including "gate control" theory, increased release of nitric oxide, suppression of the sympathetic nervous system and release of endogenous opioids-like peptides.[7] A Cochrane review by Ubbink and Vermeulen in 2005 (and updated in 2013) concluded that SCS led to fewer amputations, better pain relief and fewer side effects than conservative therapy.[5] Review of evidence by the Neuromodulation Appropriateness Consensus Committee (NACC) in 2014 recommends SCS for critical limb ischemia with level B evidence (recommends with moderate evidence of effectiveness and minimal risk of harm).[5] They also note that the evidence for sympathectomy is poor and SCS is recommended prior to sympathectomy.[5] Another review of published literature was conducted by Deogaonkar and Slavin in 2014, which concluded that SCS improves pain control, circulation, claudication, quality of life and limb survival in patients with critical limb ischemia.[7] A retrospective case-controlled study was performed by Liu and colleagues[8] in 2017 showed that the use of SCS for the treatment of critical limb ischemia improved patient's walking ability, pain severity and sleep quality. In addition, a prospective cohort study with 56 patients was conducted by Klinkova and colleagues[9] in 2020 and showed generally good outcomes for patients with critical limb ischemia who were treated with SCS.

Several factors have been investigated as predictors of response to SCS for patients with CLI.[9] Transcutaneous oxygen pressure (TcPO^2) is a noninvasive method used to measure tissue oxygenation.[9] A study performed by Klinkova and colleagues[9] investigated whether the baseline or change in TcPO^2 with standing was predictive of response to SCS. Results showed that the baseline value was less important and even patients with poor baseline TcPO2 were responsive to SCS if TcPO2 increased by > 10mmHg with orthostatic testing.[9] Orthostatic testing was conducted by measuring the change in TcPO2 from sitting to standing.[9] This is thought to be a marker for functional status of the peripheral microvasculature.[9] Study results found that an increase in TcPO2 by > 10 mm Hg during orthostatic testing associated with positive outcomes with spinal cord stimulation.[9] Another study used lower limb Tl scintigraphy and SPECT to diagnose lower limb perfusion insufficiency.[8] This was found to be an accurate tool for the diagnosis of CLI, evaluation of the microcirculation and was useful as a predictor of response to SCS therapy.[8] Factors associated with poor response to SCS included increased age and increased degree of comorbid conditions (diabetes, hypertension, cerebral vascular disease, atherosclerosis).[9]

ANGINA

Chronic refractory angina (RA) is chest pain caused by reversible ischemia in the setting of coronary artery disease that cannot be treated by medications, angioplasty or coronary artery bypass grafting.[10] The number of patients suffering from chronic refractory angina in the US is thought to be approximately 1.2 million.[11] The data available for the effectiveness of pharmacological therapy for chronic RA are very limited and clinically, treatment mirrors that of chronic stable angina.[11] First-line pharmacological therapy includes a beta-blocker or calcium channel blocker.[11] Second and third-line pharmacological therapy include nicorandil, ivabradine, ranolazine, trimetazidine, perhexiline, allopurinol, and molsidomine.[11] Additional treatment options that may be available through cardiologists include coronary sinus reducers, cell therapy, external enhanced counterpulsation, extracorporeal shockwave revascularization therapy and are beyond the scope of this article.[11] Treatment by the pain specialist should be multimodal and may include cognitive behavioral therapy, stellate ganglion blocks, transcutaneous electrical nerve stimulation (TENS), and SCS.[11] The evidence available for SCS as a treatment of chronic RA is level 2a according to a recent evaluation of all available data by the NACC.[5] Neuromodulation is also supported as a therapy for chronic RA by the American Heart Association and the European Society of Cardiology.[5] Although the evidence supporting the use of SCS for the treatment of RA is strong, there is limited evidence comparing SCS to usual care. The RASCAL Study was conducted in an attempt to address this gap in the literature.[10] Although the results showed a general improvement in the primary and secondary outcomes (Seattle Angina Questionnaire score and frequency of angina attacks), the study was not adequately powered, and further research is needed in this area.[10]

THORACIC OUTLET SYNDROME

Thoracic outlet syndrome (TOS) involves a group of disorders that cause pain and paresthesias in the ipsilateral neck, shoulder, and upper extremity secondary to compression of neurovascular structures. The broad categories of TOS include neurogenic and vascular. Vascular TOS is further delineated into arterial and venous. For the purposes of this article, we will focus on vascular TOS.

Less than 10% of cases of TOS are of vascular etiology.[12] Typical sites of compression include the scalene triangle, costoclavicular space, and retropectoralis minor space. Anatomical variants that contribute to the pathogenesis of TOS include a congenital cervical rib, altered anatomy of the clavicle and or first rib such as callus formation postfracture, tumor, osteomyelitis, fibrous bands, abnormal insertion of the anterior scalene on first rib and muscular hypertrophy.[13]

Venous TOS is caused by compression of the subclavian or axillary veins with resultant thrombosis.[14] Associated symptoms include pain, cyanosis, and swelling of the limb. Arterial TOS is caused by compression of the axillary or subclavian artery and may present with embolic episodes.[14] Associated symptoms include pain, pallor, cold extremity, weakness, paresthesias, reduced, or unobtainable pulse. Roos and Adson's tests should be performed as part of the physical examination to evaluate for vascular etiology of TOS.[15]

Several imaging modalities including radiographs, CT, MRI, and US may be useful in the evaluation of TOS. Cervical radiographs should be obtained to evaluate for a cervical rib and bony abnormalities of the first rib and clavicle. Duplex ultrasound scanning may reveal a stenotic lesion or thrombus of the involved vasculature. Hardy and colleagues[16] revealed that MRI does have a role in the diagnosis of TOS with specificities of 82–100% for multiple sources of compression. Sensitivity was low for several areas of compression and therefore MRI was not found to be a good screening tool. MRIs with postural maneuvers have also been studied and found to be better in the identification of vascular compression in the costoclavicular space.[17,18] Contrast enhancement with MRI also improved the detection of vascular compression.[18] Computed tomography (CT) scan or catheter-directed arteriography can reveal sites of vascular compression and when a cervical rib or fracture callus is present; this modality is also enhanced with dynamic maneuvers.[19,20]

Injection treatment is not effective for venous or arterial TOS. If a cervical rib is present, resection may be recommended.[21] The primary goals of treatment in arterial TOS are addressing the embolic source and repair of proximal lesion with subsequent reestablishment of distal circulation.[19] Regarding venous TOS, catheter-directed axillosubclavian vein thrombolysis when symptom onset is recent and systemic anticoagulation is the standard course of treatment.[22] Staged operative TOS decompression may alleviate the site of compression and make future stenting a better option than without decompression.[23,24] Although, more recent natural history studies note the recurrence of axillosubclavian thrombosis has been found to be uncommon and there is concern that surgical interventions may result in worsening symptoms of venous TOS.[25,26]

Postamputation Pain (Residual Limb Pain, Phantom Pain)

Over 95% of amputees suffer from chronic pain.[5] There are multiple pain syndromes that affects this population including phantom limb pain, complex regional pain syndrome (CRPS), and residual limb pain (RLP). RLP may be somatic or neuropathic (due to neuroma formation).[5] Phantom limb pain is a central pain state and can be distinguished from the other 2 syndromes by the location of the pain, which is in the amputated limb.

There is no consensus on the treatment of phantom limb pain and treatment is limited by the complex nature of the pain.[5] Generally, a multimodal approach is considered the most effective. Common treatments may include psychotherapy, physical therapy, medications (antidepressants, anticonvulsants, N-methyl-Daspartic acid (NMDA) antagonists, calcitonin, opioids), sympathetic blocks, and SCS.[27] Complementary and alternative medicine options include hypnosis, acupuncture, mirror therapy, TENS, cognitive behavioral therapy and virtual reality.[19] A systematic review and meta-analysis by Xie and colleagues[28] in 2021 reviewed ten randomized control trials and concluded that mirror therapy is beneficial for phantom limb pain in the short term. Phantom pain is generally not improved with acetaminophen, local block, or surgical revision.[27] A prospective cohort study conducted in 2015 by Prologo and colleagues[29] showed a reduction in disability scores and pain intensity scores after the cryoablation of the amputated nerve. The data for the use of SCS in treating phantom limb or stump pain are generally limited to case series data.[5] There are several more recent technologies including dorsal root ganglion stimulation and reversible nerve block with kilohertz-frequency stimulation which have shown promise in treating this population.[5] There is also some evidence for deep brain stimulation and motor cortex stimulation to target the central pain component of phantom limb pain.[27] Targeted muscle reinnervation (TMR) at the time of major limb amputation may help prevent the development of neuromas and phantom pain postoperatively.[29] A multi-center cohort study with 489 patients published in 2019 by Valerio and colleagues[29] showed reduced phantom limb and residual limb pain in patients who underwent TMR at the time of major limb amputation as compared to the traditional amputation group. TMR is a technique in which amputated nerves are transferred to nearby motor nerves at the time of amputation to prevent neuroma formation.[29] Alternatively, there is also evidence that virtual reality treatment, which requires patients to execute motor function of the phantom limb, may benefit patients with phantom limb pain.[30] A study conducted in 2014 by Ortiz-Catalan and colleagues[30]. showed significant improvement across multiple outcomes in 14 patients.

RLP may be treated with local anesthetic injection, steroid injection, or botulinum toxin at the site.[27] RLP may arise from a variety of pain generators including heterotopic ossification, infection, tumor, neuroma, ischemia, ill-fitting prosthesis, poor surgical technique, CRPS, among others. In cases of suboptimal surgical technique with poor prosthetic fit, initially socket modification should be attempted. If this is unsuccessful, surgical revision may be considered.[31] Approximately 10%-15% of patients have neuroma pain and typically describe intermittent aching, shooting, and cramping sensations.[32] Surgical revision of the amputation site is generally only indicated if there is a readily identifiable surgical pathology at the site of the pain.[27] There is case series evidence that RLP that is responsive to local anesthetic injection may have longer lasting relief with radiofrequency or cryoneurolysis.[27] There is case series level evidence for the use of SCS in RLP.[27]

COMPLEX REGIONAL PAIN SYNDROME

Complex regional pain syndrome is a mixed neuropathic and vascular pain condition that presents with a wide array of symptoms possibly including pain out of proportion to injury, autonomic dysfunction, vasomotor, sudomotor, motor, and trophic changes. CRPS type I develops without a known nerve injury, whereas CRPS II is associated with a finite nerve injury. The Budapest criteria are the diagnostic criteria for CRPS and are listed later in discussion in **Box 1**.[33]

The treatment of CRPS should be multimodal in nature and may include therapy, medications, sympathetic blocks, sympathectomy, and SCS.[33] Strong evidence exists to support several types of therapy for patients with CRPS including aqua therapy, desensitization therapy, mirror therapy, graded motor imagery, and psychotherapy.[33] The evidence for medication therapies specifically for CRPS is limited and clinical

Box 1
Budapest criteria
Pain out of proportion to injury
Symptoms (must have at least one symptom in any of the four categories)
Sensory (allodynia, hyperalgesia)
Vasomotor (temperature/color changes)
Sudomotor/edema (abnormal sweating, edema)
Motor/trophic (limited range of motion, nail changes)
Signs (must have at least one sign in at least two different categories)
Sensory
Vasomotor
Sudomotor/edema
Motor/trophic
No other diagnosis that better explains the signs and symptoms

treatment mimics the treatment of neuropathic pain in general.[33] This may include nonsteroidal anti-inflammatory drugs (NSAIDs), corticosteroids, neuropathic agents, opioids, NMDA antagonists, and vasodilators. The evidence to support the use of NSAIDs is limited to the use of these medications for neuropathic pain in general, which is mixed.[33] There is evidence to support the use of corticosteroids in the acute phase, but not for chronic CRPS due to the severe side effect profile.[33] Evidence for the use of gabapentin and pregabalin is limited.[33] The use of opioids for the treatment of CRPS is controversial and there is a lack of evidence to support routine use.[33] A systematic review of literature conducted in 2015 by Connolly and colleagues[34] showed no high-quality evidence to support the use of ketamine for CRPS. A more recent systematic review and meta-analysis conducted by Zhao and colleagues[35] in 2018 found that there is some evidence to support the use of ketamine infusions for short-term relief (<3 months) of pain from CRPS, but agrees that additional high-quality data are needed. There is no good evidence to support the use of clonidine for CRPS.[33] Case series level data are available to support the use of nifedipine for vasoconstriction associated with CRPS.[33] Phenoxybenzamine is considered third-line therapy for CRPS.[16] Calcitonin may be used help preserve bone mass and the evidence for its use is mixed.[33] Strong evidence is available for the use of bisphosphonates to limit bone loss.[33]

Sympathetic blocks are commonly used clinically, but evidence of long-term effectiveness is limited.[33] The outcomes of chemical or surgical sympathectomies are variable and reoccurrence of pain is common.[33] There is a paucity of evidence to support long-term effectiveness of these interventions. Evidence for SCS as a treatment for CRSP remains relatively strong.[5] The most recent guidelines released by the NACC in 2014 recommended SCS for the treatment of CRPS if the disease has been present for > 3 months and has not responded to more conservative therapy.[5] The NACC also recommends that all patients should be screened with a psychological evaluation and a trail of stimulation have been successfully completed.[5] This conclusion was drawn after a review of historic literature as well as more recent review of 4 randomized control studies that were performed between 2009 and 2014.[5] More recently, a case series by Yang and Hunter in 2017 showed promise for dorsal root ganglion stimulation as a salvage therapy for patients with CRPS who have failed traditional SCS.[36] Amputation has been considered as a treatment of refractory CRPS, but remains controversial as there is high risk of recurrent CRPS or phantom limb pain, among other complications.[33]

PAIN SYNDROMES FOLLOWING CEREBROVASCULAR ACCIDENTS
Central Poststroke Pain

Central poststroke pain (CPSP) may occur following a hemorrhagic or ischemic cerebrovascular accident (CVA). Lesions resulting in CPSP occur in several identified areas including the thalamus (Dejerine Rousey syndrome), cerebral cortex, brainstem, and operculum insula.[37,38]

Associated symptoms typically develop within 6 months of the CVA, although may be reported as late as 2–3 years post stroke.[39,40] These symptoms most often occur on the contralateral side and may affect the entire hemi-body or more discreet areas of the hemi-body depending on the location of lesion. In cases involving a lateral medullary infarction, in addition to contralateral hemi-body dysesthesias, patients may also report ipsilateral facial pain.[41] Estimates of prevalence vary but may occur in up to 8% of patients following stroke.[39]

First-line agents in the treatment of CPSP include lamotrigine and amitriptyline; second-line agents include gabapentin, pregabalin, phenytoin, and carbamazepine. A multidisciplinary, multimodal, team-based approach is optimal when caring for patients with CPSP. Motor cortex stimulation in patients that have not had success with other treatment modalities has some supportive evidence.[42] Case reports and case series have shown deep brain stimulation to be effective for CPSP.[43–47]

Shoulder Pain

Shoulder pain following stroke is encountered in approximately 9% of patients.[48] Hemiplegic shoulder pain is often multifactorial and requires thorough evaluation. Contributing pathology to this pain may include central etiology, peripheral nerve injury, complex regional pain syndrome, subluxation, soft tissue injury, and spasticity. Botulinum toxin has strong evidence for treating muscular hypertonicity causing shoulder pain. Neuropathic pain medications also have strong evidence in treating shoulder pain of neuropathic origin. Less robust evidence exists in the literature for suprascapular nerve block, acupuncture, steroid injections and neuromuscular electrical stimulation.[42] Peripheral nerve stimulation (PNS) has also shown promise in treating hemiplegic shoulder pain. A pilot study revealed that PNS is superior to usual care for up to 12 weeks following 3 weeks of peripheral nerve stimulation for hemiplegic shoulder pain.[43] Wilson RD and colleagues showed in a subsequent multi-center case series that patients implanted with a pulse generator experienced significant pain relief, decreased pain interference and improvement in external rotation without pain. Pain reduction was measured at 6 and 12 months with all 5 patients that received the implantable pulse generator achieving a minimum of 50% relief. A decrease in pain was also measured at 24 months with 4 of the 5 patients that received the implantable pulse generator achieving a minimum of 50% relief.[44]

Contractures

Contractures commonly occur following CVA and may cause pain, functional limitations, and skin breakdown. Contracture formation may begin days to months following the CVA. Monitoring for and early identification of contractures and appropriate referral for orthoses, stretching, serial casting, splinting, and surgical release are important.[42]

PSYCHOLOGICAL CONSIDERATIONS IN ISCHEMIC DISEASE STATES

An important part of managing pain is identifying and addressing psychological barriers to improvement. According to the Guidelines for Adult Stroke Rehabilitation and Recovery, standardized evaluation of mood and cautious antidepressant use are recommended. Patient education, behavioral health evaluation and counseling, support, and a minimum of 4 weeks of regular exercise may also be beneficial in poststroke depression.[42] Increasingly evidence reveals that preexisting mental health disorders may be associated with risk factors for cardiovascular disease both through biological pathways and through health behaviors that increase risk of CVD.[49,50]

GENERAL CONSIDERATIONS FOR THE TREATMENT OF THE VASCULAR PAIN PATIENT

There are many factors that may influence the treatment of the patient suffering from pain secondary to vascular disease. This patient population has several demographic factors, behaviors, and coexisting pathologies that are likely to impact treatment options. These factors and behaviors include increased age and smoking, whereas coexisting pathologies include coronary artery disease (CAD), chronic obstructive pulmonary disease (COPD), obesity, diabetes mellitus (DM), and poststroke status which are listed in **Box 2**.

The incidence of vascular disease increases with age. Patients in this demographic are at a higher risk for decreased renal and hepatic function, cognitive dysfunction, and falls. These factors limit medication options as well as interventions due to the limitations of using contrast media in patients with renal dysfunction.

Smoking is also known to be a major risk factor for the development of atherosclerosis and vascular disease. Smoking predisposes patients to other medical problems, including CAD, COPD, and poor wound healing. The presence of CAD increases the likelihood that a patient will be on therapeutic anticoagulation, which may limit interventional treatment options. The presence of COPD reduces ventilation and increases the risk of pulmonary complications when combined with the respiratory depressant effects of opioid therapy.

The incidence of coexisting obesity and DM is also high in the vascular patient. Interventional treatments may be more challenging in obese patient, leading to lower success rates. Obesity also increases the risk of wound complications in the surgical patient. For this reason, many physicians have body mass index (BMI) limits for considering patients for surgical treatment. Patients who suffer from obesity may not be considered a candidate for certain interventions or surgical treatment options. DM also increases the risk of the surgical patient developing wound healing complications. Poor blood glucose control increases the risk of surgical site infection and infection after an interventional procedure. High blood glucose may also limit the use of

---

Box 2
Common coexisting pathology in the vascular patient

Coronary artery disease (CAD) and chronic obstructive pulmonary disease (COPD)

Chronic kidney disease (CKD)

Obesity

Diabetes mellitus (DM)

Poststroke cognitive impairment

therapeutic corticosteroids. This is due to the concern for worsening blood glucose levels and the potential development of diabetic ketoacidosis in type I diabetic or hyperglycemic hyperosmolar nonketotic syndrome in type II diabetic. The diabetic patient is also at risk for peripheral neuropathy, which may confound the diagnosis of vascular pain-related conditions, especially in the lower extremity.

The vascular patient may also have an increased risk of having suffered from a prior stroke. This may limit therapy for multiple reasons. This poststroke patient may have some degree of cognitive impairment, which may limit his or her ability to understand treatment options or comply with complex therapies (SCS). The poststroke patient will also likely be on therapeutic anticoagulation which may limit interventional options.

CLINICS CARE POINTS

Pearls
- When treating critical limb ischemia, note that the evidence for sympathectomy is poor and spinal cord stimulation is recommended prior to sympathectomy
- When evaluating a patient with critical limb ischemia for spinal cord stimulation, considering using lower limb TI scintigraphy and SPECT or transcutaneous oxygen pressure with orthostatic testing to evaluate the microcirculation
- Understand that the treatment of phantom limb pain and treatment is limited by the complex nature of the pain and that generally, a multimodal approach is considered most effective
- Targeted muscle reinnervation (TMR) at the time of major limb amputation may help prevent the development of neuromas and phantom pain postoperatively
- A multidisciplinary, multimodal, team-based approach is optimal when caring for patients with central poststroke pain
- In the poststroke patient, monitoring for and early identification of contractures and appropriate referral for orthoses, stretching, serial casting, splinting and surgical release is important

Pitfalls
- Phantom pain is generally not improved with acetaminophen, local block, or surgical revision
- Surgical revision of the amputation site in patients with residual limb pain is generally only indicated if there is a readily identifiable surgical pathology at the site of the pain
- Be sure to evaluate the elderly and the poststroke patient for cognitive impairment, which may limit his or her ability to understand treatment options or comply with complex therapies (SCS)
- Be sure to evaluate the vascular pain patient for coexisting disease including CAD, COPD, DM, and consider the effects of these disease processes on the patient when determining the best treatment plan

REFERENCES

1. Benjamin EJ, Muntner P, Alonso A, et al. Heart disease and stroke statistics -2019 update: a report from the american heart association. Circulation 2019;139: e56–528.
2. IASP. International Association for the study of Pain Taxonomy. 2011. Available at: http://www.iasp-pain.org. Accessed 19 March, 2022.
3. Michaelis M, Janig W. Pathophysiologische Mechanismen und Erklärungsansätze aus der tierexperimentellen Forschung [Sympathetic nervous system and pain: pathophysiological mechanisms]. Schmerz 1998;12(4):261–71. German.
4. Seretny M, Colvin LA. Pain management in patients with vascular disease. Br J Anaesth 2016;117(suppl_2):ii95–106.

5. Deer T, Mekhail N, Provenzano D, et al. The appropriate use of neurostimulation of the spinal cord and peripheral nervous system for the treatment of chronic pain and ischemic diseases: the neuromodulation appropriateness consensus committee. Neuromodulation 2014;17:515–50.

6. Novo S, Coppola G, Milio G. Critical limb ischemia: definition and natural history. Curr Drug Targets Cardiovasc Haematol Disord 2004;4(3):219–25.

7. Deogaonkar M, Slavin K. Spinal cord stimulation for the treatment of vascular pathology. Neurosurg Clin N Am 2014;15:25–31.

8. Liu J, Su C, Chen S, et al. Spinal cord stimulation improves the microvascular perfusion insufficiency caused by critical limb ischemia. Neuromodulation 2018;21:489–94.

9. Klinkova A, Kamenskaya O, Ashurkovet A, et al. The clinical outcomes in patients with critical limb ischemia one year after spinal cord stimulation. Ann Vasc Surg 2020;62:356–64.

10. Eldabe S, Thomson S, Duarte R, et al. The effectiveness and cost-effectiveness of spinal cord simulation for refractory angina (RASCAL study): a pilot randomized controlled trial. Neuromodulation 2016;19:60–70.

11. Cheng K, Sainsbury P, Fisher M, et al. Management of refractory angina pectoris. Eur Cardiol 2016;11(2):69–76.

12. Degeorges R, Reynaud C, Becquemin JP. Thoracic outlet syndrome surgery: long-term functional results. Ann Vasc Surg 2004;18(5):558–65.

13. Laulan B, Fouquet C, Rodaix, et al. Thoracic outlet syndrome: definition, aetiological factors, diagnosis, management and occupational impact. J Occup Rehabil 2011;21:366–73, 21193950.

14. Ohkawa Y, Isoda H, Hasegawa S, et al. MR angiography of thoracic outlet syndrome. J Comput Assist Tomogr 1992;16:475–7.

15. Foley JM, Finlayson H, Travlos A. A review of thoracic outlet syndrome and the possible role of botulinum toxin in the treatment of this syndrome. Toxins (Basel) 2012;4(11):1223–35.

16. Hardy A, Pouges C, Wavreille G, et al. Thoracic outlet syndrome: diagnostic accuracy of MRI. Orthopaedics Traumatol Surg Res 2019;105(8):1563–9.

17. Demondion P, Herbinet S, Van Sint Jan N, et al. Cotten imaging assessment of thoracic outlet syndrome. Radiographics 2006;26:1735–50.

18. Demirbag E, Unlu F, Ozdemir H, et al. The relationship between magnetic resonance imaging findings and postural maneuver and physical examination tests in patients with thoracic outlet syndrome: results of a double-blind, controlled study. Arch Phys Med Rehabil 2007;87:844–51.

19. Bogduk N, Copenhaver DJ, Eskandar EN, et al. Bonica's management of pain. 5th edition. Philadelphia, PA: Wolter's Kluwer; 2019.

20. Gillet R, Teixeira P, Meyer JB, et al. Dynamic CT angiography for the diagnosis of patients with thoracic outlet syndrome: Correlation with patient symptoms. J Cardiovasc Comput Tomogr 2018;12(2):158–65.

21. Brooke BS, Freischlag JA. Contemporary management of thoracic outlet syndrome. Curr Opin Cardiol 2010;6:535–40.

22. Hingorani A, Ascher E, Lorenson E, et al. Upper extremity deep venous thrombosis and its impact on morbidity and mortality rates in a hospital-based population. J Vasc Surg 1997;26:853–60.

23. Lee MC, Grassi CJ, Belkin M, et al. Early operative intervention after thrombolytic therapy for primary subclavian vein thrombosis: an effective treatment approach. J Vasc Surg 1998;27:1101–8.

24. Sanders RJ, Cooper MA. Surgical management of subclavian vein obstruction, including six cases of subclavian vein bypass. Surgery 1995;118:856–63.
25. Lee WA, Hill BB, Harris JJ, et al. Surgical intervention is not required for all patients with subclavian vein thrombosis. J Vasc Surg 2000;32:57–67.
26. Lokanathan R, Salvian AJ, Chen JC, et al. Outcome after thrombolysis and selective thoracic outlet decompression as primary axillary vein thrombosis. J Vasc Surg 2001;33:783–8.
27. Benzon HT, Raja SN, Liu SS. Essentials of pain medicine. 4th edition. Philadelphia, PA: Elsevier, Inc; 2018.
28. Xie H, Zhang K, Wanget S, et al. Effectiveness of mirror therapy for phantom limb pain: a systematic review and meta-analysis. Arch Phys Med Rehabil 2021;1–10.
29. Prologo J, Gillil C, Yamada K, et al. Percutaneous image-guided cryoablation for the treatment of phantom limb pain in amputees: a pilot study. J Vasc Surg Intetervent Rad 2016;17:183–4.
30. Ortiz-Catalan M, Guðmundsdóttir R, Kristoffersen M, et al. Phantom motor execution facilitated by machine learning and augmented reality as treatment for phantom chronic and intractable phantom limb pain. Lancet 2016;388:2885–94.
31. Cifu DX, Eapen BC, Johns JS, et al. Braddom's physical medicine and rehabilitation. 6th edition. Philadelphia, PA: Elsevier, Inc; 2021.
32. Weeks SR, Anderson-Barnes VC, Tsao JW. Phantom limb pains theories and therapies. Neurologist 2010;16:277–86.
33. Freedman M, Greis A, Marino L, et al. Complex regional pain syndrome. Phys Med Rehabil Clin N Am 2014;25:291–303.
34. Connolly A, Prager J, Harden R, et al. A systematic review of ketamine for complex regional pain syndrome. Pain Med 2015;16:943–69.
35. Zhao J, Wang Y, Wang Y, et al. The effect of ketamine infusion in the treatment of complex regional pain syndrome: a systemic review and meta-analysis. Curr Pain Headache Rep 2018;22:12.
36. Yang A, Hunter C. Dorsal root ganglion stimulation as a salvage treatment for complex regional pain syndrome refractory to dorsal column spinal cord stimulation: a case series. Neuromodulation 2017;20:703–7.
37. Klit H, Finnerup NB, Jensen TS. Central post-stroke pain: clinical characteristics, pathophysiology, and management. Lancet Neurol 2009;8:857–68.
38. Garcia-Larrea L, Perchet C, Creac'h C, et al. Operculo-insular pain (parasylvian pain): a distinct central pain syndrome. Brain 2010;133:2528–39.
39. Sadosky A, McDerrmott AM, Brandenburg NA, et al. A review of the epidemiology of painful diabetic neuropathy, post herpetic neuralgia, and less commonly studied neuropathic conditions. Pain Pract 2008;8:45–56.
40. Leijon G, Bolvie J, Johansson I. Coentral Post-stroke pains-neurological symptoms and pain characteristics. Pain 1989;36:13–25.
41. Fitzek S, Baumgärtner U, Fitzek C, et al. Mechanisms and predictors of chronic facial pain in lateral medullary infarction. Ann Neurol 2001;49:493–500.
42. Winstein CJ, Stein J, Arenaet R, et al. Guidelines for Adult Stroke Rehabilitation and Recovery: a Guideline for Healthcare Professionals from the American Heart Association/American Stroke Association. Stroke 2016;47:e98–169.
43. Wilson RD, Gunzler DD, Bennett ME, et al. Peripheral nere stimulation compared to usual care for pain relief of hemiplegic shoulder pain: a randomized controlled trial. Am J Phys Med Rehabil 2014;93(1):17–28.
44. Wilson RD, Bennett ME, Nguyen VQC, et al. Fully implantable peripheral nerve stimulation for hemiplegic shoulder pain: a multi-site case series with two-year follow-up. Neuromodulation 2018;21(3):290–5.

45. Boccard SG, Pereira EA, Moir L, et al. Long-term outcomes of deep brain stimulation for neuropathic pain. Neurosurgery 2013;72(2):221–31.
46. Lempka SF, Malone DA Jr, Hu B, et al. Randomized clinical trial of deep brain stimulation for poststroke pain. Ann Neurol 2017;81(5):653–63.
47. Owen SL, Green AL, Stein JF, et al. Deep brain stimulation for the alleviation of post-stroke neuropathic pain. Pain 2006;120(1–2):202–6.
48. Langhorne P, Stott D, Robertson L, et al. Medical complications after stroke: a multicenter study. Stroke 2000;31:1223–9.
49. Sowden GL, Huffman JC. The impact of mental illness on cardiac outcomes: a review for the cardiologist. Int J Cardiol 2009;132(1):30–7.
50. Abed MA, Kloub MI, Moser DK. Anxiety and adverse health outcomes among cardiac patients: a biobehavioral model. J Cardiovasc Nurs 2014;29(4):354–63.

UNITED STATES POSTAL SERVICE® Statement of Ownership, Management, and Circulation (All Periodicals Publications Except Requester Publications)

1. Publication Title	2. Publication Number	3. Filing Date
ANESTHESIOLOGY CLINICS	000 – 275	9/18/2022

4. Issue Frequency	5. Number of Issues Published Annually	6. Annual Subscription Price
MAR, JUN, SEP, DEC	4	$375.00

7. Complete Mailing Address of Known Office of Publication (Not printer) (Street, city, county, state, and ZIP+4®)

ELSEVIER INC.
230 Park Avenue, Suite 800
New York, NY 10169

Contact Person
Malathi Samayan

Telephone (Include area code)
91-44-4299-4507

8. Complete Mailing Address of Headquarters or General Business Office of Publisher (Not printer)

ELSEVIER INC.
230 Park Avenue, Suite 800
New York, NY 10169

9. Full Names and Complete Mailing Addresses of Publisher, Editor, and Managing Editor (Do not leave blank)

Publisher (Name and complete mailing address)

DOLORES MELONI, ELSEVIER INC.
1600 JOHN F KENNEDY BLVD, SUITE 1800
PHILADELPHIA, PA 19103-2899

Editor (Name and complete mailing address)

JOANNA COLLETT, ELSEVIER INC.
1600 JOHN F KENNEDY BLVD, SUITE 1800
PHILADELPHIA, PA 19103-2899

Managing Editor (Name and complete mailing address)

PATRICK MANLEY, ELSEVIER INC.
1600 JOHN F KENNEDY BLVD, SUITE 1800
PHILADELPHIA, PA 19103-2899

10. Owner (Do not leave blank. If the publication is owned by a corporation, give the name and address of the corporation immediately followed by the names and addresses of all stockholders owning or holding 1 percent or more of the total amount of stock. If not owned by a corporation, give the names and addresses of the individual owners. If owned by a partnership or other unincorporated firm, give its name and address as well as those of each individual owner. If the publication is published by a nonprofit organization, give its name and address.)

Full Name	Complete Mailing Address
WHOLLY OWNED SUBSIDIARY OF REED/ELSEVIER, US HOLDINGS	1600 JOHN F KENNEDY BLVD, SUITE 1800 PHILADELPHIA, PA 19103-2899

11. Known Bondholders, Mortgagees, and Other Security Holders Owning or Holding 1 Percent or More of Total Amount of Bonds, Mortgages, or Other Securities. If none, check box ► ☐ None

Full Name	Complete Mailing Address
N/A	

12. Tax Status (For completion by nonprofit organizations authorized to mail at nonprofit rates) (Check one)
The purpose, function, and nonprofit status of this organization and the exempt status for federal income tax purposes:
☒ Has Not Changed During Preceding 12 Months
☐ Has Changed During Preceding 12 Months (Publisher must submit explanation of change with this statement)

PS Form 3526, July 2014 [Page 1 of 4 (see instructions page 4)] PSN: 7530-01-000-9931 PRIVACY NOTICE: See our privacy policy on www.usps.com.

---

13. Publication Title	14. Issue Date for Circulation Data Below
Anesthesiology Clinics	JUNE 2022

15. Extent and Nature of Circulation			Average No. Copies Each Issue During Preceding 12 Months	No. Copies of Single Issue Published Nearest to Filing Date
a. Total Number of Copies (Net press run)			220	176
b. Paid Circulation (By Mail and Outside the Mail)	(1)	Mailed Outside-County Paid Subscriptions Stated on PS Form 3541 (Include paid distribution above nominal rate, advertiser's proof copies, and exchange copies)	79	68
	(2)	Mailed In-County Paid Subscriptions Stated on PS Form 3541 (Include paid distribution above nominal rate, advertiser's proof copies, and exchange copies)	0	0
	(3)	Paid Distribution Outside the Mails Including Sales Through Dealers and Carriers, Street Vendors, Counter Sales, and Other Paid Distribution Outside USPS®	94	73
	(4)	Paid Distribution by Other Classes of Mail Through the USPS (e.g., First-Class Mail®)	0	0
c. Total Paid Distribution (Sum of 15b (1), (2), (3), and (4))		►	173	141
d. Free or Nominal Rate Distribution (By Mail and Outside the Mail)	(1)	Free or Nominal Rate Outside-County Copies included on PS Form 3541	29	18
	(2)	Free or Nominal Rate In-County Copies Included on PS Form 3541	0	0
	(3)	Free or Nominal Rate Copies Mailed at Other Classes Through the USPS (e.g., First-Class Mail)	0	0
	(4)	Free or Nominal Rate Distribution Outside the Mail (Carriers or other means)	0	0
e. Total Free or Nominal Rate Distribution (Sum of 15d (1), (2), (3) and (4))		►	29	18
f. Total Distribution (Sum of 15c and 15e)		►	202	159
g. Copies not Distributed (See Instructions to Publishers #4 (page #3))		►	18	17
h. Total (Sum of 15f and g)		►	220	176
i. Percent Paid (15c divided by 15f times 100)		►	85.64%	88.67%

* If you are claiming electronic copies, go to line 16 on page 3. If you are not claiming electronic copies, skip to line 17 on page 3.

PS Form 3526, July 2014 (Page 2 of 4)

16. Electronic Copy Circulation		Average No. Copies Each Issue During Preceding 12 Months	No. Copies of Single Issue Published Nearest to Filing Date
a. Paid Electronic Copies	►		
b. Total Paid Print Copies (Line 15c) + Paid Electronic Copies (Line 16a)	►		
c. Total Print Distribution (Line 15f) + Paid Electronic Copies (Line 16a)	►		
d. Percent Paid (Both Print & Electronic Copies) (16b divided by 16c × 100)	►		

☒ I certify that 50% of all my distributed copies (electronic and print) are paid above a nominal price.

17. Publication of Statement of Ownership

☒ If the publication is a general publication, publication of this statement is required. Will be printed ☐ Publication not required.
in the DECEMBER 2022 issue of this publication.

18. Signature and Title of Editor, Publisher, Business Manager, or Owner

Malathi Samayan

Malathi Samayan - Distribution Controller

Date 9/18/2022

I certify that all information furnished on this form is true and complete. I understand that anyone who furnishes false or misleading information on this form or who omits material or information requested on the form may be subject to criminal sanctions (including fines and imprisonment) and/or civil sanctions (including civil penalties).

PS Form 3526, July 2014 (Page 3 of 4) PRIVACY NOTICE: See our privacy policy on www.usps.com.

Printed and bound by CPI Group (UK) Ltd, Croydon, CR0 4YY

08/05/2025

01864717-0003